Decision Making near the End of Life

☐ The Series in Death, Dying, and Bereavement

Robert A. Neimeyer, Consulting Editor

Beder—*Voices of Bereavement: A Casebook for Grief Counselors*
Berger—*Music of the Soul: Composing Life Out of Loss*
Davies—*Shadows in the Sun: The Experiences of Sibling Bereavement in Childhood*
Harvey—*Perspectives on Loss: A Sourcebook*
Katz & Johnson—*When Professionals Weep: Emotional and Countertransference Responses in End-of-Life Care*
Klass—*The Spiritual Lives of Bereaved Parents*
Jeffreys—*Helping Grieving People—When Tears Are Not Enough: A Handbook for Care Providers*
Leenaars—*Lives and Deaths: Selections From the Works of Edwin S. Shneidman*
Leong & Leach—*Suicide Among Racial and Ethnic Minority Groups: Theory, Research, and Practice*
Lester—*Katie's Diary: Unlocking the Mystery of a Suicide*
Martin, Doka—*Men Don't Cry … Women Do: Transcending Gender Stereotypes of Grief*
Nord—*Multiple AIDS-Related Loss: A Handbook for Understanding and Surviving a Perpetual Fall*
Roos—*Chronic Sorrow: A Living Loss*
Rogers—*The Art of Grief: The Use of Expressive Arts in a Grief Support Group*
Rosenblatt—*Parent Grief: Narratives of Loss and Relationship*
Rosenblatt & Wallace—*African-American Grief*
Tedeschi & Calhoun—*Helping Bereaved Parents: A Clinician's Guide*
Silverman—*Widow to Widow, Second Edition*
Werth—*Contemporary Perspectives on Rational Suicide*

☐ Formerly the Series in Death Education, Aging, and Health Care

Hannelore Wass, Consulting Editor

Bard—*Medical Ethics in Practice*
Benoliel—*Death Education for the Health Professional*
Bertman—*Facing Death: Images, Insights, and Interventions*
Brammer—*How to Cope With Life Transitions: The Challenge of Personal Change*
Cleiren—*Bereavement and Adaptation: A Comparative Study of the Aftermath of Death*
Corless, Pittman-Lindeman—*AIDS: Principles, Practices, and Politics, Abridged Edition*
Corless, Pittman-Lindeman—*AIDS: Principles, Practices, and Politics, Reference Edition*
Curran—*Adolescent Suicidal Behavior*
Davidson—*The Hospice: Development and Administration, Second Edition*
Davidson, Linnolla—*Risk Factors in Youth Suicide*
Degner, Beaton—*Life-Death Decisions in Health Care*
Doka—*AIDS, Fear, and Society: Challenging the Dreaded Disease*
Doty—*Communication and Assertion Skills for Older Persons*
Epting, Neimeyer—*Personal Meanings of Death: Applications for Personal Construct Theory to Clinical Practice*
Haber—*Health Care for an Aging Society: Cost-Conscious Community Care and Self-Care Approaches*
Hughes—*Bereavement and Support: Healing in a Group Environment*

Irish, Lundquist, Nelson—*Ethnic Variations in Dying, Death, and Grief: Diversity in Universality*
Klass, Silverman, Nickman—*Continuing Bonds: New Understanding of Grief*
Lair—*Counseling the Terminally Ill: Sharing the Journey*
Leenaars, Maltsberger, Neimeyer—*Treatment of Suicidal People*
Leenaars, Wenckstern—*Suicide Prevention in Schools*
Leng—*Psychological Care in Old Age*
Leviton—*Horrendous Death, Health, and Well-Being*
Leviton—*Horrendous Death and Health: Toward Action*
Lindeman, Corby, Downing, Sanborn—*Alzheimer's Day Care: A Basic Guide*
Lund—*Older Bereaved Spouses: Research With Practical Applications*
Neimeyer—*Death Anxiety Handbook: Research, Instrumentation, and Application*
Papadatou, Papadatos—*Children and Death*
Prunkl, Berry—*Death Week: Exploring the Dying Process*
Ricker, Myers—*Retirement Counseling: A Practical Guide for Action*
Samarel—*Caring for Life and Death*
Sherron, Lumsden—*Introduction to Educational Gerontology, Third Edition*
Stillion—*Death and Sexes: An Examination of Differential Longevity Attitudes, Behaviors, and Coping Skills*
Stillion, McDowell, May—*Suicide Across the Life Span—Premature Exits*
Vachon—*Occupational Stress in the Care of the Critically Ill, the Dying, and the Bereaved*
Wass, Corr—*Childhood and Death*
Wass, Corr—*Helping Children Cope With Death: Guidelines and Resource, Second Edition*
Wass, Corr, Pacholski, Forfar—*Death Education II: An Annotated Resource Guide*
Wass, Neimeyer—*Dying: Facing the Facts, Third Edition*
Weenolsen—*Transcendence of Loss over the Life Span*
Werth—*Rational Suicide? Implications for Mental Health Professionals*

Decision Making near the End of Life

Issues, Developments, and Future Directions

Edited by

James L. Werth, Jr. and Dean Blevins

Routledge
Taylor & Francis Group
LONDON AND NEW YORK

First published 2009 by Routledge

2 Park Square, Milton Park, Abingdon, Oxon OX14 4RN
711 Third Avenue, New York, NY 10017, USA

Routledge is an imprint of the Taylor & Francis Group, an informa business

First issued in paperback 2016

ISBN 978-1-138-96725-0 (pbk)
ISBN 978-0-415-95448-8 (hbk)

Library of Congress Cataloging-in-Publication Data

Decision making near the end of life : issues, development, and future directions / [edited by] James L. Werth, Dean Blevins.
p. ; cm. -- (Series in death, dying, and bereavement)
Includes bibliographical references and index.

1. Terminal care--Decision making. I. Werth, James L. II. Blevins, Dean. III. Series.
[DNLM: 1. Terminal Care--ethics--United States. 2. Decision Making--United States. 3. Terminally Ill--United States. WB 310 D294 2008]

R726.8.D43 2008
616'.029--dc22 2008018741

CONTENTS

SERIES EDITOR'S PREFACE

Whether you know it or not, you have opened the cover of a remarkable book—a professional tome that reads, in significant part, like a novel. Following a useful orientation by Werth and Blevins to the intellectual sojourn to follow, you will find yourself immersed, as I was, in four compelling stories of real people facing literal life-and-death decisions about themselves and their loved ones—the sorts of stories that prompt deep reflection on the part of any thoughtful (and emotionally sensitive) reader. Of course, case-based pedagogy might be considered a standard mode of instruction in medical ethics, but it is rare to have such riveting accounts offered with such raw honesty from the vantage point of the protagonists themselves. As a consequence of their courage in baring their personal struggles and family processes you will be challenged to pierce the sometimes comforting veil of abstraction that surrounds ethical discourse in end-of-life contexts, and imagine yourself as a professional, family member, or patient in these all-too-real scenarios in which life-sustaining treatment must be administered or withheld, a therapeutic coma induced or foregone, death hastened or prolonged in the presence of irreversible deterioration, and more. In each instance, whether the patient is young or old, the family united or riven by a troubled history, you will confront with the writers the essential ambiguity that attends critical decision making as death hovers in the wings, and one is forced to confront daunting moral and medical questions under the press of pain, the uncertainty of outcome, and the shifting motivations of key players in the drama. In other words, you—like these families—will be thrust into unanticipated situations that challenge life assumptions and compel action, even if that action is ultimately to allow nature to take its course. The result is likely to be an awakened sensibility to the genuine complexity of fateful decisions made at life's end, fostering receptivity to the rigorous reflection invited by the chapters that will follow.

Not all compelling stories are told in words, of course; some that are equally important are conveyed in statistics. Yet even the chapters that speak in this vocabulary are far from dry recitations of numbers, as the reader is coaxed to confront the hard realities of the shifting mathematics of death, as the proportion of older adults swells as baby boomers age, with a corresponding reduction in the size of subsequent generations. Among the other implications of this demographic trend will be a dramatic shrinkage in the resources available to support the growing cohort of the elderly as they (read "we") face the inevitability of infirmity and death in highly technological (read "costly") environments. Thus, at every level from the deeply personal and familial to the broadly sociological and economic, the issues elucidated by the capable contributors to this volume mandate attention by professionals of many disciplines, including those responsible for bedside care of the dying as well as journalists and policymakers who ultimately shape both public opinion and the context in which care will be rendered.

Within these broad trends, the reader will also confront the diversity of settings and situations in which dying occurs, whether defined in terms of the surprising variability in the proportion of death at home or in institution in different regions of the country, or in terms of the quite different medical and psychosocial demands that mark different end-of-life trajectories. Special analysis is devoted to the pivotal cases and associated controversies that have forced end-of-life decisions into public and professional consciousness, such as those concerning Quinlan, Cruzan and Schiavo. And virtually every relevant conceptual and practical tool for grappling with such complexities—substituted judgment, the double effect, medical futility, healthcare proxies, surrogacy laws, living wills, and more—is explicated and put to use in these and numerous other cases, bringing a modicum of order to an often disorderly societal discourse.

Finally, you will encounter in the final substantial section of this helpful handbook a series of thoughtful reflections—psychological, family systemic, spiritual, cultural and attentive to diversity of populations served—that drive home the essential multiplicity of perspective with which end-of-life decisions must be engaged, as well as the need to tailor them to the unique circumstances of the patient and family. I would predict that engaging in the inner dialogues this book will engender—or better still, sharing them with students, interns and fellow professionals—will make you a more informed and aware partner in these critical decisions, whatever your context of work. And that is substantial compensation for any reader.

Robert A. Neimeyer, Ph.D.
University of Memphis
Series Editor

FOREWORD

With the exception of a few who die immediately from an unintentional injury or a massive heart attack or stroke, most Americans will find their life's end to include challenging decisions about the best use of modern medicine and health-related technology. This book is a very timely and important contribution to the literature supporting the professionals who will help those making these choices for themselves or their loved ones, as well as providing useful information for those faced with these difficult decisions. The authors have comprehensively summarized what has already been learned and accomplished to support end-of-life decision making, and have pointed the direction toward what needs to be done next. Valuable building blocks are in place, yet important work remains to be done.

Accomplishments

Perhaps the most fundamental accomplishment to date is the legal foundation for personal health care decision making. Cerminara (chapter 8) describes the dual role of the constitutional right to private decisions and the evolution of tort law that supports the right to control what happens to one's own body. Societal opinion may not have kept up with the law, but Americans have an established legal right to refuse unwanted medical care. Just because there is the technology available to use, there is no legal requirement for an individual to apply it.

The law also provides a framework for an individual's preferences for medical care to be applied to a situation in which that individual no longer has the decisional capacity to make those judgments. Legal provisions are in place to facilitate the appointment of a proxy decision maker and to recognize the role of that proxy once an individual loses decision capacity. These important legal accomplishments set the current stage for decision making at the end of life.

In recent decades, both public and professional groups have begun important educational efforts to illuminate options and promote support for decision making as death approaches. Webb (chapter 7) describes the influence of movies and television shows in teaching us that once-rare choices could involve anyone. This public education needs to be strengthened and to be an ongoing process, but the media has helped to get a conversation started.

The many references summarized by Chang and Sambamoorthi (chapter 10) represent growth in the number of evidence-based clinical resources and research reports that help health professionals support patients' decision making in palliative care. Professional groups, educational institutions, and investigators have taken important steps to improve the understanding and application of communication skills and decision models to the care of patients near the end of life. Of course, additional research and dissemination are still needed, but the effort is under way.

Substantial progress has also been made toward the valuing of varied professional perspectives on the care and support of patients approaching the end of life. Hospice and palliative care teams consistently bring the expertise of medicine, nursing, social work, and spiritual support to the care of patients, and it is the synergy of these various disciplines' contribution that best supports patients through the complex process of decision making near the end of life.

Lessons Learned

If we have learned nothing else in recent years, we have uncovered the hard work and complex processes that represent how patients and families negotiate choices available to them in life-threatening illness. We know that they are influenced by their knowledge and understanding of the illness and of death, their past experiences with dying, and their beliefs about the role of death in the continuum of life. This complicated decision making is part not only of rational thought but also of intuition. These decision makers must try hard to balance information (or the lack thereof) with personal values. And, while religious or spiritual backgrounds (Doka, chapter 16) and cultural context (Hayslip, Hansson, Starkweather, & Dolan, chapter 17) play a very important role, there is often as much diversity within cultural and religious groups as there is among them.

Stressors that have an impact on decision making at the end of life come from many places. The physical symptoms of an illness alone can dramatically affect decisions (Spannhake, chapter 3). Cognitive decline, including but also beyond memory-based dementia, plays an important role (Volicer, chapter 18). Emotional stress greatly reduces the ability to hear things clearly (Csikai, chapter 11), and depression, anxiety, and hopelessness are serious threats to good decision making (Werth, chapter 14).

Public and professional efforts to promote the use of advanced directives have met with only limited success, suggesting that the complexity of end-of-life decision making is difficult to contain within documents that require yes/no choices to be made out of context. A *process* of advanced care planning that includes the identification of broad values and goals together with the appointment of a surrogate decision maker is a preferred model (Ditto, chapter 13), with some arguing for the additional inclusion of actionable medical orders such as the Physician Orders for Life-Sustaining Treatment (POLST; http://www.ohsu.edu/ethics/polst/) form to document the process. Furthermore, although the most dramatic stories about decision making involve the withdrawing or withholding of life support therapies, we also now see that end-of-life decision making is much broader. As Webb (chapter 7) points out, the possibility of prolonging life has gone beyond feeding tubes and respirators. Decisions about sophisticated diagnostic tests and surgical techniques once reserved for the young and hardy now face those in advanced old age, whose bodies are in delicate working order without the reserve to withstand extended periods of inactivity, unfamiliar environments and routines, or infections acquired while receiving care in an institution. Finding the right balance between seeking appropriate care and refusing unnecessary care is becoming even more and more difficult to do.

Not only are there complex decisions to be made at the end of life, but the period of time defined as the end of life has very elusive boundaries. "Dying" is often hard to recognize. There is no consensus on the meaning of *terminal* (Kleespies, Miller, & Preston, chapter 9), but even with agreement about signs and symptoms, physicians are generally unable to accurately predict the remaining length of life. This uncertainty about prognosis hugely complicates end-of-life decision making.

The legal foundation of end-of-life decision making is built on individual autonomy, yet we know that decisions are more often made by a family unit or made in consideration of family-oriented issues. As Wells-Di Gregorio (chapter 15) points out, individuals who complete advance directives may do so not so much to dictate future health care as to protect family welfare, prevent disagreement among family members, reduce guilt about difficult decisions, and prevent costly care from draining family resources.

Many factors external to the individual and family also confound decision making near the end of life. The context of health care plays an important role (Prevost & Wallace, chapter 12). The frenetic pace of an intensive care unit is not conducive to careful consideration of all available options. Yet, in contrast, time may be plentiful but the information lacking in a nursing home setting because of infrequent contact with medical staff. Furthermore, research suggests that the simple availability and distribution of health services influences how end-of-life decisions are made.

The greatest single lesson that we can take from all that we have learned about the complexity of end-of-life decision making is to approach it with patience and respect. It is hard work. It requires due diligence on the part of all players—patient, family, and providers. It is a daunting task, but a very important one.

Remaining Questions

Changes in how Americans are dying require new information to inform decision making (Field, chapter 6). How will the fact that people are dying at older ages influence the typical end-of-life experience in the future? As the number of young caregivers and taxpayers continues to diminish, how will choices change? As more and more end-of-life decisions are made in advanced old age, how will the normal age-related changes in cognition have an impact on the decision-making process?

We know that we need to better balance individual autonomy and family decision making. What more can we learn about the relative importance of trust in a proxy decision maker versus individual values and preferences? Research to date has uncovered the importance of both of these factors, but we have yet to tailor the approach to decision making to suit the personality characteristics or family dynamics that might make one factor more important to a given individual or family situation.

Research on the communication skills needed in end-of-life decision making has focused primarily on communication between healthcare providers and patients or families. We have much to learn about how healthcare providers can reduce the emotional, interpersonal, and attitudinal barriers to within-family conversations (Wells-Di Gregorio, chapter 15). Approaches to advance care planning that involve surrogates in discussions hold much promise. Yet, what are the most important tools that professionals can provide to individuals and families so that they can continue these conversations at home and help to facilitate the hard work of decision making? After all, the path of least resistance is to avoid the topic altogether.

Finally, how do we help patients, families, and providers live with—even embrace—paradox? Preventive health care and healthy lifestyles deserve all of the attention that they are now receiving. Yet, a focus on vitality in old age does not itself necessitate the current denial of death. How do we frame aging in such a way that we successfully challenge everyone to live with gusto at the very same time that they prepare to exit with grace?

Remaining Tasks

Each person who reads this book will end up with his or her own list of important next steps. Here are some suggestions to begin such a discussion.

We must get palliative care out from under the shadow of terminal care. Palliation is intended to be good symptom management and supportive care at every stage of illness, starting at diagnosis. It is appropriate care for those who go on to survive their illness. So, we must learn to better tailor and constantly alter the mix of curative, life-extending, comfort, and family supportive care (Feudtner and Kazak, chapter 19) so that the "final" approach leading to the end of life, when it does come, really is a seamless transition and not a traumatic sea change.

Misconceptions about artificial nutrition and hydration need to be reduced. We may never be able to agree about the extent of our moral obligation to care for the sick, but we can make certain that all professionals and more of the public understand the empirical evidence about risks and benefits of feeding tubes and the role of natural dehydration in the dying process. These emotional topics will continue to haunt family members long after death unless there is greater awareness of the limitations of efforts to substitute medical technology when normal body functions become impaired.

Many underrepresented voices belong at the table for us to learn how to better navigate this complex territory (Hayslip, Hansson, Starkweather, & Dolan, chapter 17). Instead of viewing various groups as disadvantaged minorities, we could learn from these diverse perspectives. For example, rich end-of-life imagery about crossing the river can be found in the songs handed down from African American slaves. The traditions and insight of different racial, ethnic, and cultural groups may provide novel ways of untangling difficult aspects of end-of-life decision making.

Finally, increasing the flexibility of the various components of our healthcare delivery system could lessen the strain on end-of-life decision making. The creation of palliative care units within acute care facilities is one important step in this direction. Facilitating the ability of chronic care facilities to handle certain types of acute care needs would also ease the strain. Instead of looking to individual decision making as the key to solving some end-of-life problems, a better solution may be to modify care delivery to address the pressure points in the process.

New Stories

The poignant stories that follow—of Laura Crow, Nicola Raye, Richard (and Maureen Lyon), and Jonathon Spannhake—will grab your attention and underscore timeless and critical issues about decision making. Yet, also consider two other stories as you move from past accomplishments to the future of decision making at the end of life.

Mr. Smith is 96 years old and has been generally independent—of sound mind and in reasonably good health. In recent years, he has lived with his daughter and her family, where he is a much-loved member of this extended household. However, lately his daughter has noticed that he seems to be detaching from life. He is no longer keen to be involved in his grandchildren's activities. He is not at all interested in eating and hardly touches anything on his plate. Should she accept these new behaviors? Or, should she insist on treatment for depression? Should she push him to eat? Is it ever possible or appropriate to just let your parent go?

Then, there is Mrs. Jones. She is 89 years old and has been in a nursing home with dementia for 8 years. She no longer recognizes her family, but she is a very cheerful person, well loved and well cared for by the nursing home staff. Prior to her cognitive decline, she had signed advanced directives and discussed them with her son. She was very clear that she would not want to have medical means used to extend her life. Still, in the past year she has periodically developed a urinary tract infection. To date, these infections have been successfully treated with a transfer to an acute care facility for one or two nights of intravenous fluids and antibiotics. She has always returned to the nursing home to her previous level of functioning. What does her family do when she aspirates some food and develops pneumonia? How do they then approach the use of antibiotics?

Ironically, perhaps, the final chapter of this book—on end-of-life decisions and children—will outline some themes that could also be paramount with a very elderly decedent population. The authors' proposed factors to differentiate a pediatric population could also be the key features to consider as the dying population ages: developmental trajectory (integrity), social network (family burden), emotions (adult orphans), prognostic difficulties (frailty and dwindling), and potential negative psychiatric outcomes (haunted sense of having failed your parents). The landscape of end-of-life decision making is graying not only in terms of the age of the affected population, but also in terms of the choices involved. As you read this book, consider how we can benefit from what we have learned and done to date as we move into a future with new questions to investigate and tasks to accomplish.

June R. Lunney, Ph.D., R.N.

West Virginia University School of Nursing

ABOUT THE EDITORS AND AUTHORS

Dean Blevins received his Ph.D. from the University of Akron and is completing a master's of public health from the University of Arkansas for Medical Sciences (UAMS). He currently holds positions as the director of implementation and qualitative research with the Veterans Affairs (VA) South Central Mental Illness Research, Education, and Clinical Center; research health scientist with the VA Center for Mental Healthcare and Outcomes Research; assistant professor at UAMS Department of Psychiatry; and adjunct faculty with University of Arkansas at Fayetteville and the University of Phoenix. Dr. Blevins's research focuses on the implementation of evidence-based practices for VA and community settings, particularly in the areas of end-of-life care, mental health treatment, and HIV prevention. He has published numerous articles and several books and has given over 50 professional talks on a broad range of topics related to health care, aging, and program implementation and assessment.

Kathy L. Cerminara, professor of law at the Nova Southeastern University Shepard Broad Law Center, received her J.D. from the University of Pittsburgh School of Law and her LL.M. and J.S.D. from Columbia University School of Law. Beginning with her work during law school with Professor Alan Meisel, she has been interested in and has written about the law governing medical treatment at the end of life. The collaboration has resulted in the third edition of the treatise, *The Right to Die: The Law of End-of-Life Decisionmaking*, coauthored by the two of them. Most recently, Professor Cerminara commented extensively on the Terri Schiavo case, including among her accomplishments coauthorship of the timeline, *Key Events in the Case of Theresa Marie Schiavo*, available at http://www6.miami.edu/ethics/schiavo/terri_schiavo_timeline.html.

Victor T. Chang, M.D., F.A.C.P., is associate professor in medicine at the University of Medicine and Dentistry of New Jersey and senior attending in the section of hematology oncology of the Veterans Affairs New Jersey Health Care System. He is a Project Death in America faculty scholar and cochair of the Symptom Management Committee of the Eastern Cooperative Oncology Group. His research interests include palliative care and symptom assessment and management.

Laura Crow has a B.A. in psychology from San Diego State University and is a full-time artist in her hometown of San Diego. She is currently on a break from volunteering with Sharp HospiceCare but plans to return when her puppy has completed therapy dog training. She has previously published articles on end-of-life issues in the journal *Death Studies* and the *Journal of Counseling and Development*. The chapter in this book is a modified version of the *Death Studies* article about her brother, Josh.

Ellen L. Csikai, M.S.W., M.P.H., Ph.D., is associate professor in the School of Social Work at the University of Alabama. She has over 11 years of practice experience, a majority of which was in the hospital setting working in trauma intensive care, emergency, orthopedics, medical/surgical units, in the community hospital setting, and in hospice prior to beginning her academic career. Her areas of teaching are social work practice in health care with the dying and bereaved, aging, crisis intervention, and research. Her area of research involves end-of-life decisions and social work practice. She is the editor of the Journal of Social Work in End-of-Life and Palliative Care.

Peter H. Ditto is a professor in the Department of Psychology and Social Behavior at the University of California, Irvine. He received his B.A. from the University of California at Los Angeles and his Ph.D. from Princeton University, both degrees in psychology. Dr. Ditto is a social psychologist whose expertise is in human judgment and decision making. His research focuses on "hot cognition"—how our emotions and desires affect (and often bias) our social, political, moral, medical, and legal judgments.

Dr. Kenneth J. Doka is a professor of gerontology at the Graduate School of the College of New Rochelle and senior consultant to the Hospice Foundation of America. A prolific author, Dr. Doka has written or edited 19 books and over 60 articles and book chapters. Dr. Doka is editor of both *Omega* and *Journeys: A Newsletter for the Bereaved*. He was elected president of the Association for Death Education and Counseling in 1993 and elected to the board of directors of the International Work Group on Dying, Death and Bereavement, serving as chair from 1997 to 1999. The Association for Death Education and Counseling presented him with an award for outstanding contributions in the field of death education in 1998. He participates in the annual Hospice Foundation of America Teleconference. Dr. Doka is an ordained Lutheran minister.

Diana C. Dolan is a doctoral student in the Clinical Health Psychology program at the University of North Texas. Her teaching and research interests deal with sleep and aging, grief and bereavement, midlife antecedents of aging attitudes, and death anxiety in adulthood.

Chris Feudtner, M.D., Ph.D., M.P.H., is an assistant professor of Pediatrics at the University of Pennsylvania and the Children's Hospital of Philadelphia who focuses on improving the lives of children with complex chronic conditions and their families.

Marilyn J. Field, Ph.D., is senior program officer, Institute of Medicine (IOM). At the IOM, Dr. Field has directed two studies and reports on palliative and end-of-life care. The first report, coedited with Dr. Christine Cassel, was "Approaching Death: Improving Care at the End of Life" (1997). The second, coedited with Dr. Richard Behrman, was "When Children Die: Improving Palliative and End-of-Life Care for Children and Their Families" (2003). She has also coauthored several articles on strategies and tools for improving the quality of care at the end of life.

Robert O. Hansson, Ph.D., served on the faculty of the University of Tulsa Psychology Department, where, as professor of psychology, he taught courses in the psychology of aging. He is a Fellow of the Gerontological Society of America, and his published research deals with grief and bereavement, families and aging, relationships in later life, and aging and work. He is coeditor of *The Handbook of Bereavement Research* (3rd edition) and *Bereavement in Later Life: Coping, Adaptation, and Developmental Influences.*

Bert Hayslip, Jr., earned his doctorate in experimental developmental psychology from the University of Akron and is a regents professor of psychology at the University of North Texas. His research interests include grandparenting, grandparents raising grandchildren, cognitive aging, grief and bereavement, and mental health and aging. He has received grants from the National Institute on Aging, the Hilgenfeld Foundation, and the National Endowment for the Humanities. His published research has appeared in refereed journals such as *Psychology and Aging, The Journal of Gerontology, The Gerontologist, Experimental Aging Research*, and *The International Journal of Aging and Human Development.*

Anne E. Kazak, Ph.D., A.B.P.P., is professor of pediatrics at the University of Pennsylvania and the director of psychology and deputy director of the Behavioral Health Center at the Children's Hospital of Philadelphia. Dr. Kazak's work focuses on child and family adaptation to serious pediatric illness and the development and delivery of evidence-based care.

Phillip M. Kleespies, Ph.D., A.B.P.P., is assistant clinical professor of psychiatry at Boston University School of Medicine/VA Boston Healthcare System and is a member of the VA Boston Palliative Care Consult Team, as well as a member of the VA Boston Ethics Advisory Committee. He is the author of the book, *Life and Death Decisions: Psychological and Ethical Considerations in End-of-Life Care* (2004). He has also presented at national conferences and published book chapters and articles on end-of-life issues.

June R. Lunney, Ph.D., R.N., is associate dean for research at the West Virginia University School of Nursing. From 1991 to 1999, she served as an extramural program director at the National Institute of Nursing Research at the National Institutes of Health (NIH), during which time she helped to develop NIH support for research on end-of-life issues. She subsequently worked with Dr. Joanne Lynn at the Center for End-of-Life Care at RAND, contributing to a study on the costs and use of care at the end of life. She was the lead author on the 2003 IOM's report, "Describing Death in America," chaired the Planning Committee for the 2004 NIH State of the Science Conference "Improving End-of-Life Care," and has published empirical support for the variation in functional trajectories at the end of life.

Maureen E. Lyon, Ph.D., A.B.P.P., is clinical psychologist and associate research professor in pediatrics at Children's National Medical Center and George Washington University. Dr. Lyon's work focuses on adolescents living with a chronic illness and the development and delivery of care to increase adherence to medication, transition to adult care, and advance care planning. Dr. Lyon has developed a family-centered program (primary investigator, National Institute of Mental Health/NIH, R34), family-centered advance care planning, to help families of adolescents with life-threatening illnesses speak directly and honestly with one another about advance care planning. Currently, the family-centered advance care planning is being pilot tested with adolescents with HIV, while medically stable, and their families. This model has been adapted from previously demonstrated efficacious interventions with adults. Dr. Lyon also has a private practice in health psychology for adults in Alexandria, Virginia.

Pamela J. Miller, M.S.W., Ph.D., is associate professor of social work and teaches health practice, health policy, and social work in end-of-life and palliative care in the master's program at Portland State University.

She has conducted research, published, and spoken to numerous groups about hospice social workers and Oregon's Death With Dignity Act.

Thomas A. Preston, M.D., was awarded his medical degree by the University of Pennsylvania School of Medicine. He is the author of the book, *Final Victory, Taking Charge of the Last Stages of Life* (2000). He has presented and published extensively on topics such as physician involvement in life-ending practices and observations concerning terminally ill patients who choose suicide. He serves on the board of directors of Compassion & Choices of Washington.

Suzanne S. Prevost, R.N., Ph.D., is a professor and the National HealthCare Chair of Excellence in Nursing at Middle Tennessee State University. She is also currently a Claire M. Fagin Postdoctoral Fellow with the John A. Hartford Foundation—Building Academic Geriatric Nursing Capacity program. She earned her Ph.D. from Texas Woman's University and her M.S.N. from the Medical University of South Carolina. Her B.S.N. is from Villa Maria College in Erie, Pennsylvania. Dr. Prevost is the consulting editor for *Nursing Clinics of North America*.

Nicola G. Raye, Ph.D., is in private psychotherapy practice; she works with adults and couples on developmental issues throughout the life span. She is particularly interested in mindfulness-based interventions for stress, depression, and anxiety.

Richard is a senior in high school in Washington, D.C., and a patient at the Burgess Clinic in the Division of Adolescent and Young Adult Medicine at Children's National Medical Center. Richard's life is focused on his schoolwork and his writing. He plans to take a "gap year" after high school before going to college.

Nethra Sambamoorthi, Ph.D., consults extensively in wide areas of statistical applications and is president of CRM Portals.

Jonathon D. Spannhake is currently enrolled as an undergraduate student at Ohio University for a bachelor of specialized studies in film and creative writing. Following his graduation, he hopes to obtain a master's degree in the fine arts of film. With this degree, Mr. Spannhake hopes to eventually become a screenwriter—possibly for the Writers Guild of America. His current film achievements include being one of many great heads for the comedic film group, the Morbid Caffeine Junkies. As for Mr. Spannhake's previous illness, he has recuperated fully with few-to-no side effects. He resides happily in Athens, Ohio, working as a grill cook to help pay for his schooling.

Jon D. Starkweather is a doctoral student in the experimental psychology program at the University of North Texas. His teaching and research interests deal with statistical analyses of data, individual differences in end-of-life decision making, and engaged lifestyles in later life.

Ladislav Volicer, M.D., Ph.D., F.A.A.N., F.G.S.A., is currently courtesy full professor at the University of South Florida, Tampa, Florida, and visiting professor at the Charles University, Prague, Czech Republic. Dr. Volicer was medical director of the Dementia Special Care Unit, a 100-bed inpatient unit at the Edith Nourse Rogers Memorial Veterans Hospital in Bedford, Massachusetts, where he investigated various aspects of dementia care. He has edited 5 books and published over 200 articles on Alzheimer's disease, neuropharmacology, aging, and bioethics.

J. Brandon Wallace received a Ph.D. in sociology from the University of Florida in 1990. Currently, he is an associate professor of sociology and director of the aging studies program at Middle Tennessee State University, where he teaches courses in social gerontology, family sociology, and research methods. His research focuses on quality of care in nursing homes and, most recently, has emphasized end-of-life care in long-term care settings. As a private consultant, Dr. Wallace assists long-term care centers in using MDS (Minimum Data Set) data to assess and improve the quality of care they provide.

Marilyn Webb is distinguished professor of journalism and cochair of the program in journalism at Knox College, Galesburg, Illinois. She is also the author of the Pulitzer Prize-nominated book, *The Good Death: The New American Search to Reshape the End of Life* (New York: Bantam Books, 1997 and 1999).

Sharla Wells-Di Gregorio, Ph.D., is an assistant professor of psychiatry at The Ohio State University (OSU). Dr. Wells-Di Gregorio obtained her doctoral degree in clinical psychology from Northwestern University Medical School after completing a consultation-liaison/health psychology internship at UCLA Neuropsychiatric Institute. In 2001, she was awarded the Ann and Herbert Siegel–American Cancer Society Postdoctoral Fellowship Award to examine the biobehavioral (physical, psychological, immune) responses of spouses of women with breast cancer recurrence. Dr. Wells-Di Gregorio's research interests include family decision making at the end of life, the overlap of physical and psychological symptoms with progressive disease, and supportive care interventions for patients and family members living with terminal illness. She currently works full time as a clinical psychologist with the OSU Pain and Palliative Medicine Program, where she provides psychological interventions for patients and families to reduce pain, depression, anxiety, insomnia, and other symptoms associated with advanced disease. This includes cofacilitation of the OSU Medical Center grief support group.

James L. Werth, Jr. received a Ph.D. in counseling psychology from Auburn University in 1995 and a master of legal studies from the University of Nebraska–Lincoln in 1999. From 1999 to 2000, he was the American Psychological Association's AIDS Policy Congressional Fellow, and he worked primarily on end-of-life issues in the office of Senator Ron Wyden (D-OR). He is currently professor of psychology and director of the Psy.D. program in counseling psychology at Radford University. He has written/edited/coedited 5 books, several journal issues, and over 70 other publications on end-of-life issues or HIV disease.

1

CHAPTER

Introduction

Dean Blevins and James L. Werth, Jr.

Introduction

Various segments of society have increased their attention to end-of-life issues in the past two decades. This focus can be attributed not only to vocal advocates of improving the quality of care for people confronting life-threatening conditions, but also to public reactions to the legal and politicized medical situations that have donned the front pages of many newspapers across the country, in which issues of dignity, autonomy, and the right to control the contours and length of life have been the root foundations of extremely heated debates. People such as Nancy Cruzan, Terri Schiavo, and Jack Kevorkian have contributed to the public discussion and debate regarding quality of care for people who are dying and their loved ones.

The quality of the health care *possible* in the United States is rarely disputed; however, the technological and pharmaceutical advances that typically signal progress can also add to the complexity of situations we encounter in medical decision making—sometimes compromising quality of life and the factors that matter most to patients and their loved ones near the end of life. The technologies that can save many more lives than possible 100 or even 50 years ago can ironically become a burden to those whose suffering is prolonged and exacerbated by the healthcare system. Inequities are also common, with the healthcare system and society unfairly depriving people of care that can be beneficial or necessary. The movement to improve end-of-life care requires separating the challenges stemming from the system, from society, and from ignorance to focus on what is in the best interest of recipients of care and their loved ones. Improving end-of-life care requires a multifaceted approach involving stakeholders in health care, consumers, educators, researchers, and policy makers; all facets are addressed in this volume.

Across the endless array of possible situations that can characterize end-of-life care is the increasingly complex need to make medical and psychosocial decisions that are linked to the health and well-being of the terminally ill person, loved ones, providers, and society. It is important to acknowledge that there is no universal or easy solution to make decision making simple or free from the emotions and stress that accompany end-of-life care; however, awareness of the myriad influences confronted by patients and their loved ones is an essential first step to providing appropriate health care and ensuring that the decisions made are in the best interest of all involved, most importantly for the people to whom we are providing care.

Despite the wealth of knowledge that exists to assist in improving end-of-life care, empirical attention has only occurred recently. Pioneers of the field such as Glaser and Strauss (1965) and Elizabeth Kubler-Ross (1969) were rare until the late 1980s and early 1990s. In fact, it was not until the late 1970s when the palliative care approach was introduced to North America. Thus, there is much that has yet to be understood about decision making near the end of life and the great need for interventions to educate and assist all stakeholders. This volume begins to address these problems not only by summarizing the state of the field, but also by highlighting areas for which additional research, educational outreach, and public policy making are necessary. End-of-life decision making in the future will have as much to do with medical advances and the causes of critical illnesses as it will with the interaction of psychosocial and medical issues, law, and the media. As knowledge continues to accumulate, attention to these domains will increasingly need to be targeted by interdisciplinary teams comprised of professionals such as the contributors of this volume.

□ Organization of the Book

In an earlier work (Werth & Blevins, 2006), we focused on assembling experts to discuss how to integrate psychosocial issues into the usual care provided to people near the end of life, emphasizing how greater holistic care can be fostered in direct care provision, education, and public policy—informed by the highest-quality research possible given the state of the field. In this volume we build on this earlier work to specifically address the decision-making process that falls on all stakeholders involved near the end of life.

Specifically, each of the chapters in this volume is written to be a stand-alone contribution to the end-of-life literature. However, a unique feature of the book is the integration across all chapters of a collection of personal accounts of situations that can occur near the end of life, recounting experiences spanning symptom management, family relations, communication, hastened death, and advance care planning to provide a face to the complexity and diversity of end-of-life decision making discussed by the contributing experts. After this introduction and the four personal stories, the remaining chapters are organized around three domains: (a) broad overviews on dying and death and options near the end of life; (b) the intersection of end-of-life choices and decision making; and (c) the specific contribution of psychosocial issues near the end of life to decision making.

The volume's contributors are a collection of experts from a variety of professions who we asked to focus on the extant empirical literature and theory in addition to the applied implications of contemporary knowledge regarding end-of-life decision making. Their backgrounds and experiences are as diverse as the breadth of material discussed, which we believe provides a comprehensive review of the variety of issues to be considered as the country examines how best to help people who are dying and their loved ones as they make difficult decisions near the end of life.

□ Contents

As noted, we attempt to personalize the experiences described across the chapters by soliciting several accounts of life-threatening and end-of-life situations from individuals who have confronted various decision-making challenges. Specifically, the book begins with four stories that depict several medical scenarios: adolescent decision making and advance care planning; the powerful effect of pain; surrogate decision making for an accident victim and withdrawal of life support; and hastening death. The chapter by Richard and Lyon is the only coauthored story; Lyon is a psychologist who provides context and analysis related to the personal story of Richard, an adolescent who was born with HIV disease. This chapter includes a model of family-centered advance care planning used by Richard, whose mother died of an AIDS-related condition and who is being raised by his grandparents. Richard describes his feelings and thoughts about end-of-life planning as Lyon worked with him and his family over time to ensure a mutually agreed-on plan in the event of a medical emergency.

In the second personal account, Spannhake presents a vivid illustration of the effect of persistent and untreatable pain on decision making while he was hospitalized over the course of several months. He discusses the struggle he had with family members and friends who, while consistently present, could not always relate to his experiences and state of mind.

Crow's story recounts the experiences she and her family endured while attempting to provide care to her brother, who had been critically injured in a traffic accident. Problems with physician communication and release of accurate healthcare information required her consultation with outside medical advisors in deciding to withdraw artificial nutrition and hydration when it became clear that her brother was unlikely to recover from his persistent vegetative state.

Finally, Raye assembles a collection of decades-old journal entries and additional commentary to retell how she and her family assisted in hastening her father's death. Issues of control and dignity abound in this story as her father struggled with a gradual decrease in his ability to live his life in a manner consistent with his values and sense of self.

Field begins the overview section of the book with a detailed discussion of how people die in the United States. As one of the original editors of the Institute of Medicine (Field & Cassel, 1997) report, *Approaching Death: Improving Care at the End of Life*, she updates the original statistics, discussing the characteristics of these individuals and when and where they die. She also includes discussion of the typical trajectories of dying, costs of care, and projects into the future likely changes and trends.

Webb continues the overview section by focusing on the role of the media in influencing end-of-life attitudes across the nation. She highlights the increased attention to death and dying as society has increasingly moved to institutionalized care at the end of life. She also presents a detailed analysis of how the key players in the highly publicized Terri Schiavo case have used the media to influence the perceptions of the public and politicians over the last several decades, intermingling politics, religion, medicine, and law.

The third chapter in this section focuses on the legal precedents in end-of-life care within a larger historical context. Cerminara's discussion includes a detailed accounting of the arguments used in the highest-profile legal cases that have helped to define patients' rights in medical end-of-life decision making (i.e., those of Nancy Cruzan, Karan Quinlan, and Terri Schiavo). She concludes by building on these three cases (and others) to illustrate what legislation and judicial rulings do and do not address and areas in which there are still likely questions that can arise in complex medical cases near the end of life.

The overview section concludes with a chapter by Kleespies, Miller, and Preston, who focus on the options available to persons near the end of life. The authors talk about when and how life can be prolonged or ended intentionally, as well as when hastening death can occur as a result of an attempt to manage symptoms such as pain. They conclude by presenting how medical facilities, through the use of ethics committees, have been addressing the difficult situations that can arise in electing to prolong life or discontinue treatment. They discuss a model of ethical decision making that requires the inclusion of multiple layers of consultation to ensure that the best possible decision is reached by providers and families alike.

Chang and Sambamoorthi begin the next section by reviewing the literature about medical decision making, presenting an overview of the theoretical models that can be blended over the course of care to help explain the decisions people make near the end of life. They provide some discussion of how different types of diseases and conditions can influence the medical decision-making process and the ways in which people may come to conclusions about what to do in these difficult situations.

One of the primary issues and concerns when people are making medical decisions, particularly those that have end-of-life ramifications, is receiving and understanding information regarding options and possibilities and consequences. Csikai focuses on the issue of communication when people are making end-of-life decisions and provides numerous case examples to highlight how poor communication can complicate the process and how good communication can make the dying process better for everyone involved.

Because the vast majority of deaths in the United States occur in institutions (e.g., nursing homes, hospitals), we wanted to include a chapter focused solely on the complex issues that may arise when end-of-life decisions are made for or by a person who is receiving care in a setting staffed by professionals and governed by rules and regulations and laws that may complicate the decision-making process. Prevost and Miller examine the ways in which the institutional setting can affect how people die and the choices confronted by loved ones.

The final chapter in this section, by Ditto, is an incisive and critical examination of advance directives (especially living wills but also durable powers of attorney for health care) and the degree to which they have, or have not, lived up to their promise and possibilities in terms of increasing the quality of care and decision making near the end of life. Based on his decades of research on the utility of advance directives, Ditto reviews the limitations of these documents and offers solutions that could be considered to make them more likely to achieve the goals of helping people have their end-of-life treatment wishes followed.

The fourth section of the book, on psychosocial issues, is designed to provide a context for the various variables that can affect decision making by the person who is dying, the loved ones of the person who is ill, and the professional care providers. Werth begins this set of chapters by examining psychological and psychiatric conditions that can affect the choices considered and selected by the dying person, such as depression, anxiety, hopelessness, and dignity. He also provides suggestions for the treatment and amelioration of these conditions if they appear to be present in a person who is dying.

Wells-Di Gregorio expands the focus of the discussion from the dying person to the loved ones surrounding the ill individual. Defining *family* broadly, she discusses how family members consider options and make decisions, reviews the role of family dynamics, and includes a discussion of grief and how the decisions that are made before the person dies can affect how well the family members cope after the death occurs.

One of the most important psychosocial considerations for the dying person and the loved ones is the participants' religious or spiritual beliefs concerning issues such as how life should be lived, what the dying process and death should look like, what happens after death, and what the roles of the various participants may be. Doka provides a cogent overview of the broad issues while noting that it is not possible in a brief chapter to provide adequate coverage of the variety of belief systems and all of their attendant rituals and expectations.

Similarly, Hayslip, Hansson, Starkweather, and Dolan make the disclaimer that their coverage of cultural considerations and the effects of cultural beliefs on end-of-life decision making is necessarily a general overview designed to highlight some of the issues that may be involved. These authors emphasize that one of the primary concerns near the end of life is that care providers and others will impose their beliefs on the dying person and loved ones instead of appreciating that there are very different desires for control and information and decision-making power based on a variety of cultural factors such as race, ethnicity, age, and socioeconomic status.

With Volicer's chapter the focus shifts to a discussion of one of the most difficult end-of-life issues: determining when a person has lost the ability to make decisions for himself or herself and then what to do if this capacity appears to have diminished. Focusing on dementia while also mentioning delirium and other conditions, Volicer reviews the ways in which the determination of decision-making capacity can be assessed and, if found to be wanting, ameliorated (if possible).

Finally, Feudtner and Kazak discuss the special situation of end-of-life decision making for children and adolescents. Here the issues of capacity raised by Volicer are combined with developmental considerations; the beliefs and values of parents/guardians, other family members, and the treatment team; and the general social perspective that children should not die. They provide an examination of how decisions can be made less difficult and how everyone involved in the process can be supported before and after death occurs.

Conclusion

We owe a great deal to the contributors to this book, especially the courageous individuals who opened themselves and their families up by contributing personal stories. Similarly, the entire end-of-life field owes the authors of these chapters a great deal because of the contributions they have made to conducting research, providing care, and educating the public about dying and death and the associated processes. As editors, we have learned a great deal from these authors, and we know that our own work will be improved because of the wisdom and experience the authors have shared.

Although the authors have clearly provided high-quality reviews and analyses of a great deal of literature and experience, it is also clear that much more work needs to be done. Across the chapters, we learn how to think about decision-making issues and take pointers from the contributors about how attention to research, education, clinical practice, and public policy can be directed to advance the field and ultimately improve the quality of care for patients and their loved ones.

References

Field, M. J., & Cassel, C. K. (Eds.). (1997). *Approaching death: Improving care at the end of life*. Washington, DC: National Academy Press.

Glaser, B. G., & Strauss, A. L. (1965). *Awareness of dying*. Chicago: Aldine.

Kubler-Ross, E. (1969). *On death and dying*. New York: Macmillan.

Werth, J. L., Jr., & Blevins, D. (Eds.). (2006). *Psychosocial issues near the end of life: A resource for professional care providers*. Washington, DC: APA Books.

I

SECTION

Personal Stories

2

CHAPTER

Adolescent End-of-Life Decision Making

Family-Centered Advance Care Planning

Richard and Maureen E. Lyon

Introduction

More than 30,000 adolescents in the United States die annually from the effects of all chronic illnesses (Muniño, Arias, Kochanek, Murphy, & Smith, 2002). End-of-life (EOL) care for these patients is a public health issue (Freyer, 2004; Rao, Anderson, & Smith, 2002) because of its high physical and emotional costs and potential for the prevention of suffering associated with illness in addition to the suffering caused by communication failures during a medical crisis.

The majority of adolescents want to be involved in shared decision making about their medical treatment (Alderson, 1992), including their EOL care (Lyon, McCabe, Patel, & D'Angelo, 2004). Respect for adolescent autonomy, support for family-centered care, as well as policy recommendations (American Academy of Pediatrics, 1994, 2000; American Psychological Association [APA], 2005; Field & Behrman, 2002), professional guidelines (Children's National Medical Center [CNMC], 1994; Weir & Peters, 1997), and practice and theory (Larson & Tobin, 2000) encourage the inclusion of adolescents in decisions about their EOL care. Nevertheless, such conversations are often avoided because they are sad and anxiety provoking for both healthcare providers (Mulhern, Crisco, & Camitta,

1981) and families (Bearison, 1991; Bluebond-Langner, 1978). However, open conversations when the adolescent's medical condition is stable may prevent future suffering and support shared decision making (Crawley, Marshall, Lo, & Koenig, 2002; Leikin, 1989; Sonnenblick, Friedlander, & Steinberg, 1993). Families who have discussed these issues with their dying children tend not to regret it later (Kreicbergs, Valdimarsdottir, Onelov, Henter, & Steineck, 2004).

Families often wish to protect one another from the pain of honestly discussing what the adolescents' wishes would be if they were dying and could not speak for themselves (Bluebond-Langner, 1978; Hinds et al., 2001). Furthermore, in some cultures, values and beliefs (e.g., fear that talking about death will cause death to happen) may lead to different decisions about advance care planning (Koenig & Davies, 2002). Currently, no family-centered program is available to help the families of adolescents with life-threatening illnesses speak directly and honestly with one another about EOL care (Gilban, Kumar, de Caprariis, Olivieri, & Ho, 1996; Kane, 2006). A structured model administered by a trained facilitator has the potential to regulate these strong feelings, which make deliberative decision making, even for adults, about these "hot" or emotionally laden thoughts (Hamburg, 1986; Petersen & Hamburg, 1986) even more challenging (Slovic, Finucane, Peters, & MacGregor, 2002).

This chapter briefly reviews developmental considerations when involving adolescents in medical decision making, with particular attention to new research on the adolescent brain, as well as new theories on the intuitive or nondeliberative aspects of decision making in adolescents and adults. Illustrating many of these concepts and observations, Richard, an adolescent patient, provides a first-hand account of his experience of completing an advance directive with his social worker while his grandparents were present. Next, a structured model is presented for providing family-centered advance care planning for adolescents with a life-threatening illness. Finally, we return for a postscript with Richard and his grandparents, who 2 years later agreed to participate in a research study testing the feasibility and acceptability of this family-centered advance care planning model.

☐ The Adolescent Brain

New research demonstrates that the structure of the adolescent brain is not fully formed, particularly the prefrontal cortex (Giedd, 2007; Giedd et al., 1999; Weinberger, Elvevag, & Giedd, 2005). There is rapid growth in gray matter at around age 12 to 13 and then a pruning back of this growth completed at about age 22. This is a sensitive period of "use it or lose it," in which this part of the brain is becoming more efficient in its capacity to make connections. The frontal lobes or prefrontal cortex are involved in organization in time and space, planning, control of feelings and impulses, and reasoning. This part of the brain serves an executive function, like the chief executive officer of a large organization. Although researchers have cautioned the public and policy makers not to make inferences about adolescent behavior and decision-making capacity based on these findings, the data do suggest that adolescents, as a group, are different from adults in the maturity of their brain structure. What the data mean in terms of the actual functioning or behavior of an individual adolescent is unclear. Nevertheless, these findings have stirred up legal (Hartman, 2002) and public policy debates regarding adolescent competency to be charged as adults and executed, as well as fears regarding possible reconsideration of rights granted to adolescents to have access to some medical services without parental permission. The implications for adolescent advance care planning are unclear.

□ Adolescent Development and Decision Making

Recent developments in decision-making theory and evidenced-based research challenge our former understanding of adolescent and adult decision making. We now know that decisions are not always rational or based on all available information but rather are intuitive, depending on accessibility of information and the experience or expertise of the decision maker (Kahneman, 2002; Tversky & Kahneman, 1974). Mature decision making appears to be a dual process: System 1, the *intuitive* nondeliberative process of accessibility (ease with which thoughts come to mind) based on experience is fast, automatic, effortless, associative, and difficult to control or modify; and System 2, the *rational* deliberative process of weighing costs and benefits is slower, serial, effortful, deliberately controlled, relatively flexible, and potentially rule governed (Kahneman, 2002; see Chang and Sambamoorthi, chapter 10, this volume). Contrary to past theories of cognitive development posed by psychology theorists (Ajzen & Fishbein, 1980; Bandura, 1986; Janz & Becker, 1984; Piaget, 1952; Ward & Overton, 1990), rational decision making involving the weighing of costs and benefits decreases with age, while intuitive decision making increases with age from adolescence through adulthood (Davidson, 1991; Reyna & Ellis, 1994). Thus, the theory of bounded rationality, intuitive judgment, and choice presumes that adult decisions are frequently not deliberative, but intuitive, resulting in predictable types of errors.

People are not accustomed to thinking hard and often trust a plausible judgment that comes quickly to mind (Kahneman, 2002). Although this process is adaptive and efficient in most circumstances, one error it leads to, *framing effects,* is relevant to understanding medical decision making in adolescents and adults. Outcomes that are certain are overweighted relative to outcomes of high or intermediate probability. McNeil, Pauker, Sox, and Tversky (1982) studied one famous example of the framing effect. Using a hypothetical lung cancer patient, they asked for different choices between surgery and radiation therapy by describing outcome statistics in terms of survival rates or mortality rates. The outcomes were, in fact, exactly the same. Because 90% short-term survival (i.e., probability of living) is less threatening than 10% immediate mortality (i.e., probability of dying), the survival frame yielded a substantially higher preference for surgery. This framing effect was found not only among patients but also among experienced physicians (McNeil et al., 1982). Framing effects happen because alternative formulations of the same situation make different aspects of the situation accessible. Another important finding (Finucane, Alhakami, Slovic, & Johnson, 2000) is that the efficacy of rational deliberative decision making is impaired by time pressure, a situation under which many medical decisions are made. Clinical observations suggest that the charisma of the person who approaches the patient or the eagerness of the patient to please the other also influence EOL decisions. Occasionally, a situation arises when, for example, the adolescent tells his or her physician that he or she wants everything done to prolong life no matter what, while telling the case manager of a preference to die a natural death and discontinue medical interventions that are prolonging the dying process.

Complex decisions, especially those involving life and death, may be better made using intuitive thought than conscious deliberation (Baird & Fugelsang, 2004; Dijksterhuis, Bos, Mordgren, & van Baaren, 2006; Reyna, Adam, Poirier, LeCroy, & Brainerd, 2005; Reyna & Ellis, 1994; see Reyna & Farley, 2006, for a detailed discussion of risk and rationality in adolescent decision making). Nevertheless, if a treatment choice is too complex or the results are only negative or uncertain, the more abstract and difficult the choice will be (e.g., McCabe, 1996; Tversky & Kahneman, 1974). For further guidance, McCabe's classic article (1996) as well as Rushton and Lynch (1992) provide developmental and clinical considerations in child and adolescent EOL decision making.

☐ Evidence for Adolescent Competence in Medical Decision Making

Despite the implications of brain research and decision-making theory, research suggests that under stable medical circumstances, adolescents appear to have the same medical decision-making capacity as those 18 or older, who have the legal right to make these decisions for themselves. Adolescents 14 and older do not appear to differ from adults in their competence to make informed treatment decisions (Weithorn & Campbell, 1982), and there is no reason to suspect that young adolescents have a less-mature understanding of death than those 18 or older (Doig & Burgess, 2000; Field & Behrman, 2002). Adolescents generally defer to parental influence, but when the seriousness of the decision increases, they become less deferential to parental influence (Susman, Dorn, & Fletcher, 1992).

☐ A Personal Story

There is agreement among healthcare professionals that adolescents who wish to be involved in decisions about their EOL care should be involved (American Academy of Pediatrics, 1994, 2000; APA, 2005; Field & Behrman, 2002; Leikin, 1989, 1993). It is in this context that Richard, a budding writer and adolescent living with AIDS, was invited to tell his story. At the time of his EOL decision making, Richard was hospitalized with tuberculosis and pneumonia. There was concern his life was in danger because of his severely compromised immune system. Richard relates his experience of being approached by his social worker to make his preferences known about his own EOL care; his grandparents were present in his hospital room at that time. In the year prior to this hospitalization (his fourth), a friend of Richard's died of AIDS. At the time of this hospitalization, Richard was a 10th grader in a local parochial high school where no one knew his diagnosis. Richard honored his grandparents' request that he tell no one outside the hospital/clinic setting his HIV status. Richard wrote his story while hospitalized for yet another complication of his illness. These are his own words, aside from a few minor edits.

My End-of-Life Decision Making

Salutations Dear Readers:

My name is Richard and I am 16 years old. I am an African-American male who was born HIV positive, and I was asked to share with you some of my personal experiences with end-of-life decision making. Before I begin, I would like to give you some brief background information about who I am, what I've been through in my life, and why writing something like this might not only be important to me, but why reading it may be useful for you as well. As is my style, I will write about a variety of topics in a free-form way.

I have already lost many loved ones, a few to AIDS/HIV, including my own mother when I was just an infant. I currently live with my maternal grandparents, who care for me as best they can. I love them both unconditionally through the many ups and downs we've faced and for those yet to come. I know that they care deeply about me and my well-being, and it honestly pains me to see them stress themselves out over me when I get sick. Being HIV-positive compromises my immune system, which means that I am not able to fight off viruses and colds as well as someone with a stronger immune system could, and there's a much higher likelihood of a simple cold turning into something more serious for me. Although I may not show it as much as I would like, I'd give the world to make it clear to my grandparents how much they mean to me (and not to have AIDS/HIV)—I don't want them to worry.

Death is the inevitable conclusion to life. A majority of people fear death; I know I do. Yet, we all have to go through with it eventually. I don't mean we should walk around in a miserable state of mind waiting to die, but everyone should go out and live his or her life to the fullest (responsibly). Yes, I am fearful of death; but, no, I do not (I try not to) let it limit the things I do with my life. Being HIV-positive, I am continuously reminded of death and how important it is to take my medication, stay healthy, exercise, and eat right. This type of thing adds more fuel to the fire of life. In addition to being a student at the local high school where I live, I have the typical teenage problems everyone my age probably goes through, such as getting good grades, passing my classes, and getting a date; thinking about my friends, family, love, health, and the future—just to name a few. With my delicate health, I have more to worry about than the average person my age does. I honestly hope to live a very long, fulfilling, worthwhile life. My primary goal is to become an established and critically acclaimed author/screenplay writer and I've already had several pieces of work published, but that's another story. …

End-of-life decision making. I personally try not to think of death too much; I know it's there, but the subject itself can get so depressing. I've traveled a great deal over the United States and talked about HIV/AIDS awareness, but death and end-of-life decision making are the last things on my mind. From my understanding, end-of-life decision making is sort of like a will or life insurance. Nevertheless, end-of-life decisions don't necessarily mean decisions made at the end of someone's life because no one ever really knows when their [sic] time is up. So this would really be more like precautionary end-of-life decisions, just like the rapper Kanye West says in his song "Heard 'em say": "Nothing's ever promised tomorrow today." I would plan to make arrangements with family, friends, and loved ones about what I want to happen in case such-and-such a thing were to happen; for example, if I were in a coma and wasn't responding to any medical treatment, who decides to keep me alive or "pull the plug"?

This is a pretty hard topic to discuss, not only because death is a touchy subject, but also because I don't really have any ideas as to what MY end-of-life decisions would be. When I was 15, which was only last year, my social worker called me and asked me to fill out what is known as a Five Wishes®[1] statement that documents my end-of-life desires. Although I filled it out with my grandparents, we didn't really talk about it, nor can I remember what was on it or what I put down. This is one of those moments where I honestly wish I could have something profound to say on such a serious topic, but I don't, and I guess my inexperience also adds a bit of earnestness to the issue. My awkwardness with writing about death kind of feels like I'm typing out a suicide note. If my uncertainty confuses you, then I deeply apologize.

One thing I do know is that I pray to make peace with anyone I've harmed or hurt and to those who have done likewise to me. I've lived a good life. I also know that I don't want my funeral to be long and spiritual; more like an organized party among those who know me where they share stories of me and how I've touched their lives.

I'd like to apologize if this chapter got off topic or hasn't answered questions about how to deal with end-of-life decision making. I believe it's up to the person, the individual, to deal with his or her own way of making end-of-life decisions. Some people might leave a will while others might not, but all life really offers us that's ours to keep are the thoughts and memories we hold of the loved ones who have passed on. Thoughts and memories are ours to make and ours to hold. Looking back upon my life and the places I have been, the things I've accomplished (or could have accomplished), I know there are few (if any) regrets that I hold, but I would change nothing because these experiences are what made me the person I am today.

Thank you for your time and I hope in some way, shape, or form my experiences and outlook have benefited you, as writing this has me.

Commentary

Richard is focused on living his life fully as he struggles to describe his decision-making process. Note the number of times Richard apologizes. Richard's indecision and confusion are a common part of this process, even after a decision is made. This confusion is not simply because he was 16 years old but is typical for many adults near the EOL, depending on environmental and interpersonal circumstances (Lockhart, Ditto, Danks, Coppola, & Smucker, 2001). EOL decision making is a process that needs to be reexamined as a person's stage of illness changes.

Richard is also an orphan. The impact of growing up orphaned on decision making was examined by Cournos (1999), who discussed the impact of parental loss, the trauma response, and her reflections based on her own personal experience. She concluded that adolescents who are alone probably need and want a greater level of involvement from the treating medical staff than is required by most adult patients.

Richard's story also illustrates how easy it is to avoid these hard decisions, as well as the reluctance to disclose his preferences to his family to protect them by choosing what he thinks his family wants (Bluebond-Langner, 1978; Hinds et al., 2001). This may be one of the reasons that Richard cannot remember what he chose. In a study of 10 adolescents with cancer (Hinds et al.), the most frequently considered factor by adolescents in EOL decision making across all decisions was "doing what others think I should." The adolescents were influenced by the recommendations, preferences, or opinions of the healthcare provider and family members. They were also influenced by previous experience with life support measures, defined as the adolescent being influenced by having seen or heard about others who have been on mechanical ventilation or other technical means to extend life. The latter probably influenced Richard's decision as well, although he does not make the link directly in his story.

Richard's perception that completing the *Five Wishes* was like writing a suicide note raises concerns about the safety of approaching adolescents to participate in these decisions when the adolescents are medically unstable. Furthermore, Richard was presumed to be competent, but there was no screening to determine if he had any memory impairment, perhaps caused by HIV dementia (Lyon, Marsh, Trexler, Crane, & D'Angelo, 2007;

Power, Selnes, Grim, & McArthur, 1995), which may explain, in retrospect, his inability to remember what his wishes were.

□ Family-Centered Advance Care Planning: A Model for End-of-Life Decision Making

Richard's first experience making EOL care decisions was based on the standard of care for this hospital, an informal process guided by hospital policies (CNMC, 1994). Yet, our patients' and families' experiences, research, and theory suggest that a more sensitive and structured approach is needed if families are to feel included in the process and if adolescents are to truly give their assent/consent to treatment preferences.

Postscript

Two years after the initial discussion, Richard and his grandparents agreed to participate in the family-centered advance care planning (Lyon, 2006) protocol and gave us permission to share some of the qualitative results. Richard is now 18 years old, medically stable, and a senior in high school. He now practices jujitsu, a martial art. He plans to work for a year after graduation so he can live independently before attending college. He is working with his case manager to apply for work through vocational rehabilitation services. During the family-centered advance care planning intervention, Richard and his grandparents expressed gratitude to the research staff for being given the opportunity to discuss these hard issues. Richard made it clear that under no circumstances did he want to have anyone "pull the plug." Yet, he also clearly faced his grandparents and asked them to promise not to mortgage their house, if he were dying, to pay for his medical care. They reluctantly agreed to honor this wish. He also indicated that he did not want them to follow his instructions rigidly but gave them permission to use their own judgment if a time came when he could not speak for himself. Richard said his greatest fear was being alone, and that the most difficult part of one of his hospitalizations was being on the isolation unit. "Being on isolation was tough. Everyone was waving." When asked during the respecting choices interview, "What do you know about the possible complications that may occur because of your HIV infection?" he responded that the greatest complication of his illness is the feeling that it is a secret.

Richard also described being plagued by guilt, "Why did I outlive someone else? When is my time going to come?" The family described many experiences with taking care of dying family members, including the experience of in-home hospice. His grandfather and grandmother described how they are the ones who take care of dying family members in their home when this choice is made. Wakes for deceased family members are traditionally held at their home. Each of them expressed the wish for a natural passing that is as dignified as possible, not perceiving any discrepancy between this and Richard's wish that they not "pull the plug." Richard is comforted by his belief that his mother is waiting for him to join her. He said, "I am not afraid to die." Although not clearly articulated here, Richard's religious belief in a God and the certainty of life after death probably influenced his decisions, as is the case with many adolescents (Koenig & Davies, 2002; Lyon, Townsend-Akpan, & Thompson, 2001). Each of them expressed gratitude for the bridge this study provided for talking about these hard choices, rather than having to build the bridge themselves. Richard no longer felt confused or indecisive, and his grandparents no longer felt left out. The family left confident in the knowledge that they could go through this process again and make future decisions as the need arises.

Richard and his grandparents were able to discuss their differences and reached congruence in the decision making. In some cases, the family members and the adolescent are not able to resolve their differences (Mulhern et al., 1981) because of a belief that HIV/AIDS is a punishment from God or because of conflicting values about medical interventions near the EOL. In such an event, a referral to or consultation with the hospital chaplain or the hospital ethicist is strongly recommended.

The fear of abandonment and of dying alone is deeply felt and sometimes experienced by dying patients. The secrecy surrounding Richard's AIDS diagnosis may further contribute to his fear of dying alone as none of his classmates, neighbors, or teachers are told when he is hospitalized. They do not visit him in the hospital or send him cards, as would likely be the case if he had a nonstigmatizing disease such as cancer. Sadly, in rare instances, adolescents have been abandoned by their families (Lyon & Pao, 2006). Each of the three other personal accounts in this volume emphasizes the importance of family and friend support in life-threatening situations and care near the EOL. The treatment team then becomes like family for the patient, visiting with them, singing songs, and holding hands. Moreno and Schonberg (1999) provide an invaluable discussion of the complexities of such a situation in which an adolescent dying of cancer was alone, while Futterman and Millock (1999) discuss another adolescent whose foster parent had no legal rights yet had a long-lasting and meaningful relationship with the HIV-positive adolescent. They argue that it is cruel for a foster parent to be excluded from the final phase of decision making after caring for someone throughout a deteriorating and fatal illness.

Unlike some families who fear that advance care planning or discussing issues related to death and dying will hasten death or that involving children in decision making is not appropriate (Koenig & Davies, 2002), Richard and his family had the courage to face these hard choices together. Their relationship strengthened, and in gratitude to the research staff, Richard's grandfather said, "This [the hospital] is a 'golden place.'"

□ Note

1. *Five Wishes®* is a legal document that helps a person express how he or she wants to be treated if seriously ill or unable to speak for himself or herself. It was written with the help of the American Bar Association's Commission on the Legal Problems of the Elderly. It was developed by the nonprofit organization Aging with Dignity and its founder, Jim Towey, who was inspired by his work with Mother Teresa in India to develop this tool. Five Wishes is legally sufficient for a person over the age of 18 in most states in the United States. However, it can be used as a tool to help younger adolescents to participate in shared decision making, discussing their preferences for their own EOL care with their family. For adolescents under the age of 18, the document must be signed by their parent or legal guardian to be legally sufficient. More information is available at http://www.agingwithdignity.org.

□ References

Ajzen, I., & Fishbein, M. (1980). *Understanding attitudes and predicting social behavior.* Englewood Cliffs, NJ: Prentice-Hall.

Alderson, P. (1992). Everyday and medical life choices: Decision-making among 8- to 15-year-old school students. *Child Care Health and Development, 18,* 81–95.

American Academy of Pediatrics Committee on Bioethics. (1994). Guidelines on for-going life-sustaining medical treatment. *Pediatrics, 93,* 532–536.

American Academy of Pediatrics, Committee on Bioethics and Committee on Hospital Care. (2000). Palliative care for children. *Pediatrics, 106,* 351–357.

American Psychological Association. (2005). *Report of the Children and Adolescents Task Force of the Ad Hoc Committee on End-of-Life Issues.* Washington, DC: Author.

Baird, A. A., & Fugelsang, J. A. (2004). The emergence of consequential thought: Evidence from neuroscience. *Philosophical Transactions of the Royal Society of London, Series B: Biological Sciences, 359,* 1797–1804.

Bandura, A. (1986). *Social foundations of thought and action: A social cognitive theory.* Englewood Cliffs, NJ: Prentice-Hall.

Bearison, D. (1991). *They never want to tell you.* Cambridge, MA: Harvard University Press.

Bluebond-Langner, M. (1978). *Private worlds of dying children.* Princeton, NJ: Princeton University Press.

Children's National Medical Center. (1994, April 19). *Advance directives for health care decision-making* (Policy No. CH PC CO:10). Washington, DC: Author.

Cournos, F. (1999). The impact of growing up orphaned on decision-making capacity. In J. Blustein, C. Levine, & N. Neveloff Dubler (Eds.), *The adolescent alone: Decision-making in health care in the United States* (pp. 111–120). Cambridge, England: Cambridge University Press.

Crawley, L., Marshall, P., Lo, B., & Koenig, B. A. (2002). Strategies for culturally effective end-of-life care. *Annals of Internal Medicine, 136,* 673–679.

Davidson, D. (1991). Children's decision-making examined with an information-board procedure. *Cognitive Development, 6,* 77–90.

Dijksterhuis, A., Bos, M. W., Mordgren, L. F., & van Baaren, R. B. (2006). On making the right choice: The deliberation-without-attention effect. *Science, 311,* 1005–1007.

Doig, C., & Burgess, E. (2000). Withholding life-sustaining treatment: Are adolescents competent to make these decisions? *Canadian Medical Association Journal, 162,* 1585–1588.

Field, M. J., & Behrman, R. E. (Eds.). (2002). *When children die: Improving palliative and end-of-life care for children and their families.* Washington, DC: National Academy Press.

Finucane, M. L., Alhakami, A., Slovic, P., & Johnson, S. M. (2000). The affect heuristic in judgments of risks and benefits. *Journal of Behavioral Decision-making, 13,* 1–17.

Freyer, D. R. (2004). Care of the dying adolescent: Special considerations. *Pediatrics, 113,* 381–388.

Futterman, D., & Millock, P. (1999). Case five: Consent and an informal guardian. In J. Blustein, C. Levine, & N. Neveloff Dubler (Eds.), *The adolescent alone: Decision-making in health care in the United States* (pp. 212–219). Cambridge, England: Cambridge University Press.

Gilban, S., Kumar, D., de Caprariis, P. J., Olivieri, F., & Ho, K. (1996). Pediatric AIDS and advance directives: A three-year prospective study in New York state. *AIDS Patient Care and STDs, 10,* 168–170.

Giedd, J. N. (2007, March 28). *The teen brain.* Gallagher Lectureship presented at the annual Society for Adolescent Medicine Meeting, Denver, CO.

Giedd, J. N., Blumenthal, J., Jeffries, N. O., Castellanos, F. X., Liu, H., Zijdenbos, A., et al. (1999). Brain development during childhood and adolescence: A longitudinal MRI study. *Nature Neuroscience, 2,* 861–863.

Hamburg, B. (1986). Subsets of adolescent mothers: Developmental, biomedical, and psychosocial issues. In B. Lancaster & B. A. Hamburg (Eds.), *School-age pregnancy and parenthood: Biosocial dimensions* (pp. 115–145). New York: Aldine de Gruyter.

Hartman, R. G. (2002). Coming of age: Devising legislation for adolescent medical decision-making. *American Journal of Law & Medicine, 28,* 409–453.

Hinds, P. S., Oakes, L., Furman, W., Quargnenti, A., Olson, M. S., Foppiano, P., et al. (2001). End-of-life decision-making by adolescents, parents and health-care providers in pediatric oncology: Research to evidence-based practice guidelines. *Cancer Nursing, 24,* 122–136.

Janz, N. K., & Becker, M. H. (1984). The health belief model: A decade later. *Health Education Quarterly, 11,* 1–47.

Kahneman, D. (2002, December 8). *Maps of bounded rationality: A perspective on intuitive judgment and choice* (Nobel Prize lecture). Retrieved April 8, 2007, from http://nobelprize.org/nobel_prizes/economics/laureates/2002/kahnemann-lecture.pdf

Kane, J. R. (2006). Pediatric palliative care moving forward: Empathy, competence, quality, and the need for systematic change. *Journal of Palliative Medicine, 9,* 847–849.

Koenig, B. A., & Davies, E. (2002). Cultural dimensions of care at life's end for children and their families. In M. J. Field & R. E. Behrman (Eds.), *When children die: Improving palliative and end-of-life care for children and their families* (pp. 509–552). Washington, DC: National Academy Press.

Kreicbergs, U., Valdimarsdottir, U., Onelov, E., Henter, J. I., & Steineck, G. (2004). Talking about death with children who have severe malignant disease. *New England Journal of Medicine, 351,* 1175–1186.

Larson, D. G., & Tobin, D. R. (2000). End-of-life conversations: Evolving practice and theory. *Journal of the American Medical Association, 284,* 1573–1578.

Leikin, S. (1989). A proposal concerning decisions to forgo life-sustaining treatment for young people. *Journal of Pediatrics, 115,* 17–22.

Leikin, S. (1993). The role of adolescents in decisions concerning their cancer therapy. *Cancer, 71,* 3342–3346.

Lockhart, L. K., Ditto, P. H., Danks, J. H., Coppola, K. M., & Smucker, W. D. (2001). The stability of older adults' judgments of fates better and worse than death. *Death Studies, 25,* 299–317.

Lyon, M. E. (2006). *Lyon family centered advance care planning survey—adolescent version and patient version.* Unpublished instrument. (Available from Dr. Maureen E. Lyon, Division of Adolescent and Young Adult Medicine, Children's National Medical Center, 111 Michigan Avenue, NW, Washington, DC 20010)

Lyon, M. E., Marsh, J., Trexler, C. L., Crane, S., & D'Angelo, L. J. (2007). HIV dementia in adolescents: What's the best screening tool? *Journal of Adolescent Health,* 40, S2.

Lyon, M. E., McCabe, M. A., Patel, K., & D'Angelo, L. J. (2004). What do adolescents want? An exploratory study regarding end-of-life decision-making. *Journal of Adolescent Health, 35,* 529.e1–529.e6.

Lyon, M. E., & Pao, M. (2006). When all else fails: End of life care for adolescents. In M. E. Lyon & L. J. D'Angelo (Eds.), *Teenagers, HIV and AIDS: Insights from youths living with the virus* (pp. 215–233). Westport, CT: Greenwood.

Lyon, M. E., Townsend-Akpan, C., & Thompson, A. (2001). Spirituality and end-of-life care for an adolescent with AIDS. *AIDS Patient Care and STDs, 15,* 555–560.

McCabe, M. A. (1996). Involving children and adolescents in medical decision-making: Developmental and clinical considerations. *Journal of Pediatric Psychology, 21,* 505–516.

McNeil, B. J., Pauker, S. G., Sox, H. C., & Tversky, A. (1982). On the elicitation of preferences for alternative therapies. *New England Journal of Medicine, 306,* 1259–1262.

Moreno, J., & Schonberg, K. (1999). Case four: Saying "No" to treatment in terminal illness. In J. Blustein, C. Levine, & N. Neveloff Dubler (Eds.), *The adolescent alone: Decision-making in health care in the United States* (pp. 205–211). Cambridge, England: Cambridge University Press.

Mulhern, R. K., Crisco, J. J., & Camitta, B. M. (1981). Patterns of communication among pediatric patients with leukemia, parents and physicians: Prognostic disagreements and misunderstandings. *Journal of Pediatrics, 99,* 480–483.

Muniño, A. M., Arias, E., Kochanek, K. D., Murphy, S. L., & Smith, B. L. (2002). Deaths: Final data for 2000. *National Vital Statistics Report, 50,* 1–119. Retrieved April 8, 2007, from http://www.cdc.gov/nchs/data/nvsr/nvsr50/nvsr50_15.pdf

Petersen, A. C., & Hamburg, B. (1986). Adolescence: A developmental approach to problems and psychopathology. *Behavior Therapy, 17,* 480–499.

Piaget, J. (1952). *The origins of intelligence in children.* New York: International Universities Press.

Power, C., Selnes, O. A., Grim, J. A., & McArthur, J. C. (1995). HIV Dementia Scale: A rapid screening test. *Journal of Acquired Immune Deficiency Syndrome Human Retrovirology, 8,* 273–278.

Rao, J. K., Anderson, L. A., & Smith, S. M. (2002). End of life is a public health issue. *American Journal of Preventive Medicine, 23,* 215–220.

Reyna, V. F., Adam, M. B., Poirier, K., LeCroy, C. W., & Brainerd, C. J. (2005). Risky decision-making in childhood and adolescence: A fuzzy-trace theory approach. In J. Jacobs & P. Klacynski (Eds.), *The development of judgment and decision-making in children and adolescents* (pp. 77–106). Mahwah, NJ: Erlbaum.

Reyna, V. F., & Ellis, S. C. (1994). Fuzzy-trace theory and framing effects in children's risky decision-making. *Psychological Science, 5,* 275–279.

Reyna, V. F., & Farley, F. (2006). Risk and rationality in adolescent decision-making: Implications for theory, practice and public policy. *Psychological Science in the Public Interest, 7,* 1–44.

Rushton, C. H., & Lynch, M. D. (1992). Dealing with directives for critically ill adolescents. *Critical Care Nurse, 12,* 31–37.

Slovic, P., Finucane, M., Peters, E., & MacGregor, D. G. (2002). The affective heuristic. In T. Gilovich, D. Griffin, & D. Kahneman (Eds.), *Heuristics and biases: The psychology of intuitive judgment* (pp. 397–420). New York: Cambridge University Press.

Sonnenblick, M., Friedlander, Y., & Steinberg, A. (1993). Dissociation between the wishes of terminally ill parents and decisions by their offspring. *Journal of the American Geriatrics Society, 41,* 599–604.

Susman, E., Dorn, L., & Fletcher, J. C. (1992). Participation in biomedical research: The consent process as viewed by children, adolescents, young adults, and physicians. *Journal of Pediatrics, 121,* 547–552.

Tversky, A., & Kahneman, D. (1974). Judgment under uncertainty: Heuristics and biases. *Science, 185,* 1124–1131.

Ward, S. L., & Overton, W. F. (1990). Semantic familiarity, relevance, and the development of deductive reasoning. *Developmental Psychology, 26,* 488–493.

Weinberger, D. R., Elvevag, B., & Giedd, J. N. (2005). *The adolescent brain: A work in progress.* Washington, DC: The National Campaign to Prevent Teen Pregnancy. Retrieved April 8, 2007, from http://www.teenpregnancy.org/resources/reading/pdf/BRAIN.pdf

Weir, R. F., & Peters, C. (1997). Affirming the decisions adolescents make about life and death. *Hastings Center Report, 27*(6), 29–39.

Weithorn, L. A., & Campbell, S. B. (1982). The competency of children and adolescents to make informed treatment decisions. *Child Development, 53,* 1589–1598.

CHAPTER 3

The Grip of Pain

Jonathon D. Spannhake

Death is inevitable. Everyone can say this and understand it from one perspective or another. However, young people such as me rarely get to comprehend it first hand. It came as a shock to me when I was told I had developed Guillain-Barre syndrome (GBS). In no way was I prepared to face anything that was coming my way, but I also realize that people rarely get a notice that they may be nearing death. Once death is put into the picture, so many things come along with it. Everyone needs to comprehend the quality of their lives. Sometimes the pain given to certain people near death is bearable, and there are times when the suffering can get so terrible that a person will wish death on themselves no matter what their religion or feelings about death may be. Also, sometimes family and friends can be a big influence on quality of life, not just how a person is feeling.

My case of GBS was rare compared to what people normally experience. GBS is a rare neurological disorder that leads to damaged nerves caused by the human body's immune system; the disorder normally originates from a previous infection or illness. Effects of the syndrome are muscle weakness, a tingling or numbness in the body, and possible paralysis. For most people, GBS attacks them slowly. At first, they would not even realize anything was wrong except that they were getting more tired every day for up to several years. I had never experienced that. My first symptoms were when the tips of my toes and the tips of my fingers began to go numb. Normally, the toes would go numb and then spread from there, which made my case even more rare because my hands were going numb at the same time as my toes. After my feet and hands went numb, my mouth began to go numb as well. It was then that I was admitted to a hospital and diagnosed with GBS. From there, the numbness spread throughout my body.

When doctors originally told me that I had GBS, the first thing they mentioned to me was that recovery was normally 100%. There was no discussion of other possibilities or worst-case scenarios. For several weeks into my hospitalization, I did not expect to experience the thought process of a man about to die.

I had been transported to a rehabilitation center from the hospital. At that time I had become almost completely paralyzed. I could move my arms and legs only slightly, and I had a rapid buildup of phlegm in my lungs from the pneumonia I had developed only days before. Through all of this I could not stand the feeling of people touching any part of my body because of neuropathy, which is a problem with nerve functions that make certain parts of a human body develop sharp, shooting pains, numbness, tingling, and weakness in the affected area (which was especially dreadful around my feet and ankles).

On the third night of my stay, I woke up around 1:00 in the morning with the perception that I was being strangled. My breathing had halted. Seconds passed, and I realized what had happened. I had slid down my inclined bed, and my throat had filled up with phlegm from the pneumonia. The phlegm was strangling me. This sensation was followed by a burning, stabbing feeling in my chest. I tried throwing my body side to side with panic trying to take in a single breath of air. When I was finally able to thrust my body forward, I realized my windpipe would open up a bit, and I was able to take in short, painful breaths. I fell back and instantly thrust my body forward again for another breath. As I fell back down, I looked over at the suction machine the day nurses had given me to place in my mouth to suck out all of the unwanted phlegm and saliva. My mother had laid the tube on my stomach in case I had needed it for an occasion such as this. However, in my squirming attempts to catch my breath, it had slid to the edge of the bed, luckily still plugged in. All I had to do was grab the tube and place it into my mouth to release the pressure in my throat and breathe again.

Finally, the thought that I may die entered my mind. I was not fighting for breath because I wanted to breathe; I was fighting to stay alive. I was trying to exist. I think that deep down in the psyche everyone believes that they are immortal, whether through religious faith or just the denial of death as an inevitability in one's life. Maybe through time and aging a person would come to the realization that he or she would die, but not at the age of 20—not when death meant eternal nothingness, as it did for me, a long-time atheist. As I lay in the bed—quickly confronted by the knowledge that I was going to die, choking on my own phlegm—death changed from something that would eventually happen to something that was happening.

I did not want to believe it, but when death finally revealed its inevitable presence, I had little or no choice but to face it. My mind skipped everything I had always thought I might consider when realizing that death is imminent. The panic, sorrow, and fear were gone. Quickly, my mind went to what it wanted to do as I came close to death—leave this world connecting with life. There was a picture of my girlfriend and me at my brother's wedding taped to the side of my bed. I looked intently at the picture. I stared at my girlfriend, gazing at something that resembled what living was all about. All I wanted was to die while still connected to life, even if only a picture of it.

As I stared at the picture, a nurse walked past the room. My mind freed itself from death's grip, and I tried to call out for help. Just like that, my mind went from the darkest place it could go and back to the denying world where immortality is the truth. The nurse heard my scratchy whispers through the phlegm and helped me up. My phlegm was released through violent coughs, each one more painful than the last.

My lung had collapsed, and that is what had started the massive phlegm buildup. That was why it was so painful to breathe. So, I was brought to the intensive care unit (ICU), where they put me on a respirator and into a chemically induced coma. The reason behind the coma was so I would be unconscious and not have any memory of anything that had to be done to keep me alive. All the physicians treating me knew I was in for a lot of pain, more pain than someone can normally handle if conscious. While in the ICU, I came to face death many times, but because of the drugs being pumped into my body and because of my state of mind, I was unable to grasp how close I was to death, unlike when I was choking at the rehabilitation center.

However, the real pain came after my time in the ICU. I had been on many painkillers, skeletal muscle relaxants, antibiotics, antiseizure medications, antidepressants, steroids, laxatives, and blood thinners. After a while, the nurses and medical doctors discovered that I had developed an allergic reaction to all of the medication I was taking. Thus, I had to begin the weaning process, which consisted of slowly lowering a dose or stopping a medication cold turkey. I remember the greatest degree of pain came when I was taken off of Dilaudid, an opioid pain medication. This medication was also giving me terrible hallucinations (at the time, the physicians did not know why, but later found out it was because I was allergic to it).

At first, the medical doctors talked about putting me into another chemically induced coma to alleviate the pain I was going through so I would not develop an aneurysm from the intense pain that was keeping me awake no matter how many other shots and pills they pumped into my body. I had definitely developed a tolerance to Dilaudid, and it seemed that I was allergic to all other painkillers that worked for me. The problem with being put back into a chemically induced coma was that the chance of coming out of it again was very slim.

At that point, my mind was unable to make a single decision. I was willing to agree to anything that the physicians were offering as long as there was promise in the near future of the pain ceasing. After all, they were the ones with the medical degrees who knew what would be best for me. However, my family's and friends' opinions were different. Because they could not feel the pain and could only assume what my quality of life was at that moment, they assumed that having me put back into a coma would be worse than my taking the chances with the incredible pain.

There was a problem with all of their opinions though; they were not mine. Everyone kept telling me to keep fighting, to work through all of it. Then, I watched them leave the hospital room. They would come in, tell me to fight, and then go about their day. I had to stay in the hospital bed, writhe in pain, and do the fighting. To be completely honest, I think part of my decision to want to be put back into a coma was from the loathing of everyone else's freedom. They were fortunate enough to take a break from the hospitals, the physicians, the drugs, and the pain.

Yet, for me, the grief was ever present and uncontrollable. There was a chance that I would never be conscious again versus the chance of dying. I wanted to end this somehow, but there was no easy answer. This was just something I was going to have to learn to live with. The problem that constantly arose was that I would have done anything for the pain to end while my family wanted for me to attempt to fight this awful syndrome. There was a lot of conflict about how the situation should be handled given the fact that I felt very angry with my family and friends for having the ability to live in the normal world.

What continued to amaze me and helped me love my family as much as I could at the time was seeing just how much my entire family and group of friends cared about me. Most of my close family came to see me on a regular basis. My distant relatives still came to visit me monthly, if not weekly. My friends came to visit as often as they could. I would have never thought my relatives and companions cared about me as much as they showed during my stay in the hospital. They all helped me more than I could have ever imagined during this time. When I saw how much everyone cared, it definitely influenced me to try to keep fighting for my life. There were so many people who cared about me, and I did not want to disappoint them. That was the main reason I kept on fighting: I did not want to die disappointing those around me.

Because I was not ready to risk becoming a "vegetable" for the rest of my life, and everyone else I knew did not want me to be put back into a drug-induced coma, enough time passed by for the physicians finally to make their decision. Eventually, they decided it would be best for me to try to struggle through the pain. I was brought from the step-down hospital back to the rehabilitation center where I had been residing previously.

The pain slightly decreased after a few weeks from the new medication they had given me. Other problems occurred from this new medication regimen, including thick, full-body rashes and high body temperatures, up to 107.3°F. I was brought back to the step-down hospital, where they tried to get me off of all of my medications to see which medication was causing my body to react so awfully.

It was when I was taken off of all of my medication that I began to become mentally unbalanced. The pain was far more intense than I could have ever imagined. During the few moments when I eventually exhausted myself to sleep, I experienced disturbing nightmares. There even came a point at which I began to have unsettling hallucinations of Death incarnate. I never looked at Death, but I knew he was there because I could see darkness in the corner of my eye. I saw this hallucination many times, and each time he would tell me that it was my time, and I should have lived a better life. He told me I deserved to die. With everything else happening at that time, I would collapse under Death's words every time, thinking he was right, that I did deserve to die. Through it all, my friends and family kept telling me to fight and beat this disease. They told me to beat the GBS. My problem was that my *body* was beating the sickness, but my *mind* was losing the battle.

The time I began to see Death and hold conversations with him was around the time I also began to think about my own death. Between the conversations I had with Death and what my friends, family, and the medical doctors were telling me, I had began to contemplate the idea that dying was not as horrendous as everyone was making it out to be. Nobody wants to die, so no one wants other people they care about to die. Nevertheless, I wanted to end the pain I was feeling. I needed the pain to stop because living was much more difficult than what I started to think about death. Dying was an easy way out. Everything would finally come to an end. Not just the pain, but the smaller aspects that people thought I was coping with: the hallucinations, the nightmares, the constant starving sensation because I could not hold down any food given to me, and—of course—being cooped up in the hospital for what seemed near an eternity.

My mind, numbed from everything happening over the past couple of months, was faced with a decision. I could continue suffering, or I could die. Thinking back on everything I had wanted to cling to before all the pain began, I knew what my decision was. I did not care about connecting with life or disappointing my family anymore. In my mind, they had lost their closeness. They were not family anymore; they were just people, people who were not experiencing what I had to experience. They were not in agony every waking second of their lives, and they had not been in the company of Death.

I find it amazing looking back on my experiences in the hospital, how I felt about dying before the pain and how I viewed it completely differently when the constant, intense pain began. I had gone from clinging to life as much as I could to not even wanting to fight death if and when it would come. It was as if both thoughts had come from polar opposite people, but both thoughts had come from me in the matter of a month or two. The only fear I had of dying at the time was my beliefs in life after death.

I believe "the spirit world" or "heaven" does not exist. My largest fear, other than living the rest of my life in utter pain, is facing the end of my life. I believe that after life there is nothing, not even blackness. Blackness indicates that there is at least something, darkness after life if nothing else. Nothingness is what I fear. I did not want to exist, but I did not want to become nonexistent either.

After being moved from the step-down hospital to an infectious disease floor and then to a specialty hospital, I woke up one day to know Death was in the room with me. It was my time to go, and I had to tell people that. I could not stand the pain. Everyone needed to be told that it was my time to go. That was all I wanted to do before I died. The first person I told was my mother. When she came in that day and constantly kept telling me to fight, I told her about Death, about my decision to leave, and about how I could not live in pain anymore. It did not help when she told me that I just had to keep fighting. I was tired of fighting. It was time to give up.

The physicians believed that I was able to get better. They noticed my mentality was unstable and attempted to fix that through medication and psychotherapy. Through psychological interviews and testing, I was informed that what I had was delirium from being confined in a hospital bed too long and in response to all the different medications I was taking at the time. I was then told that it would get better with treatment and the pain would go away, but I just had to last a while longer. No one would tell me how much "a while longer" would be, but they were talking in terms of years rather than months or days. This was just something with which I had to come to terms.

Looking back at that time, I cannot really think of any way things could have gone better in my treatment. The medical doctors were always there for me and so were the nurses, personal care assistants, and other hospital staff. As for pain management, I believe I received the best care possible in that area as well. There was an entire team of pain physicians, nurses, and a psychologist who tried to help me through these troubling times. The problem is, while in an intense amount of pain, there is nothing someone can say to make it go away; time and death are the only cures for that. However, I am not saying that pain management is something that is expendable. It helped me deal with the pain and still try and keep as sane as possible in this situation.

During my stay in the hospitals—a total of 89 days—the staff tried to help me as much as possible, with the pain management group constantly trying to find ways to relieve me from the hurt to the little necessities the nurses brought into my hospital room to make my life a little easier. The difficult thing about this is that the hospital staff kept asking me what they could do to help. The problem is that there was not much they could do beyond doing their jobs and keeping up with the pain medication, whenever I was able to take it. The pain management department did help me with my decision to try to keep fighting through GBS for the majority of my stay at the hospital, although a lot of their help was putting me into a chemically induced coma or putting extreme amounts of painkillers into my body so I would not be able to feel anything, let alone pain. And, I thoroughly believe that the reason why I was losing my mental capabilities was because of all of the medications I was having pumped into my system. I had lost a sense of reality and time because of these pills, which gave me an entirely new perspective on life. However, these lost senses were something that had to happen to keep me alive. I needed all of these medications flowing through me. So being taken off all of them during my severe allergies threw me off my senses once again while I was experiencing incredible amounts of pain, and that is why I was not able to take the pain any longer.

While the hospital staff worked to help me, I also had my entire family supporting me. The problem was, with my lost senses, I had no feeling of compassion around my relatives. There were times when they would even anger me by saying the smallest things, such as "I know what you're going through" or "I'm sorry." My thoughts back then were that no one could possibly know this pain, and why were so many people sorry? The GBS was not their fault. Those two sentiments people kept telling me would constantly aggravate me. I would become angry and not be able to calm down for hours because the pain would only fuel the anger.

My family and friends still helped me out a lot. They would push me when I needed to be pushed, even if all I wanted to do was die. They cared for me when all I wanted was to be left alone. They sat next to me through my hardest times while I could not stand having anyone look at me. Even though my mind was filled with hatred for the most part, these few things helped a lot. My family and friends were there for me.

Experiencing GBS was by far the hardest thing my body and mind has ever tried to overcome. It amazes me how this disease can just one day appear into someone's life with no real medical explanation regarding what happened. I would have never thought that a disease could strike so quickly and suddenly and have such an impact on a person's life. GBS is a rough road to go down, but the outcome is almost always complete recovery. Sometimes the pain is unbearable. The help and opinions from family, friends, and physicians can only go so far before the mind can finally decide what it really wants. With all the pain, I had thought that death was better than living, even if it meant that I would be gone forever. Pain can be a powerful influence on how a person can look at end-of-life decisions, sometimes even overpowering those who mean everything to you and more.

4

CHAPTER

Decision Making in the Absence of Advance Directives

A Personal Story of Letting Go

Laura Crow

□ Introduction

Shortly after noon on November 4, 2001, my brother Josh was riding to work on the back of his best friend's Harley motorcycle. Two blocks from their destination, while stopped for a red light, the bike was struck at an estimated 48 miles per hour by a Ford Explorer. The strap on Josh's helmet broke free, and he landed head first on the pavement. Twenty minutes later, he arrived at a leading medical center, where he barely survived emergency surgery.

The shock of the phone call, which I did not receive until 7:30 that evening, chills my skin even today. My brother was gravely injured, and I lived 120 miles away in San Diego. It was the call no one expects but silently dreads, for somewhere deep inside we know that terrible things *can* happen to us and to those we love. By the time I reached intensive care, it was 11:00 p.m.

Five years prior, I had seen a dear friend die of AIDS in the very same hospital and was braced for the sight and sound of life support. I had ridden with paramedics and knew that sometimes injuries looked worse than they really were. My biological psychology course had instilled in me a deep respect and awe for the intricacies of the human brain, but nothing could have prepared me for that intensive care unit (ICU) resident's words: "Massive swelling." "Craniotomy." "Temporal lobectomy." "The prognosis is very bad." As my father awaited news in Washington, D.C., desperately searching for a flight, I began to realize the severity of our situation. I dialed his number with the weight of the world on my chest.

Josh made it through the night, and my dad made it to Los Angeles. We met the neurosurgeon who had performed my brother's surgery; he was a young, energetic, self-proclaimed optimist—the dose of hope we needed. He marveled at just how swollen Josh's brain was. The ventricles were completely effaced. It was the worst injury he had ever seen. How we found solace in that, I will never know. Everyone in our camp agreed that Josh was alive because he was a fighter, that he would have the last say, that no amount of medical expertise could hold a candle to his tenacity. I did not sleep for 3 days, surviving on adrenalin, coffee, and fear.

We waited every morning for neurosurgical updates, but after the first 72 hours it became evident that Josh's physicians were not talking. Perhaps our anguish overwhelmed them, and they feared handing out false hope, or maybe their caseloads prevented any semblance of intimate contact with patients' families. My own loss of faith in the medical system began when we asked Josh's neurosurgeon to detail the areas of injury, and he replied, "You wouldn't possibly understand. That's a seminar-level medical school discussion." End of conversation.

□ System Failure

Josh spent 71 days in the ICU. He suffered multiple hospital-acquired antibiotic-resistant infections, pneumonia, 106°F fevers, foot drop (permanent loss of ability to flex the foot), and bedsores. He endured three more brain surgeries. His limbs contracted to the point at which physical therapy harmed rather than helped. Although he emerged from the coma, he was unresponsive to commands and incapable of conscious engagement. I kept a journal for him so that he would not miss anything.

During the preceding years, I had occasionally asked myself this silly question: Who do I love the most? Invariably, the answer was Josh. As the weeks swept by, I sensed my brother slipping away. The pain felt too big to hold, but letting go terrified me. Anything other than stoic determination meant giving up, and I could not allow it. I would not. One afternoon, while Josh was still in the ICU, I asked his nurse if she believed he could recover any function. For the first time, I got an honest answer. She had assisted in the original surgery, during which that bright young neurosurgeon exclaimed to her, "My God, his brain is all over the place!" Her best-case scenario for him was 5 years in a hospital bed, then death by infection. I listened because she risked her job to tell me, and I needed to hear the truth. Once Josh was safely breathing on his own and weaned off the narcotic drip, his medical team transferred him to the floor. I hated the term *persistent vegetative state*, but it fit with the antiseptic and impersonal treatment we had experienced for over 2 months. I scolded care partners for turning and cleaning him without saying a word to him. Whether he could answer was not the point—Josh was still my beloved brother.

I felt abandoned by the medical system and painfully aware of my ignorance about Josh's injury. The neurosurgeon's assumption regarding my capacity for understanding traumatic brain injury (TBI) made me think that he knew what Josh's future held but was refusing to divulge the information. Had he simply taken the time to explain what had occurred during the accident and the consequent surgeries, even if prognostication was futile, I would have been given the chance to focus on accepting our terrible situation rather than fighting for answers that did not exist. I was explicitly asking for open disclosure and getting nowhere. Because of previous circumstances, my knowledge of health issues and hospital protocol probably exceeded that of many individuals in my position; however, I still felt as if I were grasping at air. Without the cooperation of Josh's physicians, my only choice seemed to be to wait.

We were not the only family on the unit experiencing a long-term medical crisis. I watched people like us come and go and saw tempers and tension eat away at constructive communication. My father and I argued openly only once that I recall, but struggled, often in silent bewilderment, to adapt to our situation and each other. He had lived either on the opposite coast or in a foreign country since I was 16. Suddenly, we found ourselves thrust into catastrophe, living under the same roof, and forced to make serious decisions regarding my brother's care. Fortunately, both of us were there for the same reason: to support Josh. We kept our personality conflicts bridled for the most part. The mainspring of our frustration was the inaccessibility of my brother's medical team, which we, as family members in limbo, interpreted as disinterest. Through my best friend's mother, I contacted the Brain Injury Research Center (BIRC) at the University of California at Los Angeles (UCLA), a state-of-the-art facility dedicated to the study of TBI. The lead investigator there extended an invitation to Josh's neurosurgeon to discuss my brother's injury and possible treatments, which was refused on the basis of lack of qualification—the BIRC researcher had a Ph.D. rather than an M.D. Except following surgeries, the neurosurgeon never addressed us again. Coincidentally, he was hired at a prestigious university hospital across the country just before Josh was discharged from the ICU and left without notifying us. Had he accepted the BIRC scientist's offer, my father and I probably would have been given the option to withdraw life support immediately. Months later, on studying my brother's medical chart and computed tomographic (CT) scans, BIRC researchers determined that a massive stroke and midline shift (Josh's brain twisted), both of which occurred within 12 hours of the accident, had wiped out any possibility for recovery.

On February 2, an ambulance transported Josh back to San Diego to a subacute nursing home on Coronado Island. No rehabilitation centers would accept him, despite our pleas. Every program required a consistent response to basic commands. There were times when we saw flashes of cognizance or what we interpreted as such. Looking back, I believe those behaviors—blinking, tracking, sticking out his tongue—were more reflexive than meaningful, and over the months they ceased to occur altogether; however, living in those moments, I would have sworn that he was trying to communicate. Any sign of life gave us something to hold on to, a ray of hope to make our grief more bearable.

We came together as Josh's family and friends to organize visitation schedules so that he would never have to spend a day alone. His pain continued to be grossly undermanaged; he often clenched, grimaced, sweated, and hyperventilated for hours at a time. By the end of the month, he had lost 55 pounds despite caloric increases in his feedings, which were dispensed around the clock through a percutaneous endoscopic gastrostomy (PEG) tube. Not a single physician had been able to give us anything close to an accurate picture of Josh's future, and when we requested magnetic resonance imaging (MRI), it took weeks for the order to go through. Because of his posturing and contractures, he would need an open scan; in other words, they could not fit him into a normal device, and the only hospital that owned one was across the city. I began to lose hope.

At first, I felt tremendously guilty for that. What if it were me? Would Josh give up? In truth, I had done everything but give up. My greatest fear, the one that haunted my dreams and occupied my every waking thought, was that I could not save him. So, I read medical textbooks on head injury and spoke at length with the BIRC director. The research on and statistics for severe TBI indicated that the odds were overwhelmingly stacked against Josh and us. He was only 30 years old, but his injury was diffuse. The mortality rate for patients in his state was a staggering 75%. Literally adding insult to injury, the vast majority of case studies revealed that patients with trauma like Josh's never moved beyond his level of consciousness and had a life expectancy of less than 5 years.

As I attempted to reconcile this information and my own observations of his declining condition, I journeyed through a lifetime of memories. Josh and I grew up in the same household and had never strayed very far from each other, but our experiences were far from identical. Sometimes, a simple fleeting moment can alter one person's existence while remaining virtually imperceptible to another. We are made of such moments—tiny capsules of being, private snapshots from which mind and memory are formed. I did not know these parts of Josh, and he did not know those parts of me. It was the most alone I had ever felt, for the one person I needed to talk to could not hear me.

□ Unwritten Wishes

Josh was 2 years my junior. We bonded closely as children, and our relationship deepened into adulthood. Underlying this kinship was a fierce loyalty and a need to protect one another. We were great friends. It is impossible for me to fully describe Josh to those who did not have the good fortune of knowing him personally. I have yet to meet another human being as vibrant, clever, and passionately spirited as my brother. He cherished his loved ones and treated strangers as long-lost friends. He possessed both physical and mental strength as well as a side-splitting sense of humor. Josh cared little for material wealth but treasured instead his connection to others. In his eyes, "bums on the corner" had stories worth hearing, and "little old ladies" needed traffic stopped while they ambled across the street. That was Josh.

Up until this point, I had been on a quest for his cure, but I turned a corner in late February, when the tragedy of my brother's loss of quality of life, for me, eclipsed whatever breath was left in him. No head scan or neurological scale could have provided me with more proof than what my heart was already saying. Josh would not have wanted to live in a persistent vegetative state, imprisoned in silence and crippled by atrophy. My duty to protect him now entailed releasing him from his suffering.

My responsibility to safeguard Josh also involved keeping our mother away from him. They had not spoken in many years, and prior to that she had physically and emotionally abused him. After a decade of fruitless effort to improve their relationship, Josh walked away. I supported him fully for what was an act of self-care and self-preservation. Not a month before the accident, he confessed to me that rather than be judged for his choice by those who did not know our family history (a common occurrence for both of us), he simply told everyone he met that his mother was dead. To subject Josh to her presence while he was so vulnerable would have been unfair and disrespectful. Furthermore, the lack of an advance directive could have complicated my father's and my ability to make proper decisions for Josh had my mother been involved. She could not be trusted, and there were too many loose ends.

Even if our mother felt remorse, the time for apologies and promises had passed. This was not a movie in which estranged family members get last-minute absolution at the death bed. I felt very strongly about upholding Josh's living wishes and not ceding to well-meant but inappropriate cries of, "But she's his *mother*." In Josh's eyes, he had no mother, and it was not my place to discount that. My family, including her family of origin, agreed. We told her nothing of the accident, and because Josh was not the only relative to whom she did not speak, she was none the wiser. I realize that some people might be horrified at my behavior, that for most children a mother's authority is absolute and her love is sacred. The woman they refer to is not Josh's mother. That was no fault of his; to have given her power over him without his consent would have devalued his courageous, conscious decision to leave her.

☐ The 11th Hour

The first time I audibly voiced the words "my brother is dying" was to the university registrar as I withdrew from my first semester at San Diego State University. I wished that I could shove them back inside my mouth. Hospice had not been discussed or offered by any of Josh's physicians, although he was receiving tube feedings around the clock. However, my best friend, a nursing student, had just rotated through a hospice in Los Angeles. She explained palliative care to me over the course of several long conversations, which I then shared with my father. Our concern had shifted from prolonging Josh's life to alleviating his suffering, from how to handle our own loss to honoring what we believed would be his wishes. The pain of our decision to withdraw care was devastating, not only because we would miss our family member, but also from an ethical perspective. Josh's life was in our hands, and we were choosing to end it. What if we were wrong? He had survived what should have been a fatal injury (according to his physicians), and it was impossible for us not to wonder if that was his will to live. Josh never followed anyone's rules; hearing that he "couldn't" do something only fueled his rebellious nature.

Although I knew deep inside that Josh would have vehemently protested being kept alive in his condition, I was not sure that I would find support for that belief from our family and friends. We spoke only of recovery, never of the possibility that Josh might die. I could tell that my father was struggling to remain hopeful, and part of that undertaking manifested in what I perceived as a reluctance to address the darker "what ifs." Unrestricted communication had never been encouraged by either of my parents or by theirs. That long history of family dynamics affected my ability to speak candidly and my father's capacity for supportive listening. Most of the information I had collected regarding Josh's chances of survival remained silently tucked away.

Morbidity and mortality rates for TBI are generally presented by researchers in 3- and 6-month increments. Most improvement occurs within 1 year, with the first 6 months being the most telling. Just as the 72-hour mark had meant "out of the woods" in the ICU, 6 months seemed to us a place to hang our hopes. Had Josh not been suffering, I believe that waiting for that time to pass might have allayed some of the conflict and uncertainty we felt in deciding—essentially without immediate medical counsel—whether to withdraw life support (which is what the tube feedings were). My brother's dramatic physical decline and virtually constant agitation were excruciating to witness. The future was becoming more certain as the days crept by; there would not be one for Josh.

As is the case for most young adults, my brother had no advance directives. What 30-year-old believes such precautions are necessary, especially one so enthralled with living in the moment, as Josh was? From the early days in the Los Angeles hospital, I attempted to include as many of Josh's friends as possible in discussions regarding his care. Not only was my brother extremely committed to those he loved, but also each one of those relationships was unique. Every individual in Josh's life knew him in a different way—often in ways I did not. My conversations with others allowed me a view into the intricacies of Josh's personality, revealed details about his patterns of interaction, and in a strange way eased my feelings of helplessness. At the same time, I frequently felt as if I was crossing boundaries and even breaking confidence by treading into my brother's private life without his permission. Scanning his body for bedsores or helping to bathe him was one thing; asking his friends to recount conversations and shared experiences was another. But I believed that every bit of information—trivial or not—meant something.

I do not recall ever attempting to imagine myself in Josh's position in order to make decisions for him. His fate was becoming my father's and my responsibility, yet no events in either of our lives remotely compared with what Josh was going through. The only option—at the risk of sounding too scientific or intellectual—required a methodical, thorough investigation into my brother's psychological, social, and spiritual makeup.

This is how I "substituted judgment" for Josh. Had my father and I relied solely on our own understanding of who my brother was, I believe that our frame of reference would have been significantly constrained. Through speaking with Josh's friends, I discovered that he had discussed his wishes, should he ever become incapacitated, with one person. That person recounted the conversation, in which Josh stated that he would rather die than live in such a state. Hearing those words both affirmed my intuition and tested my courage like nothing had during the preceding months. For me, the question of withdrawing life support was no longer hypothetical. My father and I decided together to allow Josh's death because keeping him alive would have been our choice, not his.

Unfortunately, head injuries pose a difficult problem for hopeful caregivers and loved ones. Deep brain activity frequently manifests as behaviors associated with higher cortical function. As I mentioned, Josh showed signs of alertness at times, and we found ourselves wrapping all of our faith around those random occurrences. Still, he seemed to be truly present on a more spiritual level, one that, to this day, I cannot deny. One evening in early March I stood at his bedside, watching as he clenched and perspired, eyes wide as saucers. I choked back tears and said:

> Josh, I know that you are dying, that you are suffering, and that you need to go. You have fought hard to live, but there is nothing left for you here. I am scared to go on without you, but I'll be OK and so will Dad. Just a little longer. We'll get you out of here.

A hush fell over the room, and when I looked up at my brother, he was sleeping.

On March 12, 2002, Josh's tube feedings were discontinued. The following day, he was transported to Lakeview Home, a four-bed hospice residence only 2 miles from my house. True to what our intake nurse had promised, the staff immediately administered pain medication as well as an antianxiety drug. On reviewing Josh's medical chart, they affirmed our suspicion that his agitation and facial contortions were in all likelihood an expression of pain. The shift nurse on duty icily commented, "He wasn't getting enough meds to treat my grandma."

I was amazed at how, although no one at the facility had met Josh before the accident, everyone there spoke to him as if he were an old pal. The ladies fawned over his handsome face and stunning green eyes. Bob, who quickly became our favorite nurse, kept up Josh's goatee, always teasing that this would be the last time. At the first hint of discomfort, more medication was dispensed without question. Because he could not protect his airway, the tracheotomy tube remained in place, which meant frequent suctioning—the only time I ever witnessed my brother in distress. The hospice team carefully described the dying process to us and anticipated that Josh would live for 5 to 10 days. Using my house as a staging area, my father, his wife, several friends, and I moved into Lakeview Home, alternating nights on the couch adjacent to Josh's bed. We encouraged him to let go and assured him how much he was loved. We laughed about old times and cried for our immense loss. And we waited.

Up until this point, my attempt to keep my mother from Josh had been successful. However, several days after he entered hospice, my grandmother, out of guilt, divulged his location. I was livid. After three visits, during which my mother brought strangers to his bedside and draped her body over his, the hospice staff had her removed and forbade her return. Josh had required double his usual medication to treat anxiety that seemed to be caused by her actions.

On March 31, Easter Sunday, Josh passed into mystery quietly and without struggle. He had outlived the hospice staff's predictions by 9 days and had the last say after all. My father and I chose to donate Josh's brain to UCLA in the spirit of our son and brother, who always gave to others whatever he could. Today, that gift is used to train bright young neurosurgeons and pioneering researchers. Somewhere, Josh is certainly grinning—he would have thought it "profoundly cool" to have his brain in a jar. That brain, the BIRC scientists verified, had withstood the worst-survived injury in the history of their program and could not have recovered function but for a miracle. Our miracle happened over the course of 30 years, while Josh kept us company here on this earth.

☐ Terri Schiavo: A Familiar Stranger

Three years to the day of Josh's death, Terri Schiavo passed on in front of millions of American viewers. Politicians, activists, attorneys, and religious leaders argued for and against the "right to die" in this country. Her family's private pain became everyone's business, including mine. Like Josh, Terri had suffered a severe brain injury at a young age and was in a persistent vegetative state. Like Josh, she had no advance directive. But my brother died peacefully up the street, without fanfare or feud.

I found myself reliving much of my grief through the nightly news. As the frenzy to "save Terri" mounted, as appeals for the reinsertion of her feeding tube were filed, and as the media swarmed to Woodside Hospice, I grew frustrated with what I saw as a vulgar distortion of both hospice care and end-of-life issues. The dying process my brother had gone through did not look like this—barbaric, gruesome, excruciating. Palliative medicine, by definition, means comfort. Before my father and I withdrew life support, we needed an explanation of what Josh would be feeling. Of course, the question of hunger arose. We drew from our own experience of unpleasant hunger pangs and projected that outward. Both Terri and Josh were severely compromised; neither of them possessed the capacity to feel hunger or thirst any longer. The body protects itself in that way, as it has for thousands of years.

Beneath my anger at the media and my government, I felt deeply empathetic toward Terri's husband and parents. I understood both sides because I had explored them within myself. As I watched those few seconds of home video in which Terri appears to smile and track the Mickey Mouse balloon, I recalled my desperate longing for my brother, and my subsequent translation of his behaviors into something that made sense to me. The nature of diffuse brain injury is to be ill defined and hard to understand, even for specialists and experts. The family that faces losing a loved one or is already experiencing living loss by sitting helpless at the bedside will find hope wherever it can. For me, letting go of Josh required cleaving my own needs from his best interest. I had to accept that allowing him to die did not mean that I loved him less or that I killed him.

I cannot speak for Terri's family, but from my standpoint, living loss played a major role in how I dealt with both Josh's final months and the aftermath of his death. In essence, he died twice—first, when he could no longer communicate with us and for the final time on Easter. During his hospitalization, I struggled to integrate my feelings of sorrow and loneliness with those of hope and courage, to very little avail. While Josh was suspended in partial consciousness, I dangled between conflicting emotions without reprieve. Ultimately, I had to abandon myself to provide for him. I found myself forgetting who Josh had been before the accident, perhaps as a way to cope with my role as caretaker and my abysmal sense of loss. For 5 months, my singular purpose in life was to look after my brother. After his death, I did not know what to do with myself; I had acclimated to the bedridden Josh, lost sight of the walking-around Josh, and was facing a future without either.

When President Bush declared that, in the face of uncertainty we must err on the side of life, I think he missed a key element of humanity. How a person lives, and the degree to which that state of being reflects his or her unique spirit, is critically important. My father and I certainly had the choice to prolong Josh's life—or death—but we believed that my brother was more than the summation of his respirations and heartbeats. Could he have ever again engaged in his favorite activities? Would he have felt whole and productive? Would he have settled for life at its bare bones or felt deprived of quality of life, with all its marvelous wonders? During Josh's stay at the nursing home, I approached our social worker with a request for hospice. Her response? "He is not actively dying. We have patients here who have lived 10 years in his condition." My reply: "Exactly." She did not know Josh and the president did not know Terri Schiavo. My father's and my decision to allow Josh's death was made out of love and is probably the one purely altruistic act either of us has ever performed.

Had my family been refused the option to withdraw life support, Josh would have succumbed eventually, but it would not have been a good death. Our final gift to my brother was to grant him his freedom. Letting Josh go was the hardest thing I have ever done ... and it was the right thing. There are no regrets or doubts, just a resonant sense of peace in knowing that Josh was unconditionally loved and honored. I still ask myself that silly question: Who do I love the most? The answer never changes, and I suspect it never will.

☐ Acknowledgment

This chapter is a slightly revised and expanded version of an article originally published in *Death Studies*.

5
CHAPTER

A Hastened Death

Nicola G. Raye

Introduction

What follows is the story of my father's hastened death, which occurred about 20 years ago. It incorporates some of the entries in the journal I kept at the time (the excerpted text). I have also added some explanatory material (the regular text). Because our family was living in a state where hastened death was (and still is) illegal and assisting in a suicide is considered a felony, I have reluctantly decided to use a pseudonym and alter a few nonessential details to protect the identities of everyone involved. I regret this because I believe that there is nothing shameful to hide, and that these stories need to be told. It is my conviction that much of the negative impact on those who help a loved one hasten death is caused by the lack of personal, social, and professional support and the need for secrecy due to the illegality. It is my hope that this situation will change. I dedicate this story to my courageous, beloved parents and family and to the friends who gave us such incredible support, all of whom for the time being shall have to remain anonymous, but not unsung, heroes in my life.

July 11

> Last Thursday, I got a voice mail from Mom saying that Dad had been asking to talk to me for several days about "getting pills." I cleared my calendar and went over the next day.

My sister and I had been anticipating this call with dread for nearly 2 years. More than 2 years earlier, at the age of 74, our father had a major stroke. After a month in rehab, he showed some improvement: His speech was no longer slurred like that of a drunk, and he was able to transfer himself from the wheelchair to the toilet or bed and support himself in the shower, but he was wheelchair bound and could no longer do the things he had been so passionate about. An inveterate walker, he had walked miles each day of his life, roaming the streets of the city where he lived. He was a self-taught classical musician and played three instruments. He had reviewed books for a living and had written seven novels (one published) and numerous short stories (several published). He was a voracious reader. A true intellectual, he loved to talk, to argue, to lecture, to debate, to philosophize. He had a small stroke at age 62 that had a relatively minor impact, but after this one he could not walk, play his instruments, manipulate the computer keyboard, and read with ease. His speech was labored because of the difficulty coordinating his breathing and his vocal chords, which sometimes made the lives of those around him a little easier because we could get a word in edgewise, but for him removed yet another of life's pleasures. After 6 months of physical therapy, speech therapy, and occupational therapy, with no further improvement in his functioning, he announced he wanted to die.

My parents were intellectuals, atheists, and lifelong political activists. They had always believed that hastening death was an acceptable option when life no longer had value for the person living it because of irreversible deteriorating physical (not emotional) health. However, at the time of my father's initial request, my mother was not ready and did not believe he was either. She got their physician to prescribe an antidepressant, and my father accepted the situation for another year and a half. I sometimes think he was giving my mother time to accept his dying, but I am sure he also maintained some hope for improvement.

During this period, my father consulted several highly regarded neurologists, who examined and tested him extensively. Each concluded that because of his exceptional intelligence and extraordinary vocabulary and memory, it was difficult to gauge the damage to his cognitive functioning. But, they all agreed that he was continuing to have small imperceptible strokes that explained his inability to recover his physical functioning and his progressive deterioration. Each said nothing could be done and recommended that he enjoy life as much as he could. His two worst fears were that at any time he could have another stroke that either (a) would incapacitate him mentally but leave his body strong so that he would continue to live, but not as himself; or (b) would not affect his mental capacity but paralyze his body completely. Both scenarios would leave him unable to take action to end his life. For him, either case would be a state far worse than death, and this caused him tremendous anxiety, which is why he wanted to be sure to die first. He also was depressed, not in the clinical sense, but because there was simply very little joy left in his life, and his personality was rigid enough that he could not or would not adapt to his constraints as some other personality types might have. We were all committed to supporting his wishes and knew it was just a matter of time before he would make the request again, but we were very ignorant about what that would entail or what would be required of us.

When my father felt unwilling to hold out any longer, we had a family meeting, and my mother and sister and I agreed, with great sadness, to support his wish. My sister and I took on the responsibility of exploring our options.

July 15

So far we have hit dead ends. P [a physician friend] is supportive but doesn't want to be directly involved, a caution that is entirely warranted. P suggested talking to Dad's doctor but at this point I'm afraid to box her into a corner; what if she were very opposed and took some kind of action? P suggested talking with other docs, but that seems delicate to me too. Dear F [a friend], who loves the whole family, said if he could kill Dad for us he would! His own mother was furious with him for calling 911, which led to her lingering a week longer than she otherwise would have. What would I do without my supportive loving friends?

I am scared and stressed. My sister and I are working well together but this is hard! What's right, what's too soon, what's crazy, etc. Meantime my house is being roofed and painted, and I am trying to clean my den and play the piano and walk and enjoy the summer! Whew!

July 18

So much has happened. The key seems to be to talk with Dad's doc, which we plan to do, though with great trepidation. Miraculously, G [a friend] called early Sunday to say that his father-in-law died peacefully of the flu and they still had his batch of unused barbiturates, Valium, and Codeine! He'd wanted a hastened death after some very severe strokes but one family member objected and he spent the next 3 years becoming mentally incapacitated and surrounded by dishonest and irresponsible caretakers; ugh. The pills are three years old so it is not clear if they are still potent. That's scary.

I spent a very pleasant afternoon with M&D [our childhood names for Mom and Dad], not telling them about this yet because it might be dead (hah!), but suggesting they call some old friends who also might have access to drugs. Mom said Dad woke up saying he wanted to take Benadryl to help him die; he didn't want to wait to accumulate the proper medications. I said that was ridiculous, it wouldn't work. She said she had told him there were things to do first. What, I asked? Make sure the will is in order and figure out what to do with the body, she said! We both started crying. I said I would contact an attorney about updating the will and get information about what to do with the body. Then we went to the park and walked around a bit and it was sweet but I could see what an effort everything is for Dad, who gets exhausted even from driving around in the car or being pushed in the wheelchair. Seems like stimulus overload, and just being present is an effort. I left them and went off to swim and cry at R's [a friend]; there's a heat wave here and it was quite wonderful.

Monday I got a message that S [an old family friend] could get hold of barbiturates from a friend of hers who is stockpiling it for her own use just in case. I also spoke with B [a colleague] and was very moved—his family wouldn't agree to help his mother who was dying of cancer and wanted to hasten her death. Now, months later, he tells me, "I feel terrible that I couldn't help my mother." Made me appreciate how lucky we are that the family is in agreement. Also made arrangements for a no-frills, low-cost cremation.

My sister and I itemized what needs to be done. We ended up spending an incredible hour with Mom and the doc, without Dad. We were all very indirect but I am pretty sure she was checking us out and seemed to be letting us know that she will be minimally supportive or at least not obstructive. It's so hard, though, because everything is so ambiguous.

We can't get the stuff from our two sources until next week. A time line is starting to fall into place. M&D see the doc next Tuesday to complete an Advance Directive. I think this will allow her to check Dad's mental competence, etc. We think she is trying to do everything possible to make Dad more comfortable. Meantime Mom will meet with the attorney and review the will.

I had thought it might take months to get the meds and that we would have a lot more time to plan and to reflect. But given Dad's condition and personality I think his sense of urgency is totally understandable. He doesn't want a nursing home, neither of them wants a caretaker in the house with them, Mom can't do the work much longer, and his quality of life is shit. He can hardly read, can't write, can't walk, can't play music, is totally dependent, and has trouble talking. What's left? Not much other than love, and I guess that's not enough.

I feel sad and awed and I respect both of them for their courage and strength and love. I think that's what this is about: love and family and friends and what's most basic and important in life, and I'm getting tremendous love and support and help all around. Death happens, and I'm trying to focus on how fortunate we are to have this choice and for Dad to not be in pain or mentally incapacitated, like B's mother or N's father. This keeps me going, because I am scared, and there's a part of me that doesn't really want to get to the end point. But my hope is that with all the love and caring and thoughtfulness around it will be okay and even beautiful and reassuring.

July 20

Dad is worse; more immobilized and so hard to transfer that it sometimes takes two people; Mom has hurt her back again and I am practically begging her to get help. My sister and I are taking turns being there to help them in the morning and the evening. Has he had another small stroke?

We're all letting go in our own ways, and I am overwhelmed at various times of day and night with emotion, pure emotion that is hard to label. I suppose it's sadness, but it mainly feels like just very profound depths, like I'm in a deep well or deep water that's the well of life, and this is about life ebbing, and about deep attachment at the very roots, and awe and recognition of connectedness, and the unpredictability and unknowability of death.

A little jewel: Tuesday night I was with M&D and he was joking about his idea of heaven. We asked how old he'll be there and he said nineteen. I asked why and he said, gazing at Mom, "Because that's when I met her and it was the happiest year of my life." She reached over and they held hands. (Sob) Then I asked what kind of memorial he'd like; he of course said no fuss. I joked and said that since he couldn't do anything about it we'd sit shiva [a Jewish mourning ritual], and he laughed [because we were all atheists and had no traditions for death].

The family is quite amazing. All the stuff I used to hate or complain about or suffer over is gone and irrelevant. We are so open and present with each other; nothing is under wraps, we discuss everything, we laugh and cry and plan. My sister and brother-in-law are great. M&D show tremendous courage and love, beyond conception. I will keep recording and doing and loving and being and who knows how long this will take? Can I actually mix up the chocolate pudding concoction? Will I ever be able to eat chocolate pudding again?

Another jewel: I'm sitting at dinner with M&D and my sister and brother-in-law, talking about editing lousy books with bad sex [several of us have been editors]. M asks D what to do with the ashes. He says, put them down the garbage disposal. Brother-in-law says you can't, there are too many of them, they'll clog it up. D laughs and shrugs and we go on to the next topic.

Another jewel: Dad and I had great morning ablutions Friday (I am going over most days to help him out of bed in the a.m. to give Mom a break). He asked if I remember him pretend-shaving my face when I was little. I said of course, it was one of my fondest memories. How did he ever think of it? Because, he said, I was always hanging around him watching him shave. Just like I was right at that moment! As always he was meticulous in his grooming, carefully putting the toothpaste away after using it, cleaning the razor: everything in its place, neat and organized. It must drive him crazy to have snot running out of his nose, food spilling on his shirt, needing a bib, choking in front of everyone, but he bears it with remarkable dignity and without complaint.

Yesterday, we found out from a sympathetic doctor acquaintance that because D is still very strong physically, the meds might not work, which would be absolutely terrible, because it would cause the very brain damage he fears so much, so we might have to use a plastic bag to suffocate him. I am struck with horror; I don't want to do this part. I am now very worried that we might need to do more than we thought and this is going to be ghoulish.

Mom and I agreed that if this were happening to either of us we'd handle it differently—be more flexible and adaptive to the situation. But he is who he is. They say people die the way they live. Well, he is stubborn, determined to do things his way, impatient, proud, independent, and has no idea of his impact on others; a true narcissist.

July 26

Every day is new and difficult. My partner and I went over to G and N's to get their stash. It was very sweet and deep and poignant. She is mainly just still very relieved that her father has finally died. When I thanked her as she put the vials in my cupped hands, she said, Thank YOU. She feels wonderful that at least she can help relieve someone else's suffering. They told us the story of when they had to put their first dog to sleep. The dog was quite ill but still quite conscious and very affectionate, and they kept holding on until they finally realized, what were they waiting for, for him to be in agony before they would let him go? Quite apropos.

Last night we all went to see Dr. T. Dad came right out, despite our advice not to be direct with her. T asked him how he's doing, and he said with a smile, I'm feeling very good because I've decided to bring my life to an end, I'm very tired of living this way. T then asked if he had a method and D said (as I groaned inwardly), yes, we have pills. T said she'd never dealt with this situation before, could not help us, but would not make notes about our discussion; this after she'd asked more questions and we'd answered quite satisfactorily. It's clear D is not depressed; if anything he's happy now that he knows the end is in sight; we all expressed our support; there is no disagreement in the family; he's not going to get better and can only get worse; and he and M have told us for years that this is what they would want. She said she would sign the death certificate and we breathed a sigh of relief; it addressed the last fear.

Dad is still anxious that something could happen at any time that would make him unable to carry this out, e.g., a stroke that would wipe out his swallow reflex entirely [it had already been somewhat compromised, and he would sometimes have difficulty swallowing or would choke on his food]. Other than that, however, his depression is totally lifted; he has been happy ever since he knew medications were available. He doesn't want to wait until the rest of the family arrives, but we will all need each other for support after he's gone and I refuse to hurry. I am prepared to fight him over this, even though I do understand his sense of urgency. My anger at his lack of concern for the living is partly appropriate but also I suspect a part of distancing and letting go. I am very fatigued, emotionally drained; I sense depression creeping in like the incoming tide, very slow and imperceptible at first but then it gathers momentum and it comes in pretty fast, and if you aren't paying attention you can get caught!

My Buddhist teacher and friend sent me a great quote from the Dalai Lama that has become my mantra: GREAT COMPASSION IS THE ROOT OF ALL FORMS OF WORSHIP. And I found some beautiful lines in a Robert Bly poem:

We did not come to remain whole
We came to lose our leaves like the trees,
The trees that are broken
And start again, drawing up from the great roots.

I have been racked with sensations of grief. It is hard to verbalize the feeling, which is very physical and profound. Deep deep pain, a sense of a tremendous pulling away at the roots, roots that are either inside of me way deep down in the depths of my being or roots that are even deeper, in the ground, underground, that I am attached to, and there is a tearing away. I assume it is my attachment to him, and that through him I am attached to the earth, to all life, and when he dies, as he dies, as he separates out, I feel this pulling away of a life force from our shared roots, and it is huge, broken roots, leaving a gaping hole that over time will heal over and put out new roots but the scar will always be there.

July 28

The family attended a wonderful outdoor concert. When we got home everyone except Mom tried on plastic bags to see how porous they might be! Gallows humor continues. I took Dad to the dentist to glue his bridge and when we left he said he felt badly he couldn't tell the dentist and say goodbye! As I wheeled him to the van, down a slight incline, I said maybe we should find a long hill with a body of water at the bottom and I could just send him down it; we laughed uproariously and then went out for pancakes.

I was overcome last night after I left them with waves of deep emotion. The thought of Dad's brilliant magnificent brain dying seemed unbearable; the idea of not seeing his face, still so compellingly handsome and beautiful to me after all these years, breaks my heart. Since I can remember, I have gazed at his face, from his baby pictures to the photo of him as a soldier to the picture of him on the back cover of his novel to pictures of him in the backyard digging up huge tree roots to the one I took of him and Mom smiling in their new kitchen.

July 30

Moved in to camp out here until "D-Day," now set for Aug. 1. We [my partner and I] went yesterday to get the second stash of pills from S, who cried and said she hadn't had a chance to talk to D. I said no one really has, he's as obstinate and impossible as ever. Same with my aunt; he said he couldn't understand why she came here to see him die, he wouldn't do it for her! She said she came to be with Mom and my sister and me and him, and teared up. Later we agreed he's a jerk, a narcissistic asshole, always has been, why do we all love and tolerate him? But we do. His heart is locked away, but it is there and somehow we love him despite the padlocks and spikes.

I'm scared—I hate the idea of having to use the bag. But I have to deal with whatever happens, just hoping I don't have nightmares afterwards. I worry terribly about Mom, as we all do, as she does. I want to surround her with love, I want her to know she is surrounded by loving friends, that there is a wonderful rich life waiting for her to join and participate in that she has been shut out of for years now. She can at last be free, and I want so much for her to experience that freedom, to taste its sweetness, and for the taste to not be ruined by the sadness.

MAY WE ALL BE OKAY, AT PEACE, SPACIOUS, FREE FROM SUFFERING, LIVE IN LOVE.

August 1, 3:45 p.m.

About two hours to go. All the other family members are on their way over except my son, who is out of the country; Dad won't wait for him. Yesterday friends visited, including R with her adorable 9-month-old granddaughter, who sat happily on Dad's lap for about half an hour; to my surprise he was delighted by her. It was touching to see this older man in the last days of his life with a new being at the very beginning of hers. People called all day to say love and goodbye; my son was first and Dad said, "When you were little I wanted to murder you, but you turned out to be a very nice boy. I love you very much, and I only wish I could stay around so I could vote for you for President."

Ritual and ceremony are out of the question in this family, but this afternoon we spent an hour or so looking through family pictures and documents. Earlier I'd gone out to get soda [to mix with alcohol] and chocolate pudding [to mix with the drugs]. People at Safeway kept saying, "How are you, have a good day." I'm fine, my father is going to die in 4 hours and I am helping to poison and perhaps suffocate him. I'm mainly pretty numb, or calm, or accepting, or all of the above, though I teared up when I looked at some of the photos, him as a small boy, him as a young man, him with me as a young father, Mom looking absolutely beautiful and pure and innocent, what could she know then of all this?

I just hope we don't have to use the bag, and if we do I hope he doesn't struggle. I would love my last experience of him to be drifting off to sleep and just gradually slowing down and going out, a flickering candle, an ember. Poor Mom is holding on with the help of Valium. I want to live fully, without holding back, without fear, boldly and honestly and richly. It is beautiful out; I want to be out in it.

August 4 [Three Days After the Death]

Well, so much has happened I'm not sure I can retrieve it all. Dad said, "You should go out for a walk." Mom was on the couch, my aunt on the deck, others not arrived yet. So I walked down to the Native American shop. I told the owner I was taking a break from being with my father who was very ill. He said, "That's interesting, you're the third person in two hours to come in mentioning someone nearby who's dying" (though I hadn't exactly!). He recommended I get a packet of three candles blessed by elders and told me they are prayer candles, to bring the light toward you. I returned to the house feeling momentarily calmed.

Dad was watching TV; he wanted to see the second episode of a two-part TV show to see how it ended! The rest of the family finally arrived. My sister and aunt and I went to make up the concoction, emptying dozens of capsules of barbiturates and grinding Valium and Codeine tablets in the coffee grinder. When we emptied it all out into the bowl it had some dark flecks in it; when we wondered what it was my aunt said, "So what's it going to do, poison him?" We were all crying and laughing the whole time. A cloud of yellowish powder wafted up as we mixed it all together; a true witch's brew. At 5:30 Dad took the Dramamine and the beta blockers and was sipping on a vodka tonic, which I think was good both for the alcohol content and for the calming effect, and most of us joined him for drinks.

Mom took Dad's blood pressure, and someone noticed that he had his right arm around her waist as she held his left hand and arm to take the reading. It was very emotional; I think we all were in suspended animation. I wondered why she was taking it; the last time, I suppose. Finally we took him into the guest room. All day he'd been quite subdued and tired but now he was somewhat animated, and as we brought in cushions to prop him up we joked that he looked like an emperor or the head of the seder. Then we went to mix up the pudding; the taste was overwhelming, vile and bilious. We kept adding chocolate syrup and sugar; it was still bitter but edible. At this point Mom asked to be left alone with him for a few minutes.

We all started to cry, and we were all holding on to each other in the living room. Then Mom came out and said to me, "Dad wants you to take his picture because he's looking so good!" I laughed and went in; he was indeed looking very happy, relaxed, and rosy cheeked. I took two of him and then two of them together. It was so powerful: He was so happy to finally be getting free, and she looked utterly stricken, about to lose her mate of over 50 years. Then they said they were ready. So we went out and got the pudding and everyone came in and we asked him who should be there and he said grandly, "Everyone can stay if you like!" Then he ate the pudding very eagerly as if he couldn't get enough, and he finished every last drop. Then he took a sip of soda (with vodka) and said, "Yuck," so I went and got him fresh soda, and he still said yuck, which I understand because I still had the bitter taste in my throat from the tasting earlier, and he asked for some bread, and there was a lot of good energy and humor and spirit in the room. So I went into the kitchen to get bread, and I took about 45 seconds to get two different kinds because I wasn't sure which he would prefer, and when I came back they'd all been laughing at something he had said. My sister had lit a cigarette for him and he took a puff, and then he give a big yawn, and his head fell gently to the right, and he was fast asleep. They told me he had offered to share his dessert with anyone who wanted some and asked for a cigarette, and it was at that point that I came back. So within less than five minutes of eating the pudding he was asleep.

We removed all but one of the pillows and gently laid him down, and he was in a deep sleep, and started snoring. The breaths were very very slow and far apart almost immediately. My brother-in-law was timing them, and people were talking, and I don't think we were fully aware of what was happening; it was so fast, so gentle, there he was joking one minute and asleep the next.

We milled around for the next hour, in and out of the room, playing sweet native flute music, talking, telling stories, laughing, crying, etc. I think he died within 60–75 minutes. His body stayed warm for a very long time, and I kept worrying that he'd come out of the sleep and we'd still have to use the bag, but we didn't. He looked incredibly peaceful, mainly the color drained out of his face pretty quickly, but his face relaxed into a very handsome eagle-like pose. I stroked him and kissed him and held his hand many times, but my one regret is that I didn't have the presence of mind to say anything to him. I guess I'd imagined the right words would come as he was falling asleep, and somehow I never got to it. I hope it's that I'd said everything, but had I? He made it very difficult to say much, would usually cut me off after a couple of minutes, I think he knew as much of my feelings as he was able to let in, but who will ever know?

I cried a lot that night, and in the morning when they came to take his body away; that was very hard, I kind of liked having him in the house with us. I'd slept in their bedroom with Mom and my aunt and kept thinking I was hearing him moving in the other room, and dreamt twice that he woke up looking normal and healthy and I was trying to figure out whether I should use the bag or not. But he was still there in the morning, much colder and a little stiff, and I snuck some pictures of him lying there, and he was really dead, but not scary at all. I kept wanting to say, "My daddy's dead, my daddy's dead."

Later we went to the funeral home and I was upset to learn they won't cremate him until next week. I am a little paranoid about this but mainly I don't like thinking of him lying in a refrigerator all alone. I will miss his presence when I go to the house; he could be funny, informative, obnoxious, and was always welcoming with me, allowing my kisses and strokes. He said very little directly though I know he loved me. A few days ago he said, "Thank you very very much for everything." That was all!

> Dad was unafraid of death; he welcomed it, saw it as freedom and release, and did not seem to mourn the end of his life. We asked him every day if he wanted to change his mind and he always said no with utter conviction. He chose to die before his worst nightmares came true, and his death was peaceful and free of suffering. He died with his integrity and dignity totally intact. He was unwavering, knew exactly what he wanted and what he was doing, and really went out in style—his own style. I believe that if he'd gotten emotional or allowed us to it would have been harder for him to carry through, and watching TV until half an hour before he took the meds was his way of saying, This is business as usual, no big deal, we have a regular day and then at the end this is what we do now. He took his pills, got to have his vanity pampered by my photographs, was surrounded by love, got to have a last smoke and the last laugh, and went out like a comet, no hassle, no fuss, no nonsense, no lingering, and no mess for us.

For the first month after the death, my mother and sister and I would talk daily about what ifs: What if we had gotten different medication for mood management, a power wheelchair, different physical therapists, a different house that was easier to get around in, or more stimulating evenings, more concerts, and so on. But, we would always come back to two things. One, for a long time he had become increasingly rigid and resistant to new things, and he had been shutting down and withdrawing and participating less over a period of time that went way back, possibly to the first stroke 13 years earlier. Was this because of his rigid personality, his brain having multiple infarcts, or a combination? Second, everyone seemed to agree that this was his window of opportunity to act, and that his fear of becoming incapable of acting was reality based and understandable, and if he was going to take action this had to be the time. Every day truly brought the risk of another stroke. We would remember the effort it took him to move, to transfer, to use the toilet, to go out—he would perspire down his back, it would exhaust him, he was totally dependent on others, and he experienced very little joy. We had asked him daily if he wanted to change his mind, and his answer was always the same: No! And, we would look at the photographs I had taken of him at the very end and see how happy he looked (I have always wondered: Did he know, when he asked me to take his picture, how important it would be to us to be able to see his happiness in those photographs?). We continued to have these discussions for many months, and occasionally over the years now, and have always reached the same conclusion: It was his time, it was his choice, and out of love we chose to support him, even though my mother would gladly have taken care of him for years more, and we would have participated unquestioningly.

In retrospect, much of what we experienced would have been the same if my father had died a natural death: all the feelings associated with the loss of a loved one. The negative side of his hastened death was the result of the illegality, so that our grief was inextricably laced with tension. But there were many positives. Because we knew exactly when he would die we had the opportunity to truly be present with each other and with him. The decision making and planning brought the family together and allowed us to talk openly about everything; we had to talk about dying and death. We grieved losing him but felt good that we could support his final wishes and protect him from his worst fears. We knew he knew he was loved as he was dying. What more could one give a loved one at the end of his or her life? My last journal entry during this period reads:

> Dad had a beautiful death. If it weren't for our fears that the medications wouldn't work or that our mother would be taken off to jail (my sister and I are almost ready to go to jail so we can stand up for our beliefs!), I'd say it was a perfect death.

☐ Afterword

I am aware that my family's story may elicit strong reactions from some readers, who will likely represent the broad diversity of opinions and attitudes in the United States toward hastened death and physician aid in dying. I am writing in early 2006, just as the U.S. Supreme Court has rejected the effort to block Oregon's Death With Dignity Act, so this is a time of heightened public awareness regarding this complex issue. How we die and the legacy we leave behind are arguably among the most important and defining actions we humans can take. I champion the rights of all individuals to hold their own views on these matters, to receive excellent end-of-life care, and to make choices at the end of their lives that allow them to die in a manner consistent with their values.

My father would have met most of the criteria specified by the Oregon Death With Dignity Act, which under certain circumstances permits physician aid in dying for people who are terminally ill. He was mentally competent, his decision-making capacity was not compromised by mental illness, and he had an untreatable, degenerative medical condition that would inevitably lead to his death—an assessment agreed on by several ranking neurologists and his own physician. His wish to hasten his death before he had lost all dignity and quality of life, as he defined it, was enduring and constant over a 2-year period, and it was consistent with his lifelong values, clearly communicated to his family and friends. An

18-month course of antidepressants did not alter his attitude, wishes, or assessment of his situation in the slightest.

However, the Oregon law requires that the individual be terminally ill (i.e., predicted to die within 6 months), excluding many people with fatal degenerative neurological conditions (e.g., amyotrophic lateral sclerosis [ALS], Parkinson's, atherosclerosis of the arteries of the brain), who may live a long time while experiencing progressive and irreversible deterioration. My father was suffering from a severely compromised quality of life and from extreme mental anguish related to fears of a fate he considered far worse than death. But, even if he had been living in Oregon today, he would not have been able to receive physician aid in dying.

It is not my intention to debate the pros and cons of legalizing physician aid in dying here or to discuss the details of the Oregon law, but I do sometimes wonder whether if my father had known that physician aid in dying would be available if he were to become incapacitated and unable to carry out his own wishes, he might have chosen to live longer. As it was, the risk felt too great to him, and he was unwilling to take it. However, I do not consider my father's hastened death to be a suicide because rather than ending his life out of shame, guilt, or despair about his life as a whole, he was actively choosing to end a life that was inexorably approaching death anyway and to end that life in a manner that allowed him to maintain his dignity and sense of self. He could have not accomplished this without the support of the family, and out of love we agreed to help, even though it meant losing him.

The beginning and ending of life are great mysteries. Who can confidently say they know the answers? I hope that readers will reflect on my father's choices and actions with compassion for his situation, regardless of their own views, and that our family's story will stimulate meaningful reflections on the universal conundrum of death.

II

SECTION

Overview of Major Issues

6

CHAPTER

How People Die in the United States

Marilyn J. Field

Introduction

That death comes to us all is a fact of life. How death comes to us, however, has changed in the past 100 years. The average age at death, the major causes of death, and the sites and surroundings of death have changed. This chapter reviews these changes and some of their implications for decision making about care near the end of life.

When We Die: The Aging of Death

In 2002, approximately 2.4 million people died in the United States (National Center for Health Statistics [NCHS], 2005, Table 31). Children under the age of 15 accounted for 1.6% of these deaths, and infants (children under the age of 1) accounted for more than half of child deaths. In contrast, adults aged 65 and over accounted for 74.1% of deaths. As the post-World War II baby boom generation enters this age bracket, the proportion of the population over age 65 will grow from approximately 12% in 2000 to almost 20% in 2030—or from almost 35 million people to over 69 million (U.S. Census, 2005). The proportion of deaths accounted for by this group will likewise increase.

With the increase in the proportion of older Americans will come a decrease in the proportion of younger people available to serve as paid or unpaid caregivers and to pay taxes to support Medicare, Social Security, and other public programs. The Social Security Administration (SSA, 2005) estimates that in 2031 there will be 2.1 workers for each Social Security beneficiary compared to approximately 3.3 today. The result may be increased pressure on both healthcare providers and family members caring for people living and dying with serious illnesses and functional limitations. If policy makers and the public continue to defer responses to projected shortfalls in funding for Medicare and Social Security, changes may be more severe and abrupt when they do come. Changes in Medicare and Medicaid policies, in particular, need to consider the implications for care at the end of life (see, e.g., Hogan, Lunney, Gabel, & Lynn, 2001; Lynn & Adamson, 2003).

As the distribution of deaths by age suggests, the average American can today expect to live a long life and to die at an advanced age (see Figure 6.1). Estimated life expectancy is over 77 years (NCHS, 2005, Table 27). In contrast, at the turn of the previous century, life expectancy was only 47 years. Just since 1950, life expectancy has increased by 9 years. For women, life expectancy is now nearly 80 years, but for men the figure is just under 74.5. Among those who survive to age 65, women may expect to live, on average, 19.5 additional years, whereas men can expect to live 16.6 years longer.

The other side of increasing life expectancy is decreasing death rates. In 1900, the crude death rate was about 1,720 per 100,000 population (U.S. Department of Commerce, 1975) compared to 964 per 100,000 in 1950 and 847 per 100,000 in 2002 (NCHS, 2005, Table 35). (Given fears of another flu pandemic, it is notable that the downward trend in death rates during the early years of the 20th century was interrupted by the influenza epidemic of 1918, when life expectancy dropped below 40 years; Brim, Friedman, Levine, & Scotch, 1970.) Between 1950 and 2002, age-adjusted death rates dropped from 1,446 per 100,000 to 845 per 100,000 (see Figure 6.1).

The decrease in death rates has been most dramatic for infants. In 1900, infants (children under the age of 1) died at a rate of 162 per 1,000 live births (U.S. Department of Commerce, 1975). By 1950, the death rate for infants had dropped to 29 per 1,000 live births, and in 2002, the rate stood at 7.0 per 1,000 live births (NCHS, 2005, Table 22). As many others have noted, a number of countries have lower infant mortality rates than the United States. Among 37 countries ranked by the Centers for Disease Control and Prevention, the United States ranked 28th in infant mortality, just ahead of Hungary (7.2 deaths per 1,000 live births) and just behind Cuba (6.5 per 1,000) (NCHS, 2005, Table 25). Hong Kong had the lowest infant death rate at 2.3 per 1,000, with Sweden next at 2.8 per 1,000.

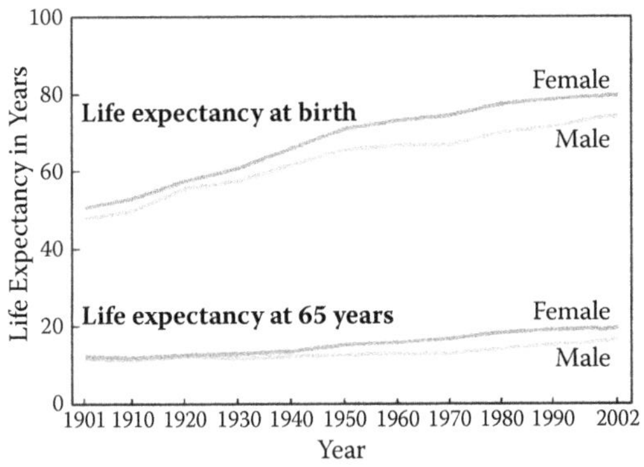

FIGURE 6.1 Changing life expectancy at birth and at age 65. *Note*: Source data spreadsheet is behind Figure 26 at http://www.cdc.gov/nchs/data/hus/hus05.pdf#summary.

Increases in life expectancy and decreases in death rates have affected all segments of the U.S. population, but significant disparities continue to exist. Life expectancy at birth for White U.S. residents was 71.7 years in 1970 compared to 77.7 years in 2002; for Black or African American residents, the corresponding figures are 64.1 years and 72.3 years, respectively (NCHS, 2005, Table 27). A similar pattern holds for women, although both White and Black women live longer, on average, than males of their race.

For the years 2000 to 2002 combined, Black or African American males had an age-adjusted death rate of 1,341 per 100,000 population compared to a rate of 993 per 100,000 population for White males (NCHS, 2005, Table 35). For Black or African American females for the same years, the rate was 902 per 100,000 population compared to 701 per 100,000 population for White females. Even more striking, infants born to White mothers in 2002 died at a rate of 5.8 per 1,000 live births compared to a mortality rate of 14.4 per 1,000 live births for infants born to Black or African American mothers (NCHS, 2005, Table 22).

In responding to these kinds of disparities, policy makers and health care providers have focused primarily on reducing disparities in access to preventive and other services and understanding and targeting the underlying causes of differences in outcomes, service use, and treatment patterns for leading sources of mortality and morbidity (see, e.g., Smedley, Stith, & Nelson, 2002). Disparities in palliative and end-of-life care have not been a primary focus except among those providing or promoting such care. A separate section of this chapter returns to these issues.

☐ How We Die

Leading Causes of Death

The drop in death rates described can be traced in large measure to public health and medical successes in preventing and treating infectious diseases. A century ago, such diseases—notably influenza, tuberculosis, and diphtheria—were the leading causes of death in the United States (Brim et al., 1970). Heart disease, stroke, and cancer were, respectively, the fourth, fifth, and ninth leading causes of death. Although deaths from tuberculosis are often lingering, many deaths from infectious disease occurred soon after the illness was contracted.

For many decades now, chronic conditions—in particular heart disease, cancer (malignant neoplasms), and stroke (cerebrovascular disease)—have predominated as causes of death (Table 6.1). In 2002, nearly 700,000 U.S. residents died of heart disease; over 550,000 died of malignant neoplasms; and over 160,000 died of cererbrovascular disease (NCHS, 2005, Table 31). These three causes accounted for 58% of all deaths.

Not unexpectedly, causes of death vary considerably across age groups. Given that those aged 65 and over account for the majority of deaths overall, it is not surprising that heart disease, cancer, and stroke lead as causes of death in this age group (NCHS, 2005, Table 32). Unintentional injuries

TABLE 6.1 Leading Causes and Number of Deaths, United States, 2002

Causes of Death	Number
Diseases of heart	696,947
Malignant neoplasms	557,271
Cerebrovascular diseases	162,672
Unintentional injuries	124,816
Chronic obstructive pulmonary diseases	106,742
Influenza and pneumonia	73,249
Diabetes mellitus	65,681
Alzheimer's disease	58,866
Nephritis, nephritic syndrome, and nephrosis	40,974
Septicemia	33,865
Total (all causes)	2,443,387

Source: From *Health, United States, 2005* (Table 31), National Center for Health Statistics (NCHS), 2005, Hyattsville, MD: NCHS.

rank ninth in this oldest age group, accounting for almost 34,000 deaths in 2002.

In generally healthier younger populations, injury ranks higher as a cause of death. For people aged 45 to 64, cancer, heart disease, and unintentional injuries are the leading causes of death. The order is slightly different for those aged 25 to 44, with unintentional injuries leading and cancer and heart disease following as the top causes of death. The description of Josh's (see chapter 4, this volume) prolonged dying in a minimally conscious state illustrates the many difficulties that may confront families when a young adult suffers a devastating but not quickly fatal brain injury. For people 15 to 24, diseases are not among the top three causes of death. Rather, unintentional injuries (15,412 deaths), homicide (5,219), and suicide (4,010) lead—and account for three-quarters of the 33,000 deaths in this age group. Unintentional injuries are also the leading cause of death for children aged 1 to 14, followed by cancer and congenital malformations, with homicide ranking fourth. Among infants, the leading causes of death are a complex of congenital conditions, disorders related to short gestation and low birth weight, and sudden infant death syndrome.

The racial disparities that characterize life expectancy and death rates overall are noteworthy also for causes of death. For Blacks or African Americans but not Whites, 2 of the top 10 causes of death are homicide (6th) and HIV infection (7th) (NCHS, 2005, Table 21). Alzheimer's disease (8th) and suicide (10th) appear in the top 10 causes for Whites but not Blacks. Although death rates for HIV infection have dropped significantly (falling from an age-adjusted rate of 16.2 deaths per 100,000 population in 1995 to 4.9 per 100,000 population in 2002), rates have not dropped as sharply for Blacks or African Americans as for Whites. Among Blacks, the death rate for HIV infection dropped from 89.0 per 100,000 population in 1995 to 33.3 per 100,000 population in 2002; for Whites, the rate dropped from 20.4 per 100,000 population in 1995 to 4.3 per 100,000 population in 2002. Richard (Richard & Lyon, chapter 2, this volume) describes his experience as an African American teenager who was born HIV positive and who has faced many medical crises.

Trajectories of Dying

As originally described by Glaser and Strauss (1965), common pathways to death can be understood as trajectories that can be characterized by their duration and shape—with shape essentially determined by an individual's well-being or functioning over time. Figure 6.2 shows four prototypical pathways, each with different implications for dying individuals, their families, and health professionals and others. They highlight

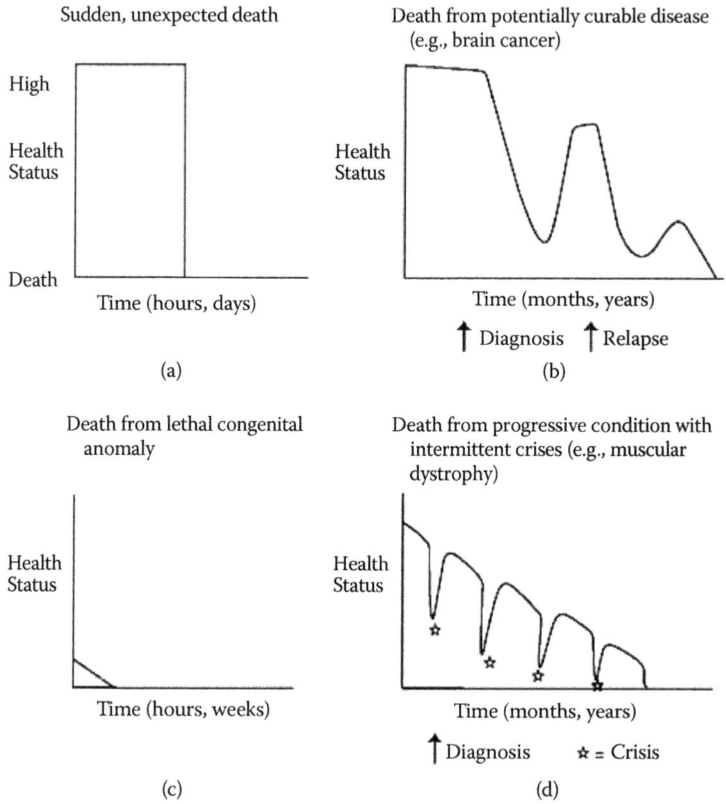

FIGURE 6.2 Prototypical trajectories of dying. *Source:* From *When Children Die: Improving Palliative and End-of-Life Care for Children and Their Families,* by M. J. Field and R. E. Behrman, Eds., 2003, p. 74, Washington, DC: National Academy Press. (See also Field & Cassel, 1997.)

the reality that no single model of care and support will apply to all dying people or their families.

As depicted in Figure 6.2a, death sometimes comes suddenly and unexpectedly to a basically healthy person, for example, when a healthy teenager dies in a car crash. In these situations, healthcare professionals can do nothing to help the person who dies; rather, their responsibility is to the shocked and bereaved survivors.

Sometimes, an injury is not immediately fatal, and families have a relatively brief forewarning of impending death. As shown in Figure 6.2c, a similar kind of brief forewarning occurs with infants unexpectedly born with problems incompatible with extended life. The demands of these medical crises can challenge professional attentiveness to confused and terrified family members, who may have little time to understand what is happening before they are asked to make difficult choices. Such situations can produce highly emotional discussions about the appropriate use of life-sustaining interventions. Tension between families and healthcare professionals can thwart or complicate efforts by physicians, social workers, or others to provide comfort and emotional support.

A different kind of devastating injury trajectory is revealed in the story of Josh (chapter 4, this volume), who had a traumatic brain injury from which recovery to aware life was impossible. Given lack of adequate information and communication from Josh's physicians, what could have been a difficult but relatively brief period leading to a family decision to withdraw mechanical ventilation turned into a months-long nightmare relieved only by the discovery of hospice as an option.

In the United States today, people who die most often have considerable forewarning of death, usually in the form of chronic illness experienced in later life. Some illnesses, including many forms of cancer, have a variable path. Some individuals who are treated and considered cured will live to die of another cause. Others have cancers that are almost always fatal within months. Yet a third group may be considered cancer free for months to years after treatment but then experience a fatal recurrence as depicted in Figure 6.2b. This part of the figure also illustrates that active treatment for cancer may significantly reduce functioning and well-being for weeks or months, depending on the regimen. Otherwise, those who die of cancer often experience only modest decreases in functioning until the last few months of life.

Although individuals and families vary in their response to life-threatening conditions, a patient's changing prognosis will usually be an important determinant of the nature and intensity of preparations for death. Figure 6.2d shows a particularly difficult trajectory for a progressive condition that is marked by periods of slow but relatively stable declines in function that are punctuated by potentially fatal medical crises, the last of which ends in death. Raye's account (chapter 5, this volume) of her father's illness illustrates this pattern, except that death did not come directly from his disease. In these circumstances, health professionals, patients, and families often face the repeated stress of weighing whether the burdens of continued active treatment exceed the benefits. As in the crisis situation associated with devastating injuries, differences in views between professionals and family members and among family members can add to levels of stress.

☐ Where We Die: From Home to Hospital and Partway Back

As a result of changes in health care, family structure, and other features of American life, death has moved out of homes and into institutions—although recent years have seen some shifting back toward death at home. In 1949, just under half of deaths occurred in hospitals, nursing homes, or other institutions (Brim et al., 1970). By 1958, the institutional percentage had risen to 61%, and data for 1980 show 74% of deaths occurring in institutions (60.5% in hospitals and 13.5% in other institutions) (Brim et al., 1970; Brock & Foley, 1996).

By 1980, advocates for dying people and their families had begun to press for changes in this institutional way of death. Hospice offered an option that also provided patients and family members with more control over decisions at the end of life. The first hospice was organized in the United States in 1974. In 1983, Congress—in a rare expansion of Medicare benefits—added coverage for hospice care (Hoyer, 1996), and private health plans also began to cover this innovation in end-of-life care. Also in the 1980s, Congress adopted a new method of paying hospitals—prospective, per-case payment based on diagnosis-related groups. This new payment method provided an incentive for reducing the length of time patients—including dying patients—stayed in hospitals. Following these changes, inpatient hospital death rates for Medicare beneficiaries dropped, and nursing home death rates increased (Brock & Foley, 1996; McMillan, Mentnech, Lubitz, McBean, & Russell, 1990; Sager, Easterlin, Kindig, & Anderson, 1989).

By 1990, deaths in residences began to be identified in national vital statistics reports. Among all those dying of chronic conditions, the age- and gender-adjusted proportion of deaths occurring in acute care hospitals dropped from 62.3% in 1989 to 51.7% in 1997 to 49.5% in 2001 (Teno, 2004). The percentage of deaths occurring in nursing homes increased from 19.2% in 1989 to 23.2% in 2001. People who experience significant functional impairment for an extended period before death are more likely to die in a nursing home than those with short periods of such impairment (Weitzen, 2004).

The percentage of people dying at home has also risen, from 15.9% in 1989 to 23.4% in 2001. Patients enrolled in hospice are more likely to die at home than others. In 2001, for those dying of cancer (the most common condition for those dying under hospice care), the home rather than the hospital was the most common place of death (38% of deaths—adjusted for age and sex—occurred at home). The story of Crow's brother (chapter

4, this volume) describes the special care provided by inpatient hospice to this young man before he died.

Analyses undertaken by the Center for Gerontology and Health Care Research at Brown University showed substantial differences in site of death among states in the United States (Teno, 2004). The lowest percentages of home deaths for cancer patients were seen in the District of Columbia (22%) and South Dakota (22%), and the highest were seen in Utah (61%) and Oregon (55%). New York, at 52%, had the highest percentage of deaths occurring in hospitals. Variation also characterizes the pattern for all chronic illness deaths with a range of 12% (District of Columbia) to 36% (Utah).

Although cancer is still the leading diagnosis for patients receiving hospice care, hospices are increasingly caring for patients with other diagnoses. In 1992, cancer was the primary diagnosis for 66% of hospice patients; in 2000, the figure was 52% (NCHS, 2005, Table 95). Patients with heart disease, the next most common diagnosis, accounted for 10% of patients in 1992 versus 13% in 2000. According to more recent data from the National Hospice and Palliative Care Organization (NHPCO, 2004), the most common diagnoses for hospice patients—after cancer (46%) and end-stage heart disease (12.2%)—are dementia (8.9%), debility (8.2%), lung disease (7.1%), and end-stage renal disease (3.1%). Over 1 million people sought hospice care in the United States in 2004, up from approximately 200,000 in 1990 (NHPCO, 2004). Many patients, however, are referred for hospice very late in their illness. One third of hospice patients do not enroll until their last week of life (Casarett, 2006).

Over 80% of those who receive hospice care are age 65 or over. Analyses of Medicare data found a significant increase in beneficiaries' use of hospice services during the 1990s. In 1998, more than half of beneficiaries with cancer used hospice services compared to 10% of those with other diagnoses (Hogan et al., 2001).

As described, life expectancy and major causes of death differ by race in the United States. Differences extend to care at the end of life. Hospice statistics indicate that blacks are less likely to use hospice services than whites (NHPCO, 2004). Studies have found ethnic and racial differences in attitudes about advance directives, disclosure of information to patients, pain, and patient autonomy (Field & Cassel, 1997). Studies suggest that a complex mix of factors appeared to be affecting attitudes and decision making about hospice and end-of-life care. These factors include lack of education about hospice, low involvement of minority health professionals in hospice care, religious and spiritual beliefs, and mistrust of the healthcare system (see, e.g., Crawley et al., 2000; Johnson, Elbert-Avila, & Tulsky, 2005).

☐ The Cost of Dying

Because most people who die are over age 65, the federal government's Medicare program is the most important source of payment for end-of-life care. Figure 6.3 shows data on source of payment for health care in the last year of life (all ages). Average spending rises sharply in the last month of life, increasing from approximately $4,000 in the month prior to the last month to approximately $8,000 in the last month. Most of this increase is accounted for by higher rates of hospital use. Concern over the high costs of care near the end of life can affect decision making, even if a person has health insurance. Richard's (Richard & Lyon, chapter 2, this volume) negotiation with his grandparents when writing his advance directive illustrated his concern that they not impoverish themselves to pay for his medical care if he were dying.

Not unexpectedly, Medicare beneficiaries who die are older (on average 78.5 vs. 70.6 years) and have higher costs and more health problems in the year before death than those who survive. One analysis of 1992 to 1999 data showed average health spending for Medicare beneficiaries during the last year of life was over $22,500 compared to $3,900 for other beneficiaries (Centers for Medicare and Medicaid Services [CMS], 2003). An analysis of 1993 to 1998 data reported that Medicare beneficiaries who died had, on average, almost four significant medical conditions in the last year of life, whereas survivors averaged slightly over one condition (Hogan et al., 2000). This analysis also found that as age at death increases, Medicare expenditures decrease, in part because nursing home use and Medicaid payments are higher. For deceased beneficiaries aged 65 to 74,

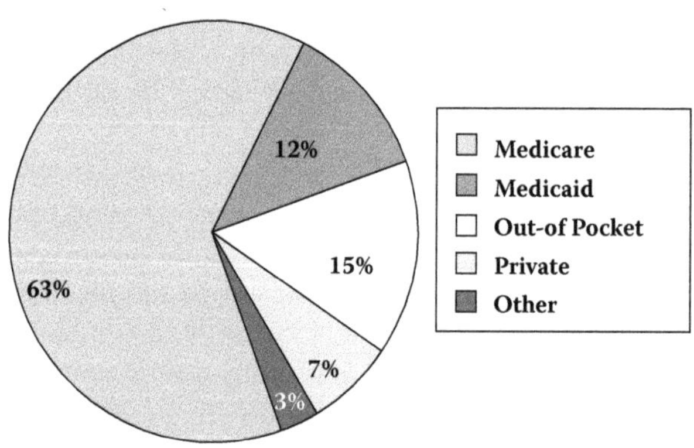

FIGURE 6.3 Source of payment for health care during the last year of life, 1992–1999. *Source:* From Last Year of Life Expenditures, *MCBS Profiles,* by Centers for Medicare and Medicaid Services (CMS), 2003, retrieved February 26, 2006, from http://www.cms.hhs.gov/mcbs/downloads/issue10.pdf.

per capita Medicare payments were $31,800, whereas payments for the group aged 85 and over were $18,800.

One implication of the difference in costs of care for those who die versus those who survive is that schemes to encourage enrollment of Medicare beneficiaries into competing health maintenance organizations and other managed care plans should take cost differences into account in designing plan payment policies. One recent analysis suggested that current methods for risk-adjusting payments are inadequate and provide strong incentive to avoid enrolling beneficiaries with terminal illnesses (Buntin, Garber, McClellan, & Newhouse, 2004).

Although Medicare spending on care at the end of life is high, this spending is not a major factor in rising Medicare costs. Costs for care in the last year of life have stayed relatively stable over a 20-year period (Hogan et al., 2000). The 5% or so of beneficiaries who die account for approximately one quarter of Medicare spending. As described, beneficiaries are sicker than other beneficiaries, so high costs are not surprising. Per-beneficiary costs for Medicare survivors with characteristics similar to decedents are also much higher than average. Some analyses suggest that hospice care may reduce costs for younger Medicare beneficiaries dying of cancer but increase costs for those dying of other causes (Campbell, Lynn, Louis, & Shugarman, 2004).

□ Conclusion

When, how, and where people die in the United States—and how much the dying process costs—have changed significantly over the past 100 years. Although racial and gender differences remain, people are living longer and dying of more chronic illnesses, with death occurring in institutions, where individuals and their families may incur significant expense. As the other chapters in this book attest, decision making near the end of life has been complicated by these changes. The legal, ethical, and moral implications as well as the impact on the dying person and loved ones are profound and deserve careful consideration. How people die and the decisions they must make at the end of life should be of concern to us all.

□ References

Brim, O. G., Jr., Friedman, H. E., Levine, S., & Scotch, N. A. (Eds.). (1970). *The dying patient*. New York: Russell Sage Foundation.

Brock, D. B., & Foley, D. J. (1996, April 30). Demography and epidemiology of dying in the U.S., with emphasis on deaths of older persons. In *A good dying: Shaping health care for the last months of life.* Briefing book for symposium sponsored by The George Washington University Center to Improve Care of the Dying and the Corcoran Gallery of Art, Washington, DC.

Buntin, M. B., Garber, A. M., McClellan, M. B., & Newhouse, J. P. (2004). Costs of decedents in the Medicare program: implications for payments to Medicare + Choice plans. *Health Services Research, 39,* 111–130.

Campbell, D. E., Lynn, J., Louis, T. A., & Shugarman, L. R. (2004). Medicare program expenditures associated with hospice use. *Annals of Internal Medicine, 140,* 269–277.

Casarett, D. (2006). Understanding and improving hospice enrollment. *LDI Issue Brief, 11*(3), 1–4. Retrieved February 26, 2006, from http://www.upenn.edu/ldi/issuebrief11_3.pdf

Centers for Medicare and Medicaid Services (CMS). (2003, May). Last year of life expenditures. *MCBS Profiles.* Retrieved February 26, 2006, from http://www.cms.hhs.gov/mcbs/downloads/issue10.pdf

Crawley, L., Payne, R., Bolden, J., Payne, T., Washington, P., & Williams, S. (2000). Palliative and end-of-life care in the African American community. *Journal of the American Medical Association, 284,* 2518–2521.

Field, M. J., & Behrman, R. E. (Eds.). (2003). *When children die: Improving palliative and end-of-life care for children and their families.* Washington, DC: National Academy Press.

Field, M. J., & Cassel, C. K. (Eds.). (1997). *Approaching death: Improving care at the end of life.* Washington, DC: National Academy Press.

Glaser, B. G., & Strauss, A. L. (1965). *Awareness of dying.* Chicago: Aldine.

Hogan, C., Lunney, J., Gabel, J., & Lynn, J. (2001). Medicare beneficiaries' costs of care in the last year of life. *Health Affairs, 20,* 188–195.

Hogan, C., Lynn, J., Gabel, J., Lunney, J., O'Mara, A., & Wilkinson, A. (2000). *Medicare beneficiaries' cost and use of care in the last year of life. Final report submitted to the Medicare Payment Advisory Commission.* Retrieved February 26, 2006, from http://www.medicaring.org/educate/download/medpac.pdf

Hoyer, T. (1996, April 30). A history of the Medicare Hospice Benefit. In *A good dying: Shaping health care for the last months of life.* Briefing book for symposium sponsored by The George Washington University Center to Improve Care of the Dying and the Corcoran Gallery of Art, Washington, DC.

Johnson, K. S., Elbert-Avila, K. I., & Tulsky, J. A. (2005). The influence of spiritual beliefs and practices on the treatment preferences of African Americans: a review of the literature. *Journal of the American Geriatric Society, 53,* 711–719.

Lynn, J., & Adamson, D. M. (2003). *Living well at the end of life: Adapting health care to serious chronic illness in old age.* Rand Health White Paper WP-137. Retrieved February 26, 2006, from http://www.medicaring.org/educate/download/wp137.pdf

McMillan, A., Mentnech, R. M., Lubitz, J., McBean, A. M., & Russell, D. (1990). Trends and patterns in place of death for Medicare enrollees. *Health Care Financing Review, 12,* 1–7.

National Center for Health Statistics (NCHS). (2005). *Health, United States, 2005.* Hyattsville, MD: Author. Retrieved February 26, 2006, from http://www.cdc.gov/nchs/data/hus/hus05.pdf#summary

National Hospice and Palliative Care Organization (NHPCO). (2004). *NHPCO's 2004 facts and figures.* Retrieved February 26, 2006, from http://www.nhpco.org/files/public/Facts_Figures_for2004data.pdf

Sager, M., Easterlin, D. V., Kindig, D. A., & Anderson, O. W. (1989). Changes in the location of death after passage of Medicare's Prospective Payment System. *New England Journal of Medicine, 320,* 433–439.

Smedley, B. D., Stith, A. Y., & Nelson, A. R. (Eds.). (2002). *Unequal treatment: Confronting racial and ethnic disparities in health care.* Washington, DC: National Academy Press.

Social Security Administration (SSA). (2005). *Social Security basic facts.* Retrieved February 26, 2006, from http://www.ssa.gov/pressoffice/factsheets/basicfact-alt.pdf

Teno, J. (2004). *The Brown atlas of dying.* Brown University Center for Gerontology and Health Care Research, Providence, RI. Retrieved February 26, 2006, from http://www.chcr.brown.edu/dying/BROWNATLAS.HTM

U.S. Census Bureau. (2005). *2004 American community survey.* Washington, DC: Author. Retrieved July 17, 2007 from http://factfinder.census.gov/servlet/DatasetMainPageServlet?_program=ACS&_submenuld=&_lang=en&_ts=

U.S. Department of Commerce. (1975). *Bicentennial edition historical statistics of the United States colonial times to 1970, Part 1.* Washington, DC: Bureau of the Census.

Weitzen, S. (2004). *Functional decline predicts site of death.* PowerPoint presentation. Retrieved February 26, 2006, from http://www.chcr.brown.edu/dying/downloads/apha20002.pdf

7

CHAPTER

The Media and End-of-Life Choices and Decisions

Marilyn Webb

The Academy Awards are noteworthy for more than just their star power. Winning movies set the tone for cultural consciousness. Naïve as it sounds, movies first made me realize that death happens to everyone, that dying was more than a private sorrow that only my family endured. And, the movies also taught me there is room for choice in how we die. There it was, up there on the big screen.

Movies—along with books, plays, TV, newspapers, and magazines—have helped to affect a sea change in how we all think about our final days (Pavlides, 2007). That sea change, of course, is based on changes in medical technology, but portraying how we respond, helping us learn what others do, educating us on late-breaking medical facts is now the job of mass media, for better or worse.

Take *Ordinary People,* which was the first movie eye-opener for me. There was the usually grinning Mary Tyler Moore in 1980, showing me another family, like mine, who became mute and twisted by unspoken grief. A child had died, and no one knew how to respond to the depth of that loss.

Then in 1983's *Terms of Endearment,* there was the hyper Shirley MacLaine, screaming in all her glory, pounding on a hospital nurses' desk for someone to give her dying daughter (Debra Winger) more pain medication.

"Get my daughter her shot!" MacLaine snarled, that snarl announcing to me a new world of choice. Winger's character, a young woman dying of cancer, was suffering acute and prolonged pain in the process. Shirley's character, Winger's activist and distraught mother, heralded the possibility that patients and families could have a medical say, not just nurses and physicians. That shriek screamed out to me the possibility for a measure of end-of-life control. The issue of control is omnipresent across all of the personal stories in this volume (see Crow, chapter 4; Raye, chapter 5; Richard & Lyon, chapter 2; and Spannhake, chapter 3).

My generation—the baby boomers—was already weaned on choice. In fact, we could be called, if anything, the choice generation. We teethed on the Pill, came of age with legalized abortion, and as we aged, were moving into the brave new days of managed infertility. But, by the time *Terms of Endearment* premiered, there were other changes taking place at the end of life, and—as Debra Winger showed us—it was not just happening to those who were old (see also Crow, chapter 4, this volume).

When Shirley screamed, it had already been 7 years since Karen Ann Quinlan had lain in a New Jersey hospital bed in a persistent vegetative state (PVS). At that time, most people did not know that medicine had now passed the days of "there is nothing more we can do" to a revolutionary "we can do pretty much whatever we want." (And notice that "we" in the previous sentence—because the decision did not yet have anything to do with the "I" of patient choice.)

In 1975, Karen Ann Quinlan went into a coma after consuming a deadly mixture of alcohol and pain medication, thus resulting in long brain deprivation of oxygen (Colby, 2006). For the first year, a respirator and a feeding tube kept her alive, but no TV cameras or photographers were ever allowed at her bedside. That is why few people knew what a PVS looked like; her body would shrivel and grotesquely twist, making it seem as if she were functioning physically in terrible pain, but in reality her higher brain functions had already died.

No one knew this because the very diagnosis of PVS was still so new, just a scant 3 years in the medical literature (Colby, 2006). The public likely did not realize that when Karen's family won their legal battle to remove her from a respirator in 1976, a feeding tube still kept her alive for another 9 years. During that time, her body withered and warped, wracked by distortion and infection and blank stares, but all the public saw was her beautiful face, smiling from her old black-and-white high school photo.

In 1976, the Quinlans were vilified for wanting to let their daughter finally find some peace, to end what they viewed as intolerable and unnecessary suffering. But widespread public opinion, knowledge, state and federal law, and cultural mores had not yet caught up. Educating the public would become an essential job for the media, a job it has been tackling now for more than 20 years.

In fact, when they envisioned the Constitution, this nation's founding fathers imagined the press as the Fourth Estate, not only educating voters on important issues of the day but also acting independently, performing checks and balances on the three chambers of government—the executive, legislative, and judicial branches. That was an ideal, of course, but press ownership, private interests, and the very expansion of knowledge that required more technical and comprehensive coverage have inhibited this ideal from becoming a reality, as the events surrounding Terri Schiavo so vividly illustrate. Journalists also are not always any more informed than their many readers are on a given issue, so the learning curves are steep.

Further, there is the question of the role of the media in the form of art and film. As depicted in the 1983 movie with Shirley MacLaine, adequate pain control meant enough narcotics so that Debra, her daughter, felt comfortable; it did not mean that nurses gave set doses at preestablished times—a radical idea. Remember this was 1983, a time when the government began pushing its "Just Say No" campaign. Who was a patient to ask for more drugs?

Fast forward to 2005, to *Million Dollar Baby,* in which Hilary Swank, in a life-affirming desire, becomes a feisty boxer (see also Pavlides, 2007). What once seemed radical in the 1980s now seems like "choice light" when Hilary's character becomes completely paralyzed and decides she no longer wants to live her life. Drugs in this case revolved around a decision about ending it all when permanent paralysis of an entire body is involved.

These ethical dilemmas have played well in living color and with the Motion Picture Academy, both movies winning coveted Oscars. But, more important, they have served to educate a nation on the kinds of personal options medical advances allow, including situations in which such options do not foster greater happiness.

The problem is not with the media but with the enormous and swift technological change, causing a loss of our ethical moorings that were based on principles of morality from a simpler day. Rather than acting only as the Fourth Estate, hard enough as that sounds, the media has now become a guiding moral light, albeit one that can be spun different ways depending on who is doing the spinning.

The good news is that media—TV, movies, print, Internet—have awakened us to the changing times, bringing information, individual dramas, and once-private conversations into the national spotlight. This ensures that these now-crucial conversations occur within each of our homes and make all of us far wiser about our futures.

The choice generation has now fully come of age; media is central to their lives, thereby making once-private tragedies intensely public. Consider that, in the 1980s, William Colby became the attorney for Nancy Cruzan's family, another young woman in a similar condition to that of Karen Ann Quinlan. While the Quinlan family had fought to remove Karen's respirator, Nancy was not on one. Instead, her family fought to remove her feeding tube (Colby, 2002). And, although Karen's family never wanted any photos, the Cruzan family felt differently. At various times during the nearly 8 years she lay bedridden until she died, Colby said the Cruzan family welcomed a team from *Frontline,* a prime-time television news reporting program, to document her decline. They also invited photographers from other television outlets, newspapers, and national magazines. Seeing those photos was probably the real start of America's awakening to the complex ethical and medical dilemmas that might now befall us all.

By the spring of 2005, live-action videos of brain-damaged Terri Schiavo allowed viewers an even closer look at how much medicine *could* do and forced the public to consider instead what it *should* do. Terri's blank eyes, swollen face, and awkward smile literally brought home public recognition of medicine's success over the past 30 years at prolonging biological life. But, that picture of success did not mean the resulting decisions were simple.

For example, as noted, when Karen Quinlan lapsed into a coma in 1975, the very diagnosis of PVS had only been around in medical literature for 3 years (Colby, 2006). Indeed, it had not yet been 10 years since technology had advanced far enough—through the use of emergency cardiopulmonary resuscitation (CPR) and life-prolonging apparatuses—to allow a person to live long enough for PVS even to exist. Prior to that, we either lived, or we died.

Since then, the possibility of prolonging life has expanded to other medical conditions and involves whole different sets of choices and technologies. We no longer think only of feeding tubes and respirators, but of dialysis, chemotherapy, or organ transplants; and, more generally, of fertility treatments, egg transplantations, neonatal miracles, and sperm donation.

At the same time, the public began to realize that end-of-life medical choices that were once considered rare—like Karen's or Nancy's or Terri's—could actually involve any of us, in any of a multitude of different conditions. The range of what medicine can do today has widened to such a degree that decisions run the gamut from respirators and feeding tubes to refusing even what was once viewed as a miracle—antibiotics and simple heart medications.

Media coverage created a national sophistication that never existed before, but it also spurred lay conversations on when treatment might not be useful anymore outside medical contexts. This was revolutionary but occurred with limited guidance from the medical, social, and spiritual communities.

As a consequence of the Karen Ann Quinlan case, the Catholic Church began reconsidering whether a respirator was normal for breathing or whether it was an extraordinary treatment (Richard Doerflinger, Assistant Director for Policy Development of the National Conference of Catholic Bishops' Secretariat for Pro-Life Activities, personal communication, February 21, 1996; see also a thorough discussion of this issue in Webb, 1997, pp. 136–148). Then, with Nancy Cruzan, the Catholic Church began to think about feeding tubes. With technology changing, it was not clear to those who were religious what was God's work and what could just be left to humans. Further, secular everyday citizens also had questions and concerns. Statistically, we may be a churchgoing nation, but Americans' own moral codes have historically been individually based. We were left to mull these issues on our own, within our own family experience, even whether the issues we were considering were within then-current law. Politicians and lawyers joined the fray, trying to help people understand the technological advances and medical options, but it was only when the media grew knowledgeable that the general public began to grow wiser.

Television, the arts, movies, and newspapers all gave necessary new information to guide us in our consideration of end-of-life decisions and dilemmas. Were we to consider feeding tubes as food? Should they always be used? Did they cause suffering, or did they not? When and how could they be removed, and who had the right to make that decision? Might treating pneumonia not necessarily be the right thing to do? Did the fact that we might effect a cure mean that we should? Would it be better to let someone die of pneumonia, or would it be better to treat the person if wellness meant she or he would just suffer more deterioration from Alzheimer's disease instead? When do the discomforts and side effects of kidney dialysis override the enjoyment of life? And, who is to decide any or all of these things?

During the 1990s, television programs like *ER* aired, helping Americans see the day-to-day realities of these questions, helping them ask, for example, which complications might occur with CPR or the use of other emergency treatments. People could witness the moral issues medical personnel faced in the trenches each day. People could also see the pain of patients and families when confronted with these situations.

Plays and movies, like *Wit* and *Angels in America,* appeared, and books like Anna Quindlen's (1994) *One True Thing* were made into films. They encouraged even tougher and more sophisticated discussions on pain management, on living with AIDS and cancer, on the burdens that prolonging terminal illnesses placed on patients and families, on how the benefits of treatment could be weighed against its burdens. They also raised the issue of assisted suicide similar to the situation illustrated in Raye's personal account (see chapter 5, this volume).

Screenwriters' organizations, newspaper and magazine editors, and television producers all began asking medical and bioethics experts to teach them to accurately portray end-of-life medical treatment and care. For example, as author of *The Good Death,* I was hired as a consultant for Bill Moyers's four-part PBS special in 2000 on death and dying, *On Our Own Terms.* (This has also been the experience of others affiliated with Last Acts, a national program funded by the Robert Wood Johnson Foundation.) These media experts knew they needed training if they were to perform the important social functions they had to play. So, the finer points of medical decision making became the fodder for prime-time entertainment as well as factual accounting on the nightly evening news. Although a more sophisticated generation was emerging, so was a conservative backlash.

In 1973, immediately after the U.S. Supreme Court decision on *Roe v. Wade*, a pro-life/antiabortion counterattack began to coalesce (Webb, 1997). State committees battling abortion on the grassroots level joined to create the National Right to Life Committee (NLRC). The NLRC's first mission statement, published that same year, included opposition to what would become central battlegrounds over the ensuing years—legalized abortion was labeled infanticide, and the fates of Karen Ann Quinlan and, later, of Nancy Cruzan and Terri Schiavo were labeled as euthanasia.

Laura Echevarria, deputy press secretary of the NLRC, held that "[t]here's a link between the two," in my 1997 book, *The Good Death* (p. 159). She continued by saying that:

> Once you start discriminating against one human being—like an unborn child in the womb—you're open to discriminating against another. For the most part, society recognizes that a newborn is a human being, but because of the location, an unborn child isn't. Once you start doing that, with that kind of mindset, it leads to classifying people as not quite human. That can then include the disabled or the terminally ill. (p. 159)

By 1986, some pro-life advocates had become more extreme and confrontational and launched Operation Rescue under the leadership of Randall Terry. Since that time, Terry and his backers have appeared at multitudes of often-violent demonstrations against abortion clinics, blocking clinic access; getting themselves arrested; and threatening clinic workers, physicians, and pregnant women.

In 1990, these very same backers appeared outside the hospital room of Nancy Cruzan, using those same confrontational tactics. The National Organization of Women later successfully sued Operation Rescue for their clinic attacks, resulting in the eventual bankruptcy of Randall Terry. But by 2003, Terry had moved from his home in Binghamton, New York, to Ponte Vedra Beach, in northern Florida, and had founded a new and similar organization, the Society for Truth and Justice. In spring 2005, its largest operation to date took place outside the Pinellas Park, Florida, hospice of Terri Schiavo.

Randall Terry had become the actual spokesperson for the Schindler family, Terri Schiavo's parents and her siblings, and he spoke out against Terri's husband, Michael Schiavo. He was the face of fundamentalism in the trenches, and his supporters had learned how to create, front and center, a public relations spectacle and a political stratagem for the religious right. This time, President George W. Bush, his brother Florida Governor Jeb Bush, and the U.S. Congress became involved, dismaying most of America. An ABC News poll (2005, par. 1) reported that "Americans broadly and strongly disapprove of federal intervention in the Terri Schiavo case, with sizable majorities saying Congress is overstepping its bounds for political gain." The Supreme Court was also invited but appropriately declined (see Cerminara, chapter 8, this volume).

"Our family asked Randall Terry to come, and we gave him carte blanche to put Terri's fight in front of the American people," Terri's father, Bob Schindler, told the press early on (Miner, 2003, par. 6). "He did exactly what we asked, and more. Randall organized vigils and protests, he coordinated the media, he helped us meet with Governor Bush" (Miner, par. 6).

The press covered all this for the next 3 years, but what it had not done well enough was to connect the dots. The very same people, even many of the very same names, were behind the past two decades of both anti-abortion and fundamentalist end-of-life activities. Among the most recognizable were Randall Terry; Missouri's former Attorney General William Webster, lead name on the Supreme Court's first post-*Roe v. Wade* case, *Webster v. Reproductive Health Services,* that limited abortion; even former Attorney General John Ashcroft, who was governor of Missouri during the Cruzan case. At this time, they had vast White House, congressional, and federal connections.

"I feel like a spectator," Joe Cruzan once despairingly told a TV reporter from *Frontline,* "like I'm sitting up in the bleachers in the poorest seats and two other teams are playing on the field, playing with my football and there's not a darn thing I can do" (Webb, 1997, p. 161). And that is also how Michael Schiavo may have felt while his wife, Terri, deteriorated over the course of 15 years.

While Joe Cruzan believed he could do nothing, there was a lot that pro-life advocates were doing in the years that Nancy lay silent, most particularly about the media and the press. The word on the streets always has it that "the press" is made up of that dirty word: liberals. Not only that, they do not understand religion, which is exactly what advocates paint end-of-life choice to be about. None of this really is true, especially the claims about liberals on the radio airwaves (see Shakir, Pitney, Terkel, Khanna, & Corley, 2007).

During those 15 years—from 1990 through 2005—that Terri Schiavo lived with her feeding tube, a vast conservative media conglomerate was building. Even as she lay dying, with her feeding tube removed for the third time in June 2005, the Christian Broadcasting Network News (CBN News) unveiled its glam Washington bureau near Dupont Circle. CBN was just one of many bright stars in an already-exploding Christian media universe.

According to media analyst Mariah Blake (2005), writing that same spring in the prestigious *Columbia Journalism Review:*

> Conservative evangelicals control at least six national television networks, each reaching tens of millions of homes, and virtually all of the nation's more than 2,000 religious radio stations. Thanks to

> Christian radio's rapid growth, religious stations now outnumber every other format except country music and news-talk. (p. 32)

In 2007, a report prepared for the Center for American Progress and Free Press said that a "statistical analysis of the political makeup of talk radio in the United States ... confirm[ed] the stunning lack of diversity in talk radio, and raise[s] serious questions about whether the companies licensed to broadcast over the public airwaves are serving the listening needs of all Americans" (Shakir et al., 2007, par. 1).

According to this report,

> 91 percent of the political talk radio programming on the stations owned by the top five commercial station owners was conservative, and only 9 percent was progressive. Ninety-two percent of these stations (236 stations out of 257) do not broadcast a single minute of progressive talk radio programming. In the top 10 radio markets in the country, 76 percent of the news/talk programming is conservative, while 24 percent is progressive. In four of those top 10 markets—Philadelphia, Atlanta, Dallas, Houston—the domination of conservative talk radio is between 96 and 100 percent. (Shakir et al., 2007, par. 2)

Blake claimed that this vast network was not just preaching about God but had politically packaged a highly conservative view of the daily news. Most people recognize the names of *Fox News* or Pat Robertson's *700 Club*, but those were only the tips of many giant, well-funded, and well-controlled icebergs.

"As Christian broadcasting has grown," Blake (2005, p. 32) wrote,

> pulpit-based ministries have largely given way to a robust programming mix that includes music, movies, sitcoms, reality shows and cartoons. But the largest constellation may be news and talk shows. Christian public affairs programming exploded after September 11, and again in the run-up to the 2004 presidential election. And this growth shows no signs of flagging. (pp. 32, 34)

Blake (2005) reported that although Christians have looked to radio ever since it began in the early 1900s, by the 1930s evangelicals were pushing policies that would end up giving them dominance on the airwaves. "[E]arly on," she wrote,

> the big three networks donated rather than sold airtime to religious organizations. The Federal Council of Churches, which represented the more liberal mainline denominations, favored this system, which it believed would help keep the religious message from

> getting corrupted. But evangelicals worried that networks would lavish mainline churches with free airtime while giving their own ministries short shrift. (p. 34)

In 1944, the National Religious Broadcasters (NRB) organization formed, lobbied federal legislators, and ended up with the government allowing religious organizations to purchase as much airtime as they could. Evangelical preachers invested and, by paying hard cash, elbowed mainline ministries to the radio sidelines.

"In the sixty-one years since its founding," Blake (2005, p. 34) said,

> the NRB has grown to represent 1,600 broadcasters with billions of dollars in media holdings and staggering political clout. Its aggressive political maneuverings have helped shape federal policy, further easing the evangelical networks' rapid growth. In 2000, for instance, the Federal Communications Commission issued guidelines that would have barred religious broadcasters from taking over frequencies designated for educational programming. The NRB lobbied Congress to intervene, at one point delivering a petition signed by nearly half a million people. Legislators, in turn, bore down on the FCC, and the agency relented.

"Over the last decade," Blake (2005, pp. 34–35) reported,

> Christian TV networks have added tens of millions of homes to their distribution lists by leaping onto satellite and cable systems. The number of religious radio stations—the vast majority of which are evangelical—has grown by about 85 percent since 1998 alone. They now outnumber rock, classical, hip-hop, R&B, soul, and jazz stations combined.

Although the audience share of these stations is still only a fraction of that of mainstream stations, Blake (2005) noted in particular that Salem Communications—only one of a swiftly growing number of religious radio news networks—now airs on 1,100 stations nationwide, which is about seven times as many as broadcast National Public Radio programs. And, many of these stations airing Salem's network news are mainstream stations. Evangelicals have now moved into TV as well, with a very particular news angle, one that became obvious nationwide in the coverage and tactics surrounding the life and death of Terri Schiavo.

Most of the public did not know much about the Schiavo case until its final days, but by then her family's story had been on Christian news programs for nearly 3 years. The Schindlers themselves had been on many of the Christian talk shows. They attended the NBR's 2005 convention to drum up support. They had become media savvy and trained. They took videos of Terri themselves and helped pick out the specific, ready-for-prime-time visuals. And, they had Randall Terry as their family spokesperson.

"Behind the maelstrom of press coverage surrounding the Terri Schiavo legal battle was a carefully crafted media campaign—one that persisted till the hours before her death this morning," wrote reporter Beth Herskovits (2005, par. 1) for *PR Week*, the public relations agency Christian Communication Network's religious wire service.

> Schiavo's parents, Bob and Mary Schindler, had actively taken their struggle in front of the public, setting up a website, releasing multimedia videos of her, and encouraging a constant presence outside her hospice. (par. 2)
>
> … The decision to release the videos is "one of the most powerful tools in the fight to save her life," said Gary McCullough, director of Christian Communication Network, the agency that represents Schiavo's parents, their legal team, and many of the groups supporting them. "It changed the whole dynamic." (par. 4)

On the other hand, in that same report, Jon Eisenberg, an Oakland, California, attorney working for Terri's husband Michael Schiavo, said,

> There's been no PR [public relations effort] on Michael's behalf.
>
> Michael Schiavo has received PR support from his legal team as well as the American Civil Liberties Union, but "none of these are PR people; we're all lawyers," Eisenberg said.
>
> He added that he is working pro bono on the case, while the Schindlers' message has been supported by "unlimited bottomless funding" from conservative groups. (Herskovits, par. 6–8)

Indeed, it was the very involvement of public relations firms here that spun the news in a particular way, distorting medical facts and crucial ethical issues for prime time. "Much of the coverage on Christian networks has distorted Schiavo's condition by indicating she retained the ability to think, feel, and function," Mariah Blake (2005, p. 36) reported in her *Columbia Journalism Review* article.

> Some newscasts reported as fact her parents' contested claim that she tried to utter the words "I want to live" before her feeding tube was pulled for the last time. Others, like Janet Folger, host of the radio and TV call-in show Faith2Action, described Schiavo as actually sitting up and talking. Evangelical pundits also demonized Schiavo's husband, Michael, and the Florida Judge George Greer, who presided over the case, referring to them as murderers and invoking holocaust rhetoric. Indeed, Christian broadcasters seemed

to set the tone for the emotional language that would burst into the mainstream media and the halls of Congress during Schiavo's final days. (p. 36)

At the same time, those videos allowed Americas to view Terri, brain damaged, seeming to smile at her mom or follow balloons with her eyes. And, these video clips also allowed the mainstream press to show how devastatingly complex a condition like PVS can be for patients and physicians, lawyers and judges, friends and families. The PR around these videos served to create a counter public backlash as well—one that may benefit most patients and families in the long run.

According to most medical opinions, PVS is akin to a waking coma. Terri's brain scans showed significant damage to her higher brain functions, but her lower brain functions still occurred: breathing, waking, and sleeping (Colby, 2006, pp. 9–11; Eisenberg, 2005, pp. 13, 16). The tricky part is that spontaneous movements may occur. Eyes may open in response to external stimuli, but a person cannot speak or obey commands. Although he or she may in some ways appear normal and awake—the person might grimace, cry, or laugh—he or she really is not. The longer this condition continues, the less likely it is for any hope of recovery. At 15 years, Terri was at the far end of PVS survival; her body had contorted, and any hope for significant remission was dim. In watching these videos, America got to learn what only physicians and unfortunate families had seen in the past few decades.

One result of the Terri Schiavo case was that a huge surge of Americans reported talking to their families about their own end-of-life choices (Pew Research Center, 2006). Another was that public opinion polls showed that most people finally understood how political this family's tragic private battle had become, and they also understood that PVS was not the only thing they needed to be concerned about: (a) Their own families needed to have their own wishes in writing in order to care for them well; (b) they needed to detail choices not just about PVS but about a whole panoply of various scary scenarios; and (c) they needed to worry about whether their physicians and medical treatment centers would adhere to them (see, e.g., Pew Research Center, 2006; Ditto, chapter 13, this volume).

Although the TV cameras rolled on the pro-life demonstrators, other Americans responded in horror to their visual display and to the national politics that went with it. At this point, press coverage fell down. An ABC News poll on March 21 found that 63% of the public supported the removal of Terri's feeding tube, as opposed to 28% who did not. A CBS News poll, also on March 21–22, gave similar results, with 61% saying the tube should be removed versus 28% who did not. On March 22, 2005, of respondents to a CNN/USA Today/Gallup poll, 52% agreed with that day's court decision to leave Terri Schiavo's feeding tube unattached, while just 39%

disagreed. The great majority of respondents in all these polls thought the Bushes and Congress and the U.S. Supreme Court should not intervene.

On-the-spot coverage in Florida in June, with reporters focused on demonstrators with years of experience knowing that TV needs good visuals (which they readily supplied), may have left evening news viewers with the impression that the two sides in this debate were equal in numbers. As the polls cited indicate, they decidedly were not.

But here's the rub. Reporters are professionally trained in "objectivity," a principle that means they are asked to look at—and report on—issues from both sides. But, what happens when one side is small and the other large? And, what happens when the issue is so complex that a "side" is not even the point of the story, but the depth of the complexities is what needs instead to be addressed?

How the American public actually felt a half year after Terri Schiavo had died was underscored in a major report from the Pew Research Center, which studies American opinion and the press. In a report released January 5, 2006, Pew researchers found:

> An overwhelming majority of the public supports laws that give patients the right to decide whether they want to be kept alive through medical treatment. And fully 70% say there are circumstances when patients should be allowed to die, while just 22% believe that doctors and nurses should always do everything possible to save a patient. (par. 1)

Moreover, although the overall numbers in this study had remained markedly similar to a prior Pew study in 1990, about the time that Nancy Cruzan died, this new poll showed that Americans had actually become a little more discriminating in their various distinctions and choices. In 2006, more people than in 1990 approved of ending life if a patient was suffering and in great pain with no hope of improvement. More believed the same way if patients had an incurable disease or if they were ready to die because living was a burden.

However, there was no change in those 16 years in how respondents thought about whether such a decision should be made based on the burden to the patient's family. Basically, both then and now, respondents thought family burdens should have less to do with it than patient suffering. Only 29% of people asked in each study believed ending a patient's life was appropriate if a family felt burdened (Pew Research Center, 2006).

Further, "[t]he Pew Research Center's survey," the report reads (par. 3),

> conducted November 9–27, 2005 among 1,500 adults, finds that while overall attitudes are largely stable, people are increasingly thinking about and planning for their own medical treatment in the event of

> a terminal illness or incapacitating medical condition. Public awareness of living wills, already widespread in 1990, is now virtually universal, and the number saying they have a living will has more than doubled from just 12 percent in 1990 to 29 percent today. (par. 3)

The numbers had increased in every age group, making it clear that this shift is not just because more of us are now elderly (Pew Research Center, 2006).

Although the number of living will signers is still low, it is clear it is getting progressively higher. A more telling number in this 2006 study is that 69% of those who were married said they have already had a conversation with their spouse about their end-of-life medical wishes, as compared with just 51% in 1990 (Pew Research Center, 2006). Further, among those whose parents were still alive, 57% said they have spoken with their mothers about her end-of-life choices, as compared with 43% in 1990, and 48% stated that they have now spoken with their fathers, compared with just 28% in 1990 (Pew Research Center).

A March 21, 2005, ABC News poll had already found these same results:

> The Schiavo case has prompted an enormous level of personal discussion: Half of Americans say that as a direct result of hearing about this case, they've spoken with friends or family members about what they'd want done if they were in a similar condition. Nearly eight in 10 would not want to be kept alive. (par. 4)

Returning to the issues of objectivity and sides in stories, to those who are likely curious, news reporting is structured to have two sides to represent some ephemeral idea of fairness. That is the standard taught in most journalism schools today and within most mainstream media outlets. However, not everyone plays by those same rules, especially when massive and powerful public relations campaigns are involved. The fairness principle really is neither fair nor even truthful when the sides, if there are any, are not equally balanced. From my own experience in studying the media and in teaching journalism at both the Graduate School of Journalism at Columbia University in New York and as chair of the Program in Journalism at Knox College in Illinois, the press has not adequatcly learned how to handle that situation.

The religious programming conservatives have long claimed that the mainstream press has too liberal an agenda, but in looking at coverage of the Schiavo tragedy, it seems that its concept of news is greatly skewed the other way. Conservatives have created a theoretical "other side" that includes fewer Americans, yet gets much more attention than the poll numbers—especially in this case—show that it deserves.

"The public discussion of the Schiavo case was marked and marred by incredible negativity and name-calling," wrote Nancy Cruzan's family's attorney, William Colby (2006, p. 3) in his book, *Unplugged*.

> This sad state came about in part due to the proliferation of cable outlets on television and the apparent need for confrontational coverage to attract viewers. As the legal case built to its contentious conclusion throughout the spring of 2005, I was doing a lot of interviews. Over and over, television producers asked me in preparation for an appearance on their show, "Which side are you on?" They seemed perplexed when I said, "Neither."

"Part of the problem is our culture itself," Colby said,

> where civil discourse over hard questions—and even basic civility—has faded into angry talking heads on the radio and television. Part of the blame in the Schiavo case must go to the bitterly divided family, willing after years of fighting to say anything about the other side. In the cauldron of charges and countercharges that became the public face of the Terri Schiavo story, it was hard to know an individual fact. It was even harder to learn "the truth." (pp. 3–4)

Throughout this debate, however, and after three decades of individual variations of private end-of-life tragedy ourselves, Americans—journalists and laypeople alike—have likely now learned to be far more nuanced and sophisticated about end-of-life choice and what that really means.

There have been years of living will legislation, state by state, until by 1992 all states had some kind of end-of-life law (Webb, 1997). Television programs like *On Our Own Terms*, produced in 2000 for PBS by Bill Moyers and supported with a massive national outreach effort; movies like *Terms of Endearment* or *Million Dollar Baby*; and our own family experiences have also taught us that specific choices at the end of life cannot all be contemplated ahead of time or written down.

Most of us will die by a roller coaster that eventually results in what end-of-life expert Joanne Lynn, M.D., might call *dwindling* (personal communication). It is a condition of chronic dying, living with what is eventually a fatal disease, or overcoming one illness only to fall victim later to another. If we survive a heart attack, if we beat cancer, if we weather a kidney transplant, we may be lucky enough to suffer from Alzheimer's. As we grow older, there is an increasing likelihood of developing some form of dementia and declining in tiny steps as a result of other illnesses—a small stroke, a urinary tract infection, a fall and broken bones, a touch of pneumonia.

"While medical science has grown more clear on comas and persistent vegetative states—issues that end-of-life experts focused on during the 1970s and 1980s—continued medical success has caused newer conditions of chronic dying to be a far more common circumstance," I found in reporting for my book, *The Good Death* (p. 188).

> These conditions include progressive degenerative illnesses such as Alzheimer's, Lou Gehrig's disease and multiple sclerosis, as well as slow declines from cancer or heart disease—conditions that medicine is far less certain about in determining when treatment is hopeless, when the condition is truly terminal, and in what length of time.
>
> In fact, now that we have this new body of end-of-life law, ethics and practice, more Americans are finding that these laws do not address the issues raised by their particular conditions. Questions patients and families ask today are not just about when a person is competent or on a machine from which he or she might be disconnected. They are about when to stop chemotherapy or dialysis, when to give ever higher doses of drugs that might create comfort but a foreshortened life. These situations are not addressed by living wills, health-care proxies, or surrogacy laws. (p. 189)

Yet, all of these are the specific ways that our crazy quilt of state laws have been written.

Still, more American families and physicians understand this brave new world we have now reached, a world beyond the point at which "nothing can be done," into a world of choice about what we might want done and what we actually might not. In this world, sophisticated as we have now become, is also brewing a new level of post-Terri Schiavo political battles that threaten once again to take decision making out of patients' and families' hands and mire them with actions by legislatures and courts.

Since the Schiavo debacle, conservatives have amped up their push—just as they did years ago with abortion—to limit state and federal laws (see Cerminara, chapter 8, this volume). John Ashcroft's failed attempt as U.S. attorney general to penalize physicians' prescribing practices in Oregon, where physician aid in dying has been legal for terminally ill patients now for nearly a decade, was overruled by the U.S. Supreme Court (*Gonzales v. Oregon*, 2006).

Importantly, the composition of the U.S. Supreme Court has changed, with new and more conservative appointees by President George W. Bush, which might make future rulings on these issues uncertain. Pressure is also growing in state legislatures to limit state living will laws and physicians' ability and freedom to prescribe pain medications. This political pressure might unfortunately increase the resistance that doctors already have to adhere to patients' living wills and accept their self-reports of pain and might further tie up end-of-life choice (see Webb, 1997, pp. 87–98; Cerminara, chapter 8, this volume).

In summary, there has been a swift learning curve for all Americans over the past few decades, but the slow, steady decline, the failure of one bodily organ after the next as we all creep toward the end of life is now far more complicated than it once seemed. News reporters have, unfortunately, had to learn the dynamics of these complications at the same time as they tried to pass along accurate information to their reading publics. The swiftness of medical, ethical, and legal changes, however, has sometimes hindered lay reporters' accuracy, but more often, the press is also a scapegoat for those who want to point fingers from various sides.

For example, in the Schiavo debate, those in the public spotlight who argued for Terri to live longer with her feeding tube in place assailed the press partly by saying the media did not know how to cover religion, mistaking the coverage of medical ethics for views about God. To those who hold certain religious beliefs, no one but God can decide when it is time to die. To others, any medical intervention has already changed this dynamic. And to reporters, Terri's battle was not just one of religion but of the tragedy of one human being caught in the jaws of the meteoric rise of medical success coupled with the still-looming facts that none of us will live forever, and that we all have different views of ethics, medicine, our own lives, and the place that we give to God.

Now that we have choices we never before had, who is to decide? And how? Those are the questions most Americans face today. It has come down to the media itself, novices though we are, to create what can only be seen as a massive project of cultural-medical education, an arena for continual debate, with frequent updates regarding how this might have an impact on our varying individual ethics. We are all engaged in vastly shifting moral terrain as we near the end of life in the 21st century, and it has become the media's public place in this cultural tsunami to help frame the private conversations each of us will have in our own homes.

References

ABC News. (2005, March 21). *Poll: No role for government in Schiavo case.* Retrieved March 10, 2007, from http://abcnews.go.com/Politics/print?id=599622

Blake, M. (2005, May/June). Stations of the cross: How evangelical Christians are creating an alternative universe of faith-based news. *Columbia Journalism Review,* pp. 32–39.

CBS News. (2005, March 21–22). *The Terri Schiavo case.* Retrieved March 10, 2007, from http://www.cbsnews.com/htdocs/CBSNews_polls/schiavo.pdf.

CNN/USA Today/Gallup Poll. (2005, March 22). Retrieved March 10, 2007, from http://www.pollingreport.com/news.htm#Schiavo

Colby, W. H. (2002). *The long goodbye: The deaths of Nancy Cruzan.* Carlsbad, CA: Hay House.

Colby, W. H. (2006). *Unplugged: Reclaiming our right to die in America.* New York: AMACOM Books.

Eisenberg, J. (2005). *Using Terri.* San Francisco: Harper.

Gonzales v. Oregon, 546 U.S. 243 (2006).

Herskovits, B. (2005, March 31). Schiavo PR battle persisted until final hours. *PR Week.* Retrieved March 10, 2007, from http://www.prweek.com/us/search/article/236893//

Miner, B. (2003, November 23). Randall Terry resurfaces: Christian right jumps into Terri Schiavo fray. *In These Times.* Retrieved March 10, 2007, from http://www.inthesetimes.com/article/369/

Moyers, B. (2000). *On our own terms.* New York: PBS.

Pavlides, M. (2007). Whose choice is it anyway? Disability and suicide in five contemporary films. In T. H. Lillie & J. L. Werth, Jr. (Eds.), *End-of-life issues and persons with disabilities* (pp. 62–72). Austin, TX: PRO-ED.

Pew Research Center for the People and the Press. (2006, January 5). *Strong public support for right to die.* Retrieved March 10, 2007, from http://people-press.org/reports/display.php3?ReportID=266

Quindlen, A. (1994). *One true thing.* New York: Random House.

Shakir, F., Pitney, N., Terkel, A., Khanna, S., & Corley, M. (2007, June 21). Conservatives dominate the airwaves. *The Progress Report.* Retrieved July 17, 2007, from http://www.americanprogressaction.org/progressreport/2007/06/conservatives_dominate.html

Webb, M. (1997). *The good death: The new American search to reshape the end of life.* New York: Bantam.

CHAPTER 8

Three Female Faces

The Law of End-of-Life Decision Making in America

Kathy L. Cerminara

Introduction

In the mid-1970s, the father of Karen Ann Quinlan, a young woman who lay in a persistent vegetative state (PVS), wished to authorize disconnection of his daughter's ventilator. He had to go to court because various physicians, the hospital in which his daughter was a patient, the state attorney general, and the county prosecutor, among others, objected to the withdrawal of ventilator support. The New Jersey Supreme Court's seminal ruling in 1976, authorizing the ventilator's disconnection, transformed Ms. Quinlan into the first of three famous female figures in the law of end-of-life decision making. The most commonly recognized public images of end-of-life litigation in America since then have been those of young women lying in bed as loving family members clustered around them (Miles, 1990). *Quinlan* and cases involving young women in Missouri and Florida have captured the public attention and provided three female faces to associate with end-of-life medical decision making.

This chapter explores the law of end-of-life decision making through the lenses provided by those cases. It discusses the theoretical bases for and the judicial and legislative development of this area of the law in America. It also uses those cases and the lessons learned from them to demonstrate the limits of the law and the issues that bear watching as courts, legislatures, physicians, other healthcare providers, and patients' family members and friends continually seek to improve end-of-life care through recognition of the right to refuse life-sustaining treatment.

□ The Beginning: *Quinlan*

In *Quinlan,* the New Jersey Supreme Court authorized withdrawal of ventilator support in the first reported case regarding end-of-life medical decision making. In doing so, the court affirmed and memorialized in the law practices that had developed in clinical care of dying patients as a consequence of the technological changes affording the ability to prolong life more than ever before. Its decision marked the beginning of a process of judicial and legislative development that might be likened to a pendulum swinging.

The analogy seems apt because lawyers, like historians and political scientists, to name a few, may point to pendulum swings of thought and attitudes in their respective fields. In history, one may trace rises and falls of great civilizations and magnificent empires. As a matter of political science, within any single country one may identify periods of time during which schools of thought as diverse as feudalism, capitalism, and socialism ebb and flow, interchangeably reigning supreme. In the law of end-of-life decision making, one similarly may discern a pendulum swing between the 1970s, when *Quinlan* was decided, and the beginning of the 21st century, when the Theresa Schiavo case was unfolding.

As the court deciding the *Quinlan* case noted, technology was the impetus for the beginning of this pendulum swing. In the latter half of the 20th century, technology opened new doors for medical treatment. The technological imperative encouraged extensive use of advanced machinery and chemical agents to prolong life much longer than previously had been possible (Rothman, 1997). As physicians and families attempted to deal with the effects of such technological advances, "humane decisions against resuscitative or maintenance therapy [were] frequently a recognized *de facto* response in the medical world to the irreversible, terminal pain-ridden patient, especially with familial consent" (*In re Quinlan*, 1976, p. 667). Explicit legal recognition of the validity of such decisions to discontinue or never to begin such therapy began to emerge in the mid-1970s, bolstered by the *Quinlan* decision itself.

Theoretical Basis

The *Quinlan* court considered the case as involving a constitutional right of privacy of "personal decision" under both the U.S. and the New Jersey constitutions (*Quinlan*, 1976, p. 663). In reality, both constitutional and common-law bases for the right to refuse life-sustaining treatment exist. The latter basis arises from a respect for the inviolability of a person's control over his or her own body as expressed through the law of informed consent, a subset of tort law that dates back to the early 20th century. Tort law seeks, among other goals, to compensate persons for injuries that stem from civil wrongs other than breach of contract (White, 1985, p. xv). This foundational basis thus has developed as a result of case-by-case decisions about whether individuals have wronged each other in their interactions. The other basis, the constitutional one, is a more abstract and broad respect for the ability of, or the liberty of, each person to make his or her own decisions about private matters. The U.S. Supreme Court, discussing such a liberty interest as applied to decisions whether to undertake the medical procedure of abortion, has noted:

> These matters, involving the most intimate and personal choices a person may make in a lifetime, choices central to personal dignity and autonomy, are central to the liberty protected by the Fourteenth Amendment [of the U.S. Constitution]. At the heart of liberty is the right to define one's own concept of existence, of meaning, of the universe, and of the mystery of human life. (*Planned Parenthood of Southeastern Pennsylvania v. Casey*, 1992, p. 851)

The tort law just described recognizes these core values, but the constitutional protections accorded privacy and liberty at both the state and federal levels secure them more broadly and strongly.

Although the *Quinlan* court recognized a constitutional right in both the Fourteenth Amendment to the U.S. Constitution and the New Jersey state constitution, the U.S. Supreme Court over the last several decades has chosen to focus on the law of end-of-life medical decision making as rooted in the first theoretical basis identified here (i.e., the tort law of informed consent; *Vacco v. Quill*, 1997, p. 807). Tort law has developed as follows: For a physician or other medical caregiver to touch another (to infringe on a patient's ability to remain untouched and undisturbed), that physician or caregiver must obtain consent from the patient. To fail to obtain consent is to engage in the tort of battery. This is because "[e]very human being of adult years and sound mind has a right to determine what shall be done with his own body" (*Schloendorff v. Society of New York Hospital*, 1914, p. 93). Each patient can control what happens to his or her own body by consenting or not—a task that has become more complex as medical treatment has evolved technologically. It has become clear that for a patient to truly be consenting to the touching (more broadly understood as consenting to interference with his or her bodily integrity), the patient had to receive and appreciate information about the medical condition, the treatment, and the treatment's risks and benefits. The law of informed consent, which elaborates on the rights and liabilities of parties involved in that process, evolved to say generally that, for consent to be valid, a patient who is capable of making medical decisions must be provided with sufficient information to make a knowledgeable decision and must be acting voluntarily when consenting.

Although statutes play some role in this area of the law, that role is limited. Courts, rather than legislatures, have always been and continue to be the governmental bodies in charge of developing the law in this area. Tort law generally is judge-made law, developed slowly and incrementally by the judiciary through successive decisions on individual cases. Thus, it differs vastly from areas of the law such as securities regulation and bankruptcy, to name a few, which are based entirely on statutory language passed by legislatures. It is this judge-made aspect of tort law that permits it to grow and change over the years in response to individual situations in an effort to serve underlying goals.

Goals of the Law and State Interests

In addition to the theoretical bases of the law of end-of-life decision making, there are a number of important state interests influencing law making in this area. State actors such as attorneys general, courts, legislatures, and executive branch officials commonly assert one or a combination of four traditionally identified state interests in arguing against a decision to refuse life-sustaining treatment: preservation of life, prevention of suicide, protection of third parties, and maintenance of the ethics of the medical profession (*Superintendent, Belchertown State School v. Saikewicz*, 1977). The litany of these state interests is so common that those working regularly in this area of the law can recite them without a second thought.

Although mindful of these interests (especially the strongest, the interest all of society has in preserving life), the law of end-of-life decision making arose out of a historical basis of *too much* medical care being provided. The impetus for the law's development lay in attempts to preserve life that the person in question (the person whose life it was) did not want to have preserved. When applying the law to such instances of overtreatment, courts recognized that a right to consent would indeed be a shallow and almost worthless right if there were no ability on the part of the patient to refuse consent (Meisel & Cerminara, 2004, § 2.06[A], pp. 2–23). Such recognition acknowledged that the state interest in preserving life is indeed limited by the patient's condition and desires.

Moreover, that recognition evidenced a respect for the broader theoretical basis of the right to refuse medical treatment. To say that everyone "has a right to determine what shall be done with his own body"

(*Schloendorff*, 1914, p. 93) is to recognize first that every person has the right to direct whether his or her body will or will not be touched. More deeply, however, it also is to recognize that even matters not involving touching, the very decisions about when to cease efforts to continue to live, are personal. Thus, in the United States, it is believed that the individual who will have to deal most personally with the consequences of the decision (the person who will live or die as a result of it) is the one who should make it (although a more interdependent or collectivistic perspective is considered appropriate in some subcultures within this country and in many other countries; see Hayslip, Hansson, Starkweather, & Dolan, chapter 17, this volume).

It is significant that the *Quinlan* court and other courts have recognized that this right ultimately is rooted in state and federal constitutions. Whereas tort law, generally speaking, is aimed at resolution of disputes among private parties, with compensation a major goal, the focus of the law changes when a constitutional right is at stake. Constitutional rights generally protect citizens against action by the state, not against actions by private parties. Thus, a legislature that does not agree with the way a court has decided some tort-law-based informed consent issue may, simply because it disagrees with that court decision, pass a law to ensure that future courts addressing similar informed consent issues will decide such issues differently. A legislature may not, however, restrict a citizen's constitutional rights except in a constitutionally appropriate manner, in furtherance of one or more state interests justifying such an action. Constitutional rights supersede all other sorts of law, such that no governmental actor can contravene these liberties (Baron, 2004).

Not Just a Right for the Competent Patient

The law initially began to recognize these principles in cases involving patients who had decision-making capacity, but the question arose almost immediately about whether a patient who had become unable to make healthcare decisions contemporaneously had to remain on life-sustaining treatment indefinitely once losing decision-making capacity. The answer, overwhelmingly, has been that surrogate decision makers are able to refuse such treatment on behalf of patients who have become incompetent, as illustrated by the *Quinlan* case.

The *Quinlan* court determined that the state's interests in preventing exercise of the right to refuse treatment were weak in light of Ms. Quinlan's condition and the unlikelihood of recovery in the form of a return to a cognitive, sapient state. Although recognizing that the state had interests in preserving life and upholding the professional medical judgment of the physicians who had refused to remove the ventilator, the court said:

> We think that the State's interest contra weakens and the individual's right to privacy grows as the degree of bodily invasion increases and the prognosis dims. Ultimately there comes a point at which the individual's rights overcome the State interest. It is for that reason that we believe Karen's choice, if she were competent to make it, would be vindicated by the law. (*Quinlan*, 1976, p. 664)

The court went on to rule that Ms. Quinlan's father, acting as her guardian, could assert what her father believed her choice would have been under the circumstances. State interests did not justify preventing the exercise of that choice, even though, due to Ms. Quinlan's condition, she could not exercise that choice herself.

☐ The United States Supreme Court Speaks: *Cruzan*

In the years after *Quinlan*, state courts increasingly considered end-of-life medical decision-making cases. By 1990, the U.S. Supreme Court was considering its only case thus far directly involving the asserted right to have medical treatment withheld or withdrawn. That case involved another young woman in a PVS. In *Cruzan v. Director, Missouri Department of Health* (1990), the parents of such a young woman petitioned the Missouri courts for permission to authorize withdrawal of their daughter's percutaneous endoscopic gastrostomy (PEG) tube, which was providing her with artificial nutrition and hydration after an automobile accident. The Missouri state court applied a clear and convincing evidentiary standard when deciding whether to authorize the withdrawal. In doing so, rather than looking for clear and convincing evidence of the values and prior statements of Nancy Beth Cruzan (the young female patient) to determine whether she would have wanted treatment in her condition, the state court looked for proof that Ms. Cruzan earlier had specified that she wanted artificial nutrition and hydration withdrawn if she ever entered a PVS. Thus, to support withdrawal of treatment, the Missouri state court not only required clear and convincing evidence but also required that the evidence demonstrate Ms. Cruzan's prior, actual, expressed wishes. The argument before the U.S. Supreme Court focused on whether the Missouri state court's application of such a demanding standard of proof violated Ms. Cruzan's liberty interest in refusing treatment under the U.S. Constitution.

The U.S. Supreme Court ruled that the Missouri state court's imposition of such a high procedural, evidentiary barrier in *Cruzan* did not violate the U.S. Constitution. After examining the common-law roots of the right to refuse treatment and a series of state court decisions concerning the asserted right, the Court ruled that "the principle that a competent person has a constitutionally protected liberty interest in refusing unwanted medical treatment may be inferred from our prior decisions" (*Cruzan*, 1990, p. 278). It thus assumed "that the United States Constitution would grant a competent person a constitutionally protected right to refuse lifesaving hydration and nutrition" (*Cruzan*, p. 279).

The Court ruled, however, that the Missouri state court's imposition of a stringent evidentiary burden was constitutionally permissible in an end-of-life decision-making case like *Cruzan*, involving an incompetent patient who had not designated anyone to speak for her on her incompetence. The Court decided only that Missouri could do what it had done in that case, which was to judicially impose a high evidentiary hurdle in the case of an incapacitated patient who had not previously designated a proxy decision maker when that patient's legal guardians wished to authorize withdrawal of medically supplied artificial nutrition and hydration. The Court did not determine that state courts should or must require such a level of proof, and in fact, most states do not do so, either legislatively or judicially.

The Limits of Cruzan

In the years immediately following *Cruzan*, scholars and end-of-life decision-making advocates argued that the *Cruzan* court's assumption of the existence of a constitutional right to refuse life-sustaining treatment, in the context of the Court's other Fourteenth Amendment liberty interest cases, meant that persons with terminal illnesses could exercise some control over the timing of their own deaths even if they were not dependent on life-prolonging technological measures. In 1997, however, the U.S. Supreme Court signaled that the constitutional right at the root of the law of end-of-life medical decision making does not encompass a right to make as many medical decisions as certain advocates had believed. In so signaling, the Supreme Court made clear that its decision in *Cruzan* had marked, in essence, the beginning of a swing back from broad recognition of a federal constitutional right to a narrower interpretation.

The Supreme Court thus settled, for the time being at least, the question of the constitutionality of state laws prohibiting assisted suicide. In part because of the previously mentioned state interest in the prevention of suicide, virtually every court that has decided an end-of-life decision-making case has distinguished the activity of withholding or withdrawing life-sustaining medical treatment from suicide or suicide assistance. Courts so distinguishing generally hold that withholding or withdrawing life-sustaining medical treatment differs from assisting a suicide because withholding or withdrawing merely allows a disease or terminal condition to take its natural course toward death rather than artificially preventing that disease or condition from reaching its natural conclusion. As a natural outgrowth of the patient's right to prevent others from engaging in unauthorized touching, poking, and prodding, the authorization of withholding or withdrawal of treatment represents an exercise of the right to refuse to consent to an invasion of the patient's bodily integrity. Assisted suicide, by contrast, occurs when a person other than the patient provides some sort of assistance to a patient who then uses the opportunity or the materials provided by the other person to end his or her own life.

The U.S. Supreme Court announced a constitutional distinction between withholding or withdrawal of treatment and assisted suicide in *Washington v. Glucksberg* (1997) and *Vacco v. Quill* (1997). In this pair of cases, the Court was called on to decide a constitutional challenge to state statutes criminalizing suicide assistance. Terminally ill patients and their physicians had sought the ability to end the patients' inevitable dying processes without waiting for nature to take its course. Specifically, they wanted assurance that physicians could not be prosecuted for assisting suicides if they were to write prescriptions of lethal doses of medication for terminally ill patients to take when they decided to hasten their dying process. Had the federal constitutional right the Court identified in *Cruzan* been a broad right to make decisions about personal and private matters or had the Court chosen in *Glucksberg* and *Quill* to interpret its precedent as leading to recognition of such a broad right, then the right indeed could have encompassed "a due process liberty interest in controlling the time and manner of one's death" (*Compassion in Dying v. Washington,* 1996, p. 720). Instead, however, the Court ruled:

> The right assumed in *Cruzan* ... was not simply deduced from abstract concepts of personal autonomy. Given the common-law rule that forced medication was a battery, and the long legal tradition protecting the decision to refuse unwanted medical treatment, our assumption [of the existence of a constitutional right] was entirely consistent with this Nation's history and constitutional traditions. The decision to commit suicide with the assistance of another may be just as personal and profound as the decision to refuse unwanted medical treatment, but it has never enjoyed similar legal protection. Indeed, the two acts are widely and reasonably regarded as quite distinct. ... In *Cruzan* itself, we recognized that most States outlawed assisted suicide—and even more do today—and we certainly gave no intimation that the right to refuse unwanted medical treatment could be somehow transmuted into a right to assistance in committing suicide. (*Glucksberg*, 1997, pp. 725–726)

Clearly, then, at least as far as federal constitutional matters go, the pendulum had swung, in *Cruzan*, as far as it would go toward a broad definition of an individual's constitutional right to engage in end-of-life medical decision making. Because assisted suicide does not represent an exercise of the essential ability to tell others to stop injecting substances into a patient's body or maintaining a patient through the use of equipment, the federal constitution, as interpreted in *Glucksberg*, does not protect a terminally ill patient's choice to receive assistance in ending the dying process. Assisted suicide would implicate a terminally ill patient's choice of the timing of death when the dying process already effectively had begun, but the federal constitutional right thus far recognized by the U.S. Supreme Court does not extend that far. Although states may pass laws permitting the practice, as the state of Oregon did in a statute called the Death With Dignity Act, the pendulum of judicial decision making had swung away from any possibility of recognition of a federal constitutional right to do so (*Glucksberg*, 1997).

That swing also eliminated any argument that euthanasia could be encompassed within a patient's constitutional rights. Euthanasia occurs when another person, whether a caregiver, a friend, or an acquaintance, ends a patient's life by introducing a death-producing agent, for example, by a lethal injection or by smothering the patient with a pillow. In one of the more famous euthanasia cases, a long-time advocate for physician assistance in terminally ill patients' suicides actually went one step further than assisting in suicides. Dr. Jack Kevorkian videotaped himself administering a lethal injection to Thomas Youk, who had been diagnosed as having amyotrophic lateral sclerosis (Werth, 2001). The state of Michigan, in which the activity took place, had attempted to prosecute Dr. Kevorkian several times in the past for assisting patients in ending their own lives, but such prosecutions had always failed due either to jury acquittals or to lack of sound legal basis in Michigan law. After Dr. Kevorkian administered the lethal injection to Mr. Youk, however, a jury convicted him of second-degree murder. An actor's belief that ending a patient's life serves that patient's best interests does not justify actually ending that life under the law. This applies even when videotaped evidence proves that the actor committed the act with the patient's consent, and indeed at his request, as it did of Dr. Kevorkian's actions with respect to Mr. Youk.

Raye (chapter 5, this volume) described the story of the decision-making processes surrounding an act of assisting her father in ending his life. From the discussion here, it is clear that current law would consider her actions and those of her family as illegal, not protected under current interpretations of the U.S. Constitution. If the medications had not worked, so that she or her family would have had to smother her father, it is possible that she and her family would, like Dr. Kevorkian, have been prosecuted for a crime (in his case, second-degree murder; in their cases, whatever the applicable state law would proscribe).

□ The Third Female Face: *Schiavo*

One more young female face symbolizes the difficulty that many, including family members and the medical profession, have with end-of-life medical decision making. In 1990, the same year that the U.S. Supreme Court decided *Cruzan*, a young woman in Florida, Theresa Marie Schiavo, suffered a cardiac arrest and entered a PVS. Her family initially was united in ensuring that she received the most aggressive care possible, even flying her across the country for implantation of an experimental thalamic stimulator (Cerminara & Goodman, n.d., November 1990 entry). Despite all efforts, Ms. Schiavo remained in a PVS, receiving artificial nutrition and hydration through a PEG tube just as Ms. Cruzan had, and by 1998, her family had divided on the issue of whether she would have wanted further medical treatment under the circumstances. Her husband sought a judicial determination of whether Ms. Schiavo would have wanted to continue on artificial nutrition and hydration through the PEG tube; he believed that she would have wished to stop, while her parents believed that she would have wished to continue.

Over the next 5 years, several Florida courts affirmed a trial court's ruling that Ms. Schiavo would have wished to discontinue receipt of artificial nutrition and hydration in her current condition. Then, however, the legislative and executive branches of both the state of Florida and the United States intervened, effectively extending the process for two additional years. In the spring of 2005, slightly more than 15 years after she entered a PVS and nearly 30 years after the New Jersey Supreme Court decided *Quinlan*, physicians finally removed Ms. Schiavo's PEG tube and watched her pass away.

The personal story of Josh (Crow, chapter 4, this volume) illustrates the removal of artificial nutrition and hydration on his admittance into hospice. Josh's family did not express tension and divided opinions about the course of his care, but, especially in the absence of an advance directive (similar to Ms. Schiavo), family discord could have been a distinct possibility. If Josh's mother had contested the decision made by Crow and her father, legal interjection likely would have been necessary to resolve the dispute.

The Judiciary Versus the Elected Branches of Government

Schiavo came to symbolize a number of remarkable conflicts. One of the most striking emerged between the judicial branch of government on one side and the legislative and executive branches on the other. Nearly prompting a constitutional crisis, the Florida Legislature, Florida's governor Jeb Bush, the U.S. Congress, and U.S. President George W. Bush attempted repeatedly to intervene in and reverse the results of judicial decision making (*Bush v. Schiavo*, 2005; *Schiavo ex rel. Schindler v. Schiavo*, 2005a, 2005b). It is well established in the law that neither the legislative nor the executive branches of government may retroactively change the result of a judicial decision in a particular case (*Bush v. Schiavo*, 2005). To permit otherwise would be to eliminate a major "check" the judiciary places on the legislative and executive branches in the U.S. system of constitutional government.

To appreciate this point, one must recognize the vast difference between the roles of the three branches of government. Both as a matter of federal governmental structure and as a matter of the way that most, if not all, states have chosen to organize themselves, the legislative, judicial, and executive branches have separate and distinct roles to play in the legal system. Although courts often have stated that they wish not to interfere with the private, personal area of end-of-life medical decision making unless required to do so (Meisel & Cerminara, 2004, §§ 3.19, 3.20), sometimes patients, family members, or healthcare providers find it necessary to seek judicial resolution of end-of-life disputes. When a court resolves such a case, some citizens may wish, as several did in *Schiavo*, to petition the executive and legislative branches to reverse the effect of decisions made by the judicial branch. Acquiescing to such requests is unwise and inadvisable, however, because the roles of elected officials controlling the legislative and executive branches differ from the roles of officials who are either wholly or partially insulated from election forces, such as those in the judicial branch in many jurisdictions. There are certain end-of-life medical decision-making issues that can and should be determined on the elected official playing field and others that belong in judicial hands.

Trial and appellate court judges each have unique roles, but their roles also contrast sharply with the role of legislatures in the American system of government. Trial court judges are responsible for supervising the parties' introduction of evidence into a record and for rendering the initial decision in a case, sometimes with the assistance of a jury and sometimes without it. Appellate court judges are responsible for reviewing decisions rendered by trial judges for legal issues only, not for redeciding facts. Judges at all levels are responsible only for deciding the precise cases before them. Legislatures, by contrast, are responsible for setting forth general rules to guide future conduct of citizens and institutions. They think broadly and enact rules to govern the entire citizenry from the effective date of their acts onward.

In other words, unlike legislators, judicial bodies look at a given factual situation and determine how the law applies to that precise situation. When another, slightly different, factual situation arises after one court has determined a case, the next court is responsible for determining whether the decision of the previous court should guide the decision in the case before it, and so on. The law develops in this manner slowly, over time, as it has developed since the days of medieval England, when such common-law courts first began to operate (Baron, 2004).

Thus, the outcome of an individual court case is both more and less instructive than a legislature's passage of a statute to govern future conduct. It is more instructive because the court examines the exact facts before it closely. Short of reversal by a higher court, its ruling absolutely governs those facts it has examined with such care. Attorneys and those within the jurisdiction of that court know that the court's decision also will govern a future factual situation if that situation is identical to or closely resembles the original one. The court's ruling is less instructive than a legislature's actions with respect to future matters, however, because, technically, no case binds any subsequent factual situation other than one presenting with the exact same constellation of facts (Meisel, 2005). Thus, when another case arises, the parties involved in this case, their attorneys, and the court will be attempting to determine whether the case involves any facts that are so significantly different from the previous case's facts that the latter case should be decided differently. Chief considerations in making this determination are what the reasons, or the policies, are behind the law and whether any factual differences are important for purposes of furthering those policies.

Courts exist precisely to provide checks on the legislative and executive branches because the majority view is not always the legally correct one. The most effective check against decisions made at the behest of a populace motivated by emotion or prejudice rather than reason is a judiciary that can look at what has been done against an external yardstick, such as the Constitution. The majority of the public likely do not know the actual facts of any judicial case. "Outsiders" to any litigation, including the public, legislators, and members of the executive branch of government, almost certainly were not in the courtroom and thus could not observe witnesses' actions, expressions, or mannerisms. They also probably have not examined the exhibits offered into evidence. Yet, those details determine credibility or lack thereof. Such outsiders thus are not qualified to interfere with a trial court judge's or a jury's interpretation of facts presented at trial. The fact finder is the only one who can say whether certain evidence can be believed and what was proved at trial.

Schiavo presented an instance in which many citizens, legislators, and executive branch officials seemed to forget these basic civics lessons. Legislators passed, and Florida's Governor Jeb Bush and U.S. President George Bush signed, legislation that could have had the effect of overturning the courts' multiple determinations that Ms. Schiavo was in a PVS and that her medically supplied nutrition and hydration should be withdrawn because that was what she would have wished to have done. Constitutional balance prevailed, however, and the Florida courts' rulings stood.

Medically Supplied Nutrition and Hydration

Schiavo also illustrated conflicts more specific to the law of end-of-life decision making. For example, once disagreement erupted between Ms. Schiavo's husband and parents, conflict surfaced regarding what sort of authority should be accorded a surrogate decision maker. Chief among the issues were concerns about whether anyone should be able to refuse or to authorize withdrawal of medically supplied nutrition and hydration on behalf of an incompetent patient who had not specifically stated a desire to refuse such treatment. Although such issues legally had been settled since the late 1980s, and certainly since 1990, when the Supreme Court decided *Cruzan*, disability rights groups joined with pro-life forces in *Schiavo* to open the issues for examination once again, thus "unsettling the settled" in this area of law (Shepherd, 2006).

Although not explicitly stated in the U.S. Supreme Court's majority opinion, a majority of the justices in *Cruzan* concluded that medically supplied artificial nutrition and hydration constitutes medical treatment that can be refused the same as any other treatment. The majority implied as much, and even named "lifesaving nutrition and hydration" as the type of treatment it had in mind when assuming the constitutionally protected right to refuse (*Cruzan*, 1990, p. 279). Justice O'Connor, writing in concurrence, made a point of stating, "Artificial feeding cannot readily be distinguished from other forms of medical treatment" (*Cruzan*, p. 288). Like other forms of medical treatment, artificial feeding involves intrusion and restraint, neither of which medical professionals can initiate without informed consent. Thus, Justice O'Connor concluded, "Accordingly, the liberty guaranteed by the Due Process Clause [of the Fourteenth Amendment of the U.S. Constitution] must protect, if it protects anything, an individual's deeply personal decision to reject medical treatment, including the artificial delivery of food and water" (*Cruzan*, p. 289).

The four dissenting justices in *Cruzan* (Brennan, Marshall, Blackmun, and Stevens) agreed. Justice Brennan, writing for himself and Justices Marshall and Blackmun, said bluntly that "[n]o material distinction can be drawn between ... artificial nutrition and hydration ... and any other medical treatment" (*Cruzan*, 1990, p. 307). Justice Stevens's agreement, expressed in his separate dissent, is not as easily realized. He did not expressly discuss whether artificial nutrition and hydration constituted medical treatment. He did, however, refer several times to Ms. Cruzan's condition and her "medical treatment," while displaying a familiarity with the record, implying that he could not have overlooked the fact that her "medical treatment" was artificial nutrition and hydration. When criticizing the majority's listing of precedential cases, for example, Justice Stevens noted that "none of the decisions surveyed by the Court interposed an absolute bar to the termination of treatment for patient in a persistent vegetative state" (*Cruzan*, p. 347). Clearly, in his view, the result of the case before him was an absolute bar to termination of something constituting "treatment."

Yet, many of the debates about withdrawal of treatment in *Schiavo*, nearly 15 years after *Cruzan*, reflected great concern about withdrawal of medically supplied nutrition and hydration. Religious figures retreated from previously clear principles indicating that medically supplied nutrition and hydration should be treated as any other treatment, as they urged that medically supplied nutrition and hydration constituted everyday care that could not be refused (Cerminara, 2005). Disability rights groups paired with vitalist activists in using vivid imagery, including protesters dressed as spoons, to emphasize their determination that no one should be able to authorize withdrawal of medically supplied nutrition and hydration on another person's behalf (Cerminara, 2006). Rather than focusing on the highly technological, invasive nature of the medical procedures involved in maintaining a patient on a PEG tube, the persons protesting against its withdrawal relied on images of starvation and dehydration, even though research indicates that dying due to lack of medically supplied nutrition and hydration does not result in pain (Bernat, Gert, & Mogielnicki, 1993).

□ The Issues the Next Young Woman's Case May Present

Presuming that the pattern of high-profile cases involving young women in PVS continues, it may be possible to predict which major future issues will face the family and friends of that next young woman. *Cruzan* itself left open a number of issues that have not yet been resolved on the U.S. Supreme Court level. State legislatures may act to attempt to resolve some of the conflicts raised by *Schiavo* and may be asked to revise their state laws regarding assisted suicide. State courts may see issues of state constitutional law arise more frequently. Finally, if the tenor of previous court decisions is any indication, every attempt should be made to ensure that end-of-life decision making is returned, in the main, to the private realm of patient, physician, and family. In that vein, efforts to incorporate more structured forms of alternative dispute resolution into the medical decision-making process may increase, as may efforts to ensure dissemination of knowledge about advance directives and to improve various end-of-life care options.

Issues Left Open After Cruzan

The *Cruzan* Court did not decide as many issues as people assume it did. Any of the open issues could develop into disputes that might reach a court, if not the U.S. Supreme Court itself. First, as noted, the Court in *Cruzan* did not even decide that competent patients have a federal constitutional right to refuse medical treatment. Instead, it simply assumed the existence of that right so that further analysis could take place. Second, the Court expressly stated that the question of whether an *incompetent* person had such a right was not really before it because "[s]uch a 'right' must be exercised for [the patient], if at all, by some sort of surrogate," so that the real question before it was whether Missouri's procedural safeguards, intended to ensure that the surrogate was acting in accordance with the patient's wishes, were too stringent (*Cruzan*, 1990, p. 280). Thus, even if a competent person does have the right identified by the *Cruzan* court, it is unclear whether the Supreme Court would hold as the *Quinlan* court held—that a person has a constitutional right to have the right to refuse treatment after he or she has become incompetent.

Third, though judicial head counting results in a conclusion that medically supplied artificial nutrition and hydration constitutes medical treatment that can be refused or ordered withdrawn, the majority of justices in *Cruzan* did not say this. Justices O'Connor, Brennan, Marshall, and Blackmun clearly said this, and Justice Stevens obviously meant this, so five members of the Court did, effectively, rule this way. In the absence of an affirmative statement to this effect, however, an advocate for the opposing position may attempt to explain why these five votes should not be considered a majority ruling on the issue.

Fourth, the *Cruzan* Court itself identified as unresolved the issue of "whether a State might be required to defer to the decision of a surrogate if competent and probative evidence established that the patient herself had expressed a desire that the decision to terminate life-sustaining treatment be made for her by that individual" (*Cruzan*, 1990, p. 287, n. 12). Justice O'Connor emphasized in her concurrence that the Court had not decided this issue, noting that "the patient's appointment of a proxy to make health care decisions on [his or] her behalf" would be "an equally probative source of evidence" of the patient's instructions (*Cruzan*, p. 290). She argued that following an appointed proxy's decisions "may well be constitutionally required to protect the patient's liberty interest in refusing medical treatment" (*Cruzan*, p. 289). This issue—the appointment of a person as a patient's proxy decision maker, especially if the patient provided no further instructions—is one that surely will arise more frequently as state legislation develops further.

State Legislative Attempts to Resolve Concerns Raised in *Schiavo*

One way in which a patient might provide further instructions to an appointed proxy decision maker is to detail those instructions in an advance directive. Advance directives are written or oral statements of a patient's wishes regarding future medical care, issued when the patient has decision-making capacity in anticipation of the time that he or she will become incapable of making medical decisions. One purpose of an advance directive is to designate a proxy to make future decisions. Another, however, is to specify the type of care the patient wishes to receive or refuse in the future under certain circumstances. If a patient does not appoint a proxy decision maker, the patient still may issue the latter sort of advance directive, which is sometimes termed an *instruction directive*. In that instance, state statutes generally will list, in order of priority, the persons, called *surrogate decision makers*, who are to carry out the patient's wishes. Most states have enacted statutes explaining what sort of condition a patient must be in for an advance directive to become effective, but once that advance directive becomes effective, a patient's proxy or surrogate decision maker generally must follow the patient's wishes to the extent they are known.

In the aftermath of *Schiavo*, at least two major concerns arose regarding this usual scenario of decision making near the end of life. First, concern arose about the identity of persons who might be appointed by operation of law to be patients' surrogate decision makers once patients had become incompetent to make their own healthcare decisions. Second, concerns arose about the level of information a proxy or surrogate decision maker had to have to support a determination that a patient would have refused medically supplied nutrition and hydration.

The first concern, about the identity of surrogate decision makers, arose out of debates over whether Ms. Schiavo's husband or her parents were the most appropriate decision makers in her case. Ms. Schiavo had not appointed a proxy decision maker herself in advance, so it was necessary to consult and to follow the list provided in Florida's statutes identifying, in order of priority, the persons who should serve as her surrogate decision maker. Her husband was first on the list, as her appointed legal guardian, and also was second on the list, as her spouse. Yet, her parents claimed that Michael Schiavo should not be able to serve as his wife's surrogate decision maker, at least in part because he had begun cohabiting with another woman during the years after Ms. Schiavo entered a PVS.

In the immediate aftermath of *Schiavo*, at least one state passed legislation intended to alleviate concerns of this sort. In Louisiana, beginning shortly after Ms. Schiavo died, a spouse, even though legally married to the patient, may not serve as a patient's surrogate decision maker if he or she has "cohabited with another person in the manner of married persons" (Louisiana Rev. Stat. Ann. § 40:1299.58.2(14)). It may be that other state legislatures will choose to revise their definitions of *spouse* or to revise their surrogate decision-maker lists in some way to address similar concerns as the law develops further in light of *Schiavo*.

Similarly, the law may develop further to address concerns about the emotional significance of medically supplied nutrition and hydration that arose first in *Cruzan* and then later in *Schiavo*. It is unlikely that the law will retreat from the *Cruzan* court's ruling that medically supplied nutrition and hydration is a medical treatment, but some scholars, politicians, and advocates may succeed in arguing that specific direction from the patient must be available for surrogate or proxy decision makers to refuse it. The National Right to Life Committee (NRLC), for example, promulgated model legislation, proposed in many state legislatures during and immediately after *Schiavo*, to this effect (Cerminara, 2006).

The NRLC's (n.d.) model legislation presumes that all persons desire administration of medically supplied nutrition and hydration, despite their condition, unless one of three exceptions applies:

- When, in reasonable medical judgment, it is not medically appropriate, as detailed in the statute, to administer the medically supplied nutrition and hydration.
- When the patient had executed "a written advance directive or proxy designation specifically authorizing the withholding or withdrawal of nutrition or hydration in the applicable circumstances" (NRLC, § 4(B)).
- When "there is clear and convincing evidence that the incompetent person, when competent, gave express and informed consent to withdrawing or withholding nutrition or hydration in the applicable circumstances" (NRLC, § 4(C)), when "express and informed consent" means "consent voluntarily given with sufficient knowledge of the subject matter involved" (NRLC, § 2(C)). Such a definition requires that a patient has to have known and considered, at the time of any prior statements regarding refusal of treatment, information such as the identity of the treatment or procedure eventually required, the condition for which the treatment or procedure would be required, and alternatives available and risks present at the time the treatment or procedure is required.

To know all that in advance is impossible, but *Schiavo* spawned many efforts to pass such state laws. One reason it did so was the emotional symbolism of medically supplied nutrition and hydration. A second was the unfortunate and inaccurate perception that withholding or withdrawal of medically supplied nutrition and hydration differs significantly from withholding or withdrawal of other treatments. Because of the emotion involved and the prevalence of such misconceptions, however, such efforts to change the law may continue.

State Laws Authorizing Physician-Assisted Suicide

On the other side of the coin, persons who would rather see terminally ill patients meeting their inevitable deaths without the hoopla that attends a major case such as a *Quinlan*, *Cruzan*, or *Schiavo* can be expected to continue to argue for the passage of more state laws permitting physicians to assist such patients in ending their own lives. Oregon's passage of such a law in the 1990s has met with resistance from the federal government, but advocacy groups continue to attempt to achieve passage of similar legislation in other states (Sneyd, 2007; Vogel, 2007). They use stories such as *A Hastened Death* (Raye, chapter 5, this volume) to illustrate the case for passage of such laws.

Oregon's Death With Dignity Act (1995) permits competent, terminally ill persons who are residents of that state to receive prescriptions from their physicians that can be used to end their lives. Each patient must make multiple requests for the prescription, both orally and in writing, and procedures have been established both to ensure referral to counseling when it might be needed and to ensure adequate record keeping of both requests and prescription usage. The Oregon statutory scheme also requires annual reporting on the operation of the act by the state's Department of Human Services. Each year, the reports have revealed that many more persons request prescriptions than actually use them and indicate that the primary reasons for requesting such prescriptions include concerns about a loss of autonomy and about becoming unable to engage in activities that make life enjoyable (Oregon Department of Human Services, 2007).

Because the Oregon Death With Dignity Act is state legislation, the federal government has no power directly to say that it should be repealed; that power belongs to the citizens of Oregon alone. Federal legislators and members of the federal executive branch have, however, attempted in a variety of ways to reduce the effectiveness of Oregon's law permitting physician-assisted suicide. Federal legislators have unsuccessfully attempted to pass statutes that would prohibit the use of federal controlled substances as the prescription medications that Oregonians use to achieve death under the terms of the act. In addition, although the U.S. Supreme Court has ruled that it cannot do so, the federal Department of Justice has attempted to warn physicians that they risk losing their ability to prescribe federally controlled substances if they write prescriptions in accordance with the act (*Gonzales v. Oregon*, 2006).

State Constitutional Rights

State constitutions also may prove to be fertile ground for further change. First, state courts may expect to see future litigation efforts concentrating on state constitutional rights to refuse life-sustaining treatments, given that arguments for further affirmance of such federal constitutional rights seem, at least temporarily, to be stalled. Alternatively, constitutional conventions in various states may seek to amend existing state constitutions either to expand the rights contained within them or to ensure that certain rights are not read into them.

One such argument will revolve around whether state constitutions currently protect, or should be amended to protect, the right to refuse life-sustaining treatment, especially in the form of medically supplied nutrition and hydration. Many state courts have joined the New Jersey Supreme Court in *Quinlan* in stating that their state constitutions safeguard a right to refuse life-sustaining treatment. To the extent that the state constitutional provisions at issue in those judicial decisions parallel the U.S. Constitution's Fourteenth Amendment guarantee of due process, the U.S. Supreme Court's decision in *Cruzan* likely would determine the extent to which those state constitutions currently safeguard such a right. Constitutions in some states, however, include more specific privacy protections, so that they may be read to safeguard more rights than the U.S. Constitution does. In addition, various states regularly convene constitutional conventions or otherwise consider constitutional amendments; activity could take place in those states with an eye toward either enacting more specific privacy protections or attempting to tighten state constitutional language to cut off arguments that additional state constitutional rights exist.

Another such debate may revolve around whether state constitutions grant terminally ill patients the right to physician-assisted suicide. The U.S. Supreme Court's decisions in *Vacco* (1997) and *Glucksberg* (1997) control only the question of whether the U.S. Constitution ensures such patients a constitutional right to obtain the assistance of a physician in ending their lives. Future state court cases could result in the recognition of such a state constitutional right in states where the possibly applicable constitutional provisions are drafted more broadly than the U.S. Constitution. Alternatively, the same as with the right to refuse life-sustaining treatment, state constitutions may be amended either to safeguard or to negate the existence of such a right.

Alternative Dispute Resolution

All of this presumes a certain amount of legal activity, either on the legislative front or in courtrooms. Most courts, however, and indeed most lawmakers of various sorts, have noted that end-of-life decision making ideally should not take place in either a legislative chamber or a courtroom. One important point made by the *Quinlan* court was that courts should not usually be involved in the private matters of end-of-life decision making. Thus, that court authorized the disconnection of Ms. Quinlan's ventilator so long as (a) "the responsible attending physicians conclude[d] that there is no reasonable possibility of Karen's ever emerging from her present comatose condition to a cognitive, sapient state" and (b) "the hospital 'Ethics Committee' or like body ... agrees that there is no reasonable possibility of Karen's ever emerging from her present comatose condition to a cognitive, sapient state" (*Quinlan*, 1976, pp. 671–672). It noted that it expected future cases to proceed in a similar manner, and indeed, the *Quinlan* decision led to the nationwide establishment of hospital ethics committees and similar bodies to consider such matters internally in an attempt to avoid the need to go to court.

Another way to avoid litigation is to engage in alternative dispute resolution. Ethics committees acting with defined bioethics mediation agendas have had some success in resolving disputes that might have seemed, at the outset, to present irresolvable conflicts (Dubler & Liebman, 2004). Not all end-of-life decision-making cases are amenable to mediation (Dubler, 2005), but given the courts' recognition that they should not be involved unless absolutely necessary, mediation or other forms of alternative dispute resolution should increasingly be attempted before positions become entrenched in the courts and resolution short of litigation is impossible. Other methods to resolve conflict, including pastoral counseling (Murray & Jennings, 2005) and social worker intervention, would assist in this effort.

Increased Education, Knowledge, and Understanding

Finally, to assist in effectuating the frequent statements by courts and legislators that end-of-life decision making should be a private matter, the law has begun to attempt to ensure that sufficient dialogue occurs early enough to avoid having to litigate end-of-life decision-making issues. States have begun requiring that healthcare providers take continuing education courses in end-of-life decision-making issues, and both state and federal legislatures have attempted to ensure that providers know about patient wishes regarding care at the end of life. Hospice care, enhanced recognition of the concerns of vulnerable populations such as persons with disabilities, and support for caregivers should also help improve end-of-life care in the future.

State advance directive laws and federal legislation intending to promote those laws represent steps toward some of these goals. Advance directives are rather blunt tools, at best, to use to engage in optimal end-of-life decision making, and they have not been used as much as expected (Fagerlin & Schneider, 2004). Yet, they are the best tools currently available to assist patients' families, friends, and healthcare providers in ascertaining patients' wishes once they have become incompetent. In addition to the possibility of improving the current structure of advance directives (Hickman, Hammes, Moss, & Tolle, 2005), the law can assist in ensuring that patients' wishes are followed by facilitating increased education for both patients and healthcare providers and ensuring that healthcare providers know of the existence of patients' advance directives. For example, a federal statute, the Patient Self-Determination Act (1990), requires that healthcare facilities receiving Medicare or Medicaid payments inquire whether patients have advance directives and provide patients with information about their rights under state law with regard to end-of-life decision making. Some states include continuing education courses in end-of-life ethics as part of their licensure maintenance requirements for healthcare providers. Some states have created, and the federal government has considered creating, central, Internet-based advance directive registries to ensure that healthcare providers know of patients' wishes, as expressed in advance directives, if they have been unable to ascertain those wishes in any other way. Such steps could go a long way toward improving end-of-life decision making.

Similar educational efforts should take place regarding, and additional legislative attention should be paid to, hospice care and other forms of palliative care. These areas present unique policy challenges requiring broader discourse regarding end-of-life decision-making and care options. As Murray and Jennings (2005) have said, "We must rebuild, reinforce, and reinterpret our laws, institutions, and practices around the acknowledgement that dying is an interpersonal affair, that it is not undergone strictly by individuals" (p. S54). Hospice care does just this, and laws that encourage and support the development of hospice care and strong palliative care practices (for example, by eliminating physicians' concerns that prescription of adequate pain relief will cause them legal or regulatory trouble) are essential.

Similarly, and finally, the law should develop to ensure enhanced understanding of all those affected by decision making at the end of life. The broader population involved in the process of dying also often includes communities, as illustrated by the concern expressed by persons with disabilities when the *Schiavo* case prompted questions about perceived inequities in treatment. The law should encourage increased expression of points of view from those communities as it develops further. The process of dying also draws into it numerous caregivers, including friends and family members. Such caregivers require support, and the law could develop to better provide such support. It could, for example, require or encourage employers to give paid leave to persons who are taking care of a dying friend or relative. At a minimum, it could encourage educational efforts about the burdens borne by such caregivers as patients are dying. Such laws could help round out supportive efforts to ease the process of dying for everyone, not only the person who is actually dying.

Concluding Thoughts

Although three young women in tragic circumstances have engendered much publicity while molding the law of end-of-life decision making, innumerable proxy and surrogate decision makers each day face difficult choices like those made by these young women's families. The law has developed to the point of recognizing both the right to refuse treatment as exercised by competent patients and the right for such decision makers to authorize withholding or withdrawal of treatment on behalf of incompetent patients when those patients would not have desired the treatment. The right to refuse life-sustaining treatment thus importantly recognizes competent and incompetent patients' abilities to both maintain bodily integrity and control personal affairs through private decision making. This area of law faces continual challenges, some rooted in misunderstandings about governmental checks and balances, some based on misconceptions regarding certain types of treatment, and some reflecting concerns that not all voices are heard in the debates surrounding end-of-life decision-making issues. Yet, the goal remains the same as always: to ensure that patients are not subjected to treatment they do not desire, even if that treatment would prolong the act of breathing and the function of bodily organs for a while longer. Whatever developments loom in the future, this core principle should remain constant.

References

Baron, C. (2004). Life and death decision-making: Judges v. legislators as sources of law in bioethics. *Journal of Health and Biomedical Law, 1,* 107–123.

Bernat, J. L., Gert, B., & Mogielnicki, R. P. (1993). Patient refusal of hydration and nutrition. *Archives of Internal Medicine, 153,* 2723–2727.

Bush v. Schiavo, 885 So. 2d 321 (Fla. 2004), *cert. denied,* 125 S. Ct. 1086 (2005), *aff'g* 2004 WL 980028 (Fla. Cir. Ct., Pinellas County May 5, 2004).

Cerminara, K. (2005). Tracking the storm: The far-reaching power of the forces propelling the *Schiavo* cases. *Stetson Law Review, 35,* 147–178.

Cerminara, K. (2006). Musings on the need to convince some people with disabilities that end-of-life decision-making advocates are not out to get them. *Loyola University Chicago Law Journal, 37,* 343–384.

Cerminara, K., & Goodman, K.W. (n.d.). *Key events in the life of Theresa Marie Schiavo.* Retrieved December 30, 2005, from http://www.miami.edu/ethics/schiavo/timeline.htm

Compassion in Dying v. Washington, 79 F.3d 790 (9th Cir. 1996) (*en banc*).

Cruzan v. Director, Missouri Department of Health, 497 U.S. 261 (1990).

Dubler, N. N. (2005). Conflict and consensus at the end of life. *Improving End of Life Care: Why Has It Been So Difficult? Hastings Center Special Report, 35,* S19–S25.

Dubler, N. N., & Liebman, C. B. (2004). *Bioethics mediation: A guide to shaping shared solutions.* New York: United Hospital Fund.

Fagerlin, A., & Schneider, C. (2004). Enough: The failure of the living will. *Hastings Center Report, 34,* 30–42.

Gonzales v. Oregon, 126 S. Ct. 904 (2006).

Hickman, S. E., Hammes, B. J., Moss, A. H., & Tolle, S. W. (2005). Hope for the future: Achieving the original intent of advance directives. *Improving End of Life Care: Why Has It Been So Difficult? Hastings Center Special Report, 35,* S26–S30.

In re Quinlan, 355 A.2d 647 (N.J. 1976).

Louisiana Rev. Stat. Ann. § 40:1299.58.2(14).

Meisel, A. (2005). The role of litigation in end of life care: A reappraisal. *Improving End of Life Care: Why Has It Been So Difficult? Hastings Center Special Report, 35,* S47–S51.

Meisel, A., & Cerminara, K. L. (2004 and annual supplements). *The right to die: The law of end-of-life decision-making* (3rd ed.). New York: Aspen.

Miles, S. H. (1990). Courts, gender and the "right to die." *Law, Medicine & Health Care, 18,* 85–95.

Murray, T. H., & Jennings, B. (2005). The quest to reform end of life care: Rethinking assumptions and setting new directions. *Improving End of Life Care: Why Has It Been So Difficult? Hastings Center Special Report, 35,* S52-S57.

National Right to Life Committee. (n.d.). *Model Starvation and Dehydration of Persons With Disabilities Prevention Act.* Retrieved December 30, 2005, from http://www.nrlc.org/euthanasia/modelstatelaw.html

Oregon Death With Dignity Act. (1995). *Oregon Revised Statutes* 127.800–127.995.

Oregon Department of Human Services. (2007). *Death With Dignity annual reports.* Retrieved July 17, 2007, from http://egov.oregon.gov/DHS/ph/pas/ar-index.shtml

Patient Self-Determination Act of 1990, Publ. L. No. 101-508, 4206, 4751 of the Omnibus Reconciliation Act of 1990.

Planned Parenthood of Southeastern Pennsylvania v. Casey, 505 U.S. 833, 851 (1992).

Rothman, D. (1997). *Beginnings count: The technological imperative in American health care.* New York: Oxford University Press.

Schiavo ex rel. Schindler v. Schiavo, 357 F. Supp. 2d 1378 (M.D. Fla.), *aff'd,* 403 F.3d 1223 (11th Cir.), *reh'g en banc denied,* 403 F.3d 1261 (11th Cir. *en banc*), *stay denied,* 125 S. Ct. 1692 (2005a).

Schiavo ex rel. Schindler v. Schiavo, 358 F. Supp. 2d 1161 (M.D. Fla.), *aff'd,* 403 F.3d 1289 (11th Cir.), *reh'g en banc denied,* 404 F.3d 1282 (11th Cir. *en banc*), *stay denied,* 125 S. Ct. 1722 (2005b).

Schloendorff v. Society of New York Hospital, 105 N.E. 92 (N.Y. 1914).

Shepherd, L. (2006). Terri Schiavo: Unsettling the settled. *Loyola University Chicago Law Journal, 37,* 297–341.

Sneyd, R. (2007, March 21). House votes down assisted suicide bill. *Associated Press Wire.* Retrieved July 27, 1007, from http://www.wcax.com/Global/story.asp?S=6261213

Superintendent, Belchertown State School v. Saikewicz, 370 N.E.2d 417 (Mass. 1977).

Vacco v. Quill, 521 U.S. 793 (1997).

Vogel, N. (2007, June 8). Assisted death bill fails again in Capitol. *Los Angeles Times,* p. B1.

Washington v. Glucksberg, 521 U.S. 702 (1997).

Werth, J. L., Jr. (2001). Using the Youk-Kevorkian case to teach about euthanasia and other end-of-life issues. *Death Studies, 25,* 151–177.

White, G. E. (1985). *Tort law in America: An intellectual history.* New York: Oxford University Press.

9

CHAPTER

End-of-Life Choices

Phillip M. Kleespies, Pamela J. Miller, and Thomas A. Preston

Introduction

This chapter examines the end-of-life choices available to the terminally ill. As Kleespies (2004) noted, when death is near, many in our society struggle with the dilemma of whether to fight on strenuously with the hope of a reprieve, if not a cure, or to attempt to bow out gracefully with the acknowledgment that meaningful life is essentially over. In fact, major sociocultural movements have formed around one side of this dilemma or the other. In this context, we have organized the chapter so that we first discuss the choices available to those terminally ill individuals who might wish to die, and we then discuss the choices available to those terminally ill persons who might wish to prolong life, even though their circumstances might be dire. Our discussion includes the major issues, problems, and potential conflicts related to each choice.

A century ago, the question of having some choice, or needing to make a choice, about how one might die was not as pressing an issue as it is today. The remarkable advances in biomedical science and in the treatment of acute, life-threatening illnesses have radically changed life expectancy and patterns of dying, at least in developed countries like the United States. Yet, for many in our society, these advances, as exciting as they have been, were also clearly seen as having some potentially serious and negative repercussions. These concerns were given voice in two high-profile court cases: the case of Karen Ann Quinlan (*In re Quinlan*, 1976) and the case of Nancy Beth Cruzan (*Cruzan v. Director, Missouri Department of Health*, 1990) (see also Cerminara, chapter 8, this volume). In both of these cases, the young women involved were being kept alive in a persistent vegetative state on respirators and with artificial nutrition and hydration. Their respective families asked to have treatment discontinued so that their daughters might be allowed to die.

After years of court proceedings, both families won the right to have life-sustaining treatment discontinued and to allow their unconscious daughters to die. The struggle to achieve these ends, however, sent shock waves through those who were less concerned with prolonging life (whatever the person's condition might be) and were more concerned with the individual's quality of life. Adding to this concern was the realization that modern medicine had largely transformed acute causes of death into chronic illnesses marked by a slow decline in mental and physical capacities (Lynn, 2005).

Those who shared these concerns came to be referred to as the *right-to-die* movement. Citing the ethical principles of autonomy and compassion, they advocated for greater self-determination in the dying process and for decreased control of dying by physicians and medical institutions. After the *Quinlan* and *Cruzan* cases, it appeared that they might have achieved a national consensus, at least in law and medicine, about the individual's right, when terminally ill, to refuse life-sustaining treatment and to exercise some choice in the conditions and timing of his or her death (Murray & Jennings, 2005).

The United States, however, is a multicultural society, and there are segments of the population for whom life is thought to have intrinsic value regardless of any adverse conditions and for whom hastening death is never desirable. Others hold religious beliefs that ascribe value to whatever suffering one must endure, or they hold that the time of death is not something for humans to determine (see Doka, chapter 16, this volume, for a review). They have been referred to as the *right-to-life* movement. In addition, our nation tends to maintain an optimistic perspective that, through hard work and ingenuity, we can conquer the forces of nature. In the arena of medicine and health care, this point of view is manifest in our faith in the power of empirical science and technology, a faith that, as Daniel Callahan (2005) noted, "treats death as a contingent accidental event that can be done away with, one disease at a time" (p. S6).

The voice of the right-to-life segment of our society was initially heard in cases such as that of Helga Wanglie (Miles, 1991). Mrs. Wanglie was an elderly woman who was in a persistent vegetative state with severe brain damage. The hospital's clinical team was of the opinion that treatment was not benefiting her, and the team suggested that it be withdrawn. The patient's husband, daughter, and son, however, insisted that it be continued. Their position was that physicians should not play God, that the patient would not be better off dead, that removing life support showed a moral decay in our civilization, and that miracles can happen. They opposed the hospital in a court proceeding and won the right to represent Mrs. Wanglie and to have acute care continued.

This sad and protracted case and others like it (e.g., the case of Baby K, an infant born without a major portion of the brain and kept alive on a ventilator; *In re Baby K*, 1994) were clear indications that there were radically different value systems at work in our society when it came to end-of-life issues. These value conflicts, however, were never more apparent than in the recent high-profile case of Terri Schiavo, a woman who, at the age of 27, suffered a cardiac arrest and significant brain damage because of a lack of oxygen at the time of the arrest (see also Cerminara, chapter 8, this volume). She was kept alive in a persistent vegetative state on artificially administered nutrition and hydration. Her husband maintained that, earlier in her life, she had stated that she would not wish to live in such a condition. As her legally appointed guardian and health-care proxy, he asked the court to determine what her wishes would have been and then attempted to follow the court's determination by having her removed from life support and allowed to die. Her parents opposed him and maintained that, with rehabilitative efforts, there was still hope of recovery, and that it would be tantamount to murder by starvation to remove her feeding tube. Accusations were exchanged on both sides, and the case moved through the court system. Over the course of 15 years, this intrafamilial struggle escalated to the point of involving not only multiple courts, but also the highest branches of the state and federal governments. This case has led to a reexamination of the notion of whether there ever was a national consensus on end-of-life issues (Murray & Jennings, 2005). It is in the aftermath of the Schiavo case that we examine end-of-life choices in this chapter.

□ The Choice to End Life

In this section, we discuss the choices available to those who have sought greater self-determination in the manner and timing of death. Of course, making such choices presupposes that the individual is capable of making an informed decision or, if not, that he or she has engaged in advance care planning or has a duly recognized surrogate decision maker. Space limitations preclude a discussion of the criteria for informed consent here (see Kleespies, 2004, and Ditto, chapter 13, this volume, for a discussion of informed consent).

The choices for those who are terminally ill and do not wish to prolong life can be classified under three headings: (a) the refusal of life-sustaining treatment; (b) interventions that may secondarily hasten death; and (c) assisted death. Prior to the Schiavo case, it had been thought by many that the first two categories dealt with generally accepted healthcare practices that respected the individual's autonomous wishes about the dying process. The controversy around the Schiavo case, however, has raised questions about how settled these practices really are, at least in the eyes of certain segments of the U.S. population. Assisted death, of course, remains the subject of heated national debate and is currently explicitly legal in only one state, Oregon.

The Refusal of Life-Sustaining Treatment

The right of a competent patient to refuse medical treatment is legally protected, even if that refusal may lead to death. This right is based on the ethical principle of autonomy and on U.S. Supreme Court rulings such as that of Justice Benjamin Cardozo, who in 1914 wrote that "every human being of adult years of sound mind has a right to determine what shall be done with his (or her) own body" (Nicholson & Matross, 1989, p. 234). Physicians, nurses, and other healthcare providers are ethically and legally able to follow the wishes of a person (or his or her duly appointed surrogate) to withhold or withdraw life-sustaining treatment (Meisel, 1995; Meisel, Snyder, & Quill, 2000).

Withholding and withdrawing life-sustaining treatments have long been viewed as legally and ethically equivalent. Physicians, however, seem to prefer to withhold treatment at the outset rather than to withdraw it once it has been initiated (Committee on Bioethics, 1994; Singer, 1992; Snyder & Swartz, 1993). One hypothesis about why this might be the case is that it may be easier, psychologically, for physicians to allow someone to die rather than to take the more active step of stopping treatment (McCamish & Crocker, 1993). Physician bias against withdrawing treatment, however, can make it more difficult for patients who might wish to choose a trial of a treatment near the end of life and have it discontinued if it is of little benefit.

One of the most emotionally charged issues related to refusing life-sustaining treatment has been withholding or withdrawing artificial nutrition and hydration (Boisaubin, 1993). It is an issue that reemerged in the Schiavo case as Terri Schiavo's parents accused her husband and guardian of attempting to execute their daughter by dehydration and starvation (*Statement of Schindler Family*, 2004). Having adequate food and water is necessary for life, and providing food and drink to others is linked to caring and nurturance at a very basic level. We feed infants who cannot feed themselves. It should come as no surprise then that a decision to withhold or withdraw nutrition and hydration could be seen as very disturbing.

The argument revolves around whether artificially administered nutrition and hydration are considered basic sustenance that should not be denied to any human being or medical treatments that are indistinguishable in any morally relevant way from other life-sustaining treatments (McCamish & Crocker, 1993).

In the Cruzan case, this issue, albeit not the main judicial focus, was nonetheless considered by the U.S. Supreme Court. The Court adopted the consensus opinion that artificial nutrition and hydration are life-sustaining medical interventions to be treated no differently than other such interventions. This judicial opinion, however, did not totally resolve this emotion-laden issue. A few states continued to have laws that did not permit the refusal of nutrition and hydration (Snyder & Swartz, 1993), and with respect to children, Congress felt it necessary to pass Public Law 98-457 (1984), the Child Abuse Prevention and Treatment and Adoption Reform Act, a law that contained the so-called Baby Doe Rules that required that artificial feeding be continued for children even when in terminal conditions (Boisaubin, 1993).

As Werth and Kleespies (2006) have indicated, there are several other issues related to the refusal of life-sustaining treatment that are also not entirely resolved. For the person involved in making end-of-life choices, it is important to be aware of these factors. First, if a time frame is included, there is no real consensus on a medical definition of terminal illness. Thus, it might be defined as an illness for which there is no known cure and for which life expectancy is 6 months or less. With many fatal illnesses, however, it is exceedingly difficult to predict with accuracy when someone will die (Mishara, 1999; Thibault, 1997). In a study by Christakis and Lamont (2000), for example, only 20% of physicians who referred patients to a hospice program were accurate in their predictions (with accuracy defined as between 0.67 and 1.33 times the actual length of survival). Over 60% of the physicians who participated in the study gave predictions that were overly optimistic. Such findings suggest that it is misleading if the definition of terminal illness is locked into a narrow time frame. Many treatment providers, however, are heavily influenced in their thinking by the Medicare requirement that life expectancy must be 6 months or less if the patient is to obtain coverage for hospice services.

Second, there has never been a formal agreement on the criteria for mental competence to make healthcare decisions. In terms of determining the capacity to refuse treatment, Grisso and Appelbaum (1998) noted that the following four criteria have been most often cited in legal proceedings: (a) the ability to express a choice, (b) the ability to understand information relevant to the illness and proposed treatment, (c) the ability to appreciate the significance of the information for one's own illness and treatment, and (d) the ability to reason with the relevant information and engage in a logical process of weighing treatment options. The fact that these four criteria have been most often cited, however, does not mean that all four are necessarily applied in any given case. In fact, different jurisdictions may use a combination of two or three of these criteria. Yet, whether one uses two, three, or four criteria can make a difference in the threshold for decision-making capacity. A higher threshold may mean that more people are denied autonomous decision making, while a lower threshold may mean that fewer vulnerable individuals are protected from their own impaired decision-making ability. It is clearly in the clinician's interest to be aware of which criteria are typically employed in the jurisdiction in which he or she practices.

Finally, although family members have been recognized in the judicial process as appropriate surrogate decision makers for the incapacitated patient, a problem remains in terms of how to make decisions for a patient who lacks decision-making ability and has no family or friends to serve as surrogates. A number of states have created a pool of individuals who, on judicial request, are available to act as guardians for these individuals, but many states have not developed such a resource. The institutional or hospital ethics advisory committee (EAC) has sometimes been asked to fill that void and be an advocate for the patient. Yet, as Kleespies, Hughes, and Gallacher (2000) have pointed out, EACs consist of hospital staff who, although not a part of the treatment team, may identify more with the team than with the patient and may find it hard not to be influenced by the needs, mores, and values of the institution for which they work. In an era of managed care that emphasizes cost containment, this is not a small concern. Bioethicists Beauchamp and Childress (2001) also considered this issue and concluded that, in the absence of good alternatives, an EAC review may outweigh the risks. At the least, it can foster open discussion and debate.

Interventions That May Hasten Death

In two cases heard together (*Washington v. Glucksberg* and *Vacco v. Quill*) in 1997, the U.S. Supreme Court upheld state laws making physician-assisted dying illegal, but it accepted another medical practice that can end a patient's life. The Court noted the legality of using high-dose morphine to relieve end-of-life suffering, even to the point of causing unconsciousness and hastening death (see especially Justice O'Connor's concurrence). The justices justified the practice because the medication is intended to alleviate pain, not to cause death.

For decades, physicians have administered morphine (sometimes called a morphine drip) or other narcotic medicines to relieve the suffering of dying patients. When used solely to relieve pain, these drugs rarely cause death, but there is risk because in high enough doses they can result in death by stopping lung or heart functioning, particularly in a weakened, dying patient. Physicians have always felt justified in risking a patient's life by saying the intention is not to kill but to relieve pain or suffering. This reasoning derived from the so-called principle of double effect, in which one intended effect is pain relief and the other effect—unintended but foreseen—is the death of the patient earlier than would have happened without the morphine.

The double effect has been sanctioned by virtually all religions. In 1957, a group of physicians put the question to Pope Pius XII whether the suppression of pain and consciousness by the use of narcotics is permitted by religion and morality even if it is foreseen that the use of narcotics will shorten life. The Pope reportedly answered that, if no other means exist, and if, in the given circumstances, it does not prevent the carrying out of other religious and moral duties, then it is permissible (President's Commission, 1983).

Although physicians all across the United States have used morphine drips widely in treating dying patients (Fohr, 1998), no one really knows in most cases whether the treatment has hastened dying (Quill, Dresser, & Brock, 1997). Physicians who use this treatment know they could be causing their patients' deaths, and physicians may sometimes use the drug in a way that probably does hasten dying (Preston, 1998).

The morality and legality of the practice has been justified by framing it in terms of the physician's double-effect intent. Bioethicists, however, have disputed the validity of this framing (see, e.g., Battin, 1994; Beauchamp & Childress, 2001) because physicians are perfectly capable of giving morphine for both effects—pain relief and ending life—and many physicians would probably have trouble articulating or understanding how they are dividing their intentions in a given case (Wilson, Smedira, Fink, McDowell, & Luce, 1992).

Some who oppose physician-assisted dying fear that physicians may hide an intent to kill behind the principle of double effect (Schorr, 1998), while some proponents of physician-assisted dying consider the principle a double standard by which opponents can covertly approve one means of aid in dying while opposing physician-assisted dying (Quill, Dresser, et al., 1997).

Healthcare workers on both sides of the physician-assisted dying issue appreciate the double-effect construct in practice because it allows them to give good palliative care to dying patients without guilt-laden uncertainty or ambiguity about their intent. Calling this practice double effect legitimizes it by emphasizing the first effect of the physician's act in prescribing high-dose morphine (palliation of symptoms) and, to some degree, disregarding the second effect (the physician's direct involvement in how and when the patient dies).

In its majority opinions in the *Glucksberg* and *Quill* cases, the U.S. Supreme Court also sanctioned palliative sedation as a way to relieve severe suffering in dying patients for whom conventional treatment is not effective. In this practice, a physician injects a sedative continuously to induce a constant coma. Because the patient is unconscious, he or she does not consciously experience symptoms and has no distress. No nutrition and fluids are given, and the patient then dies slowly through starvation and dehydration. The time from beginning of palliative sedation to death is usually hours to days, but it may be days or more than a week if the patient has been well nourished and hydrated before withdrawing hydration and nutrition.

This procedure is deemed allowable because the patient has the constitutional right to refuse therapy (fluids and nutrition), and the patient gives consent for the physician to induce unconsciousness for the purpose of eliminating symptoms. This procedure, however, is controversial (Quill & Byock, 2000). On one hand, some physicians disavow it because the act does lead to the patient's death, and they believe it is killing. Other physicians defend it on the basis of intent to relieve suffering, not to kill, and the patient's right to refuse treatment (artificial administration of food and fluids) (Krakauer et al., 2000; Orentlicher, 1997). However one views it, because the patient dies slowly and without a specific act by the physician in the hours or minutes before death, dying appears to be natural, and one can say the disease killed the patient. Yet, appearances aside, in palliative sedation physicians are directly involved in helping their patients die.

A death related to double effect did not occur in the situation described by Spannhake (chapter 3, this volume). Yet, had he decided to have a coma induced for a second time, it apparently was very likely that such a death would have ensued. His treatment staff were well aware of this probability. Given his mindset when in excruciating pain, he would have chosen death but for the urging of family and friends.

Another means of dying for terminally ill patients, now gaining wider understanding, is voluntarily stopping eating and drinking (VSED). Patients dying of chronic, debilitating diseases such as cancer frequently stop eating and drinking before dying. This is a natural process because of internal organ dysfunction, and death soon follows, within days or perhaps 1–2 weeks (Miller & Meier, 1998).

Any terminally ill patient can choose to copy this natural process through VSED. Hunger usually lasts only 2 or 3 days, after which the breakdown of body tissues for energy suppresses hunger. Rubbing wet swabs on the lips and inside the mouth can ameliorate thirst. Morphine or light sedatives are very effective in suppressing both hunger and thirst, and if a terminally ill patient has good comfort care, including frequent turning and eye care, symptoms are minimal and manageable (Miller & Meier, 1998; Quill, Lo, & Brock, 1997).

Two factors determine the duration from beginning of VSED to death. Duration to death of a well-nourished and hydrated patient may be up to 3 weeks, but for an emaciated patient who already has not been eating or drinking much, the duration may be 2 or 3 days. Also, the stricter the adherence to total absence of fluids or food, the shorter the time to death will be. The occasional taking of small sips of water—often offered by well-meaning loved ones—delays the process of dehydration, which is what leads to death. All in all, if done correctly and with sufficient comfort care with morphine or other medicines, this approach is effective and peaceful.

Assisted Death

Battin and Lipman (1996) discussed the definition of *assisted death* this way: "The person intentionally ends his or her own life with the means supplied by another person" (p. 3). Although this definition is not agreed on by everyone and it is used inconsistently in the literature, we use it in this chapter.

Miller (1996) and Kleespies (2004) explored at length the arguments for and against assisted death. These authors discussed two factors that support assistance with dying: compassion and self-determination. Prolonged illness can be unbearable, and often patients have little hope for recovery while living with fear and anxiety about what will happen next. Pain may not be managed despite best efforts, and suffering may be extreme. A terminally ill person may feel out of control and that dignity has been lost to the disease and to the dying process. This leads to thinking about self-determination and the person's right to control the details about his or her death, including the right to choose assistance.

There are also many arguments against the intentional termination of life as well (Kleespies, 2004; Miller, 1996). There are those whose religious and moral beliefs lead them to view assisted death as wrong and against God's will. Some may view the request for assistance with death as a "cry for help" (Miller, 1996, p. 16). There is concern that there can never be enough safeguards to allow such a choice at such a sensitive time in someone's life. Others believe that assistance with death is disrespectful to the terminally ill and a threat to the health professionals involved, and that pain and depression can be treated. There is also worry about the slippery slope (Hendin, 1995, 1999). This means that if the terminally ill have the right to choose death, then other groups deemed disposable by society may be persuaded also to end life early and possibly against their will. The question of whether physicians should prescribe medication for the purpose of death is debated within the profession of medicine. How can a person who is supposed to help and heal also be a person who can assist with dying?

There are many societal concerns as well. The United States is the only industrialized nation that does not have healthcare coverage for all citizens. This problem is felt even more acutely by citizens of color (Bodenheimer & Grumbach, 2005). How can we move forward with legalizing assisted death when the playing field for health coverage is so out of balance? The ethical, legal, and moral questions and debates will continue to ebb and flow as laws are passed and court decisions emerge that formalize choices at the end of life. Many view the arguments pro and con about assisted death as equally balanced (Quill, Meier, Block, & Billings, 1998). In the state of Oregon, however, there is an ongoing in vivo experiment with legalized assisted death from which there is much to learn.

Oregon's Death With Dignity Act

The Oregon Death With Dignity Act (DWDA) was passed by voters in November 1994 (Oregon Death With Dignity Act, 1995). Previously, both Washington in 1991 and California in 1992 had ballot measures defeated by the exact same margins, 54% to 46% (Hoefler, 1994). These initiatives, although similar to Oregon's, allowed for a lethal injection if the patient did not die from taking medications (Miller et al., 1994). Like Washington and California, Oregon's ballot measure came from grassroots efforts and from citizens who believed strongly in this choice. Ballot Measure 16 only passed by a slim margin (51% to 49%), and Oregon's law was immediately blocked by a court injunction for 3 years. During this time, there was another ballot measure sent to the voters from the legislature in 1997 asking to repeal the law passed in 1994. This ballot measure (51) was rejected by an even higher percentage of citizens, as 60% voted to keep the law.

Although DWDA has been in continuous effect since 1997, and 292 Oregonians have used a lethal prescription to end their lives (Oregon Department of Human Services, 2007), numerous federal and congressional attempts have been made to stop the law. The Assisted-Suicide Funding Restriction Act of 1997 prohibits the use of federal money for assisted death, similar to the Hyde Amendment's restriction of federal funding for abortions (Miller, 2000). Congress attempted to pass federal laws that would prohibit the use of medication for assisted death, and most recently, the U.S. attorney general declared that prescriptions written under Oregon's law violated the Controlled Substances Act (CSA). The U.S. Supreme Court subsequently decided that the CSA did not apply to Oregon's law. Some view this as the final hurdle for the law after 12 years of uncertainty, although Congress may try to look at the practice of medicine under the CSA.

Oregon's Nine Years of Experience With the Death With Dignity Act

Oregon's law allows a terminally ill adult resident of the state to obtain a lethal prescription to end life. The main tenets of the law can be seen in Table 9.1.

Of the 292 Oregonians who used the law over 9 years, 54% were men, and 46% were women. Younger people, those divorced or never married, and those with baccalaureate degrees or higher were more likely to use DWDA than others who died in the state of the same diseases and in the same years. Eighty-six percent of those who used the law were enrolled in a hospice program when the medication was ingested. Ninety-seven percent of those who used the law were white, and 2% were recorded as Asian American. The three most common illnesses were cancer at 81%, followed by amyotrophic lateral sclerosis (ALS), chronic lower respiratory disease, and HIV/AIDS. Only three patients who used the law did not have health insurance. The most cited end-of-life concerns have been loss of autonomy, lessened ability to engage in activities that make life enjoyable, and loss of dignity (Oregon Department of Human Services, 2007). A psychiatrist or psychologist must evaluate the patient if either the

TABLE 9.1 Summary of Components of the Oregon Death With Dignity (DWD) Act (1995)

(a)	The terminally ill person (with less than a 6-month prognosis) must be 18 years of age and an Oregon resident;
(b)	The request must come directly from the terminally ill person, who must have the capacity to make and communicate health care decisions;
(c)	Two physicians must agree on prognosis, diagnosis, and capacity to make decisions;
(d)	The prescribing physician must file a report with the Oregon Department of Human Services, Health Services;
(e)	The choice of DWD cannot give insurance companies a reason not to pay the patient's health or life insurance claims;
(f)	All end-of-life options, such as hospice and pain and symptom management must be discussed with patient by both physicians;
(g)	Notification of next of kin is recommended but not required;
(h)	The process can be stopped at any time;
(i)	No health professional or health system is required to participate, and a professional can be a conscientious objector and transfer care;
(j)	If either physician believes the patient may have impaired judgment, a licensed psychologist or psychiatrist must assess; and
(k)	The terminally ill person must make two oral requests separated by 15 days and sign a written request that is witnessed by two people.

prescribing or consulting physician believes that the patient's judgment is impaired. Over 9 years, 13% (36 patients) had a mental health referral and then went on to use the lethal prescription. The referrals for mental health evaluation have decreased over the years from 31% in 1998 to 4% in 2006 (Oregon Department of Human Services). Part of this decrease is explained by the fact that some health systems and agencies initially required a mental health exam for every DWDA request, and this requirement has gradually been eliminated.

Lessons Learned in Oregon

Although there are 9 years of data about the use of Oregon's law, there is still controversy over how to interpret the results and what this all means for the future of end-of-life choices. Ms. Raye's story about the death of her father (chapter 5, this volume) highlights the secrecy the family needed for an assisted death to happen in a state where the practice was illegal. That secrecy is now eliminated in Oregon, yet the impact on bereaved families remains unclear. Some initial concerns have been settled as the data emerged over 9 years: (a) There have not been any calls to the emergency medical services for intervention after the lethal medication was ingested; (b) the reporting system appears to be effective; (c) the law has remained patient driven; (d) fewer citizens have used the law than initially predicted; and (e) there has not been an influx of terminally ill from other parts of the country.

Research has underscored some knowledge about the use of Oregon's law and those who have used it. Ganzini et al. (2000) found that patients who requested a lethal prescription and had a mental disorder were stopped from pursing the option, and Ganzini et al. (2002) found that depression is one of the least-mentioned reasons for the choice of assisted death. Tolle et al. (2004) found that terminally ill persons who choose to use the DWDA provisions are generally independent, strong, and forceful. Oregon continues to have one of the highest hospice rates and lowest in-hospital death rates in the country (Tolle, Rosenfeld, Tilden, & Park, 1999).

There are still many unknowns in Oregon, and there is continued need for research about the law and the people who use it. For example, there is no provision in the law to accommodate a mental status change once the prescription is in hand. Also, 456 prescriptions have been written, and 292 people have used the law to end their life. There could be some interesting information about those who start the process but never conclude it. This information could include a wide range of factors, from becoming too ill, changing one's mind, gaining comfort from the option but not using it, death, or admission to hospice (Ganzini & Dobscha, 2004).

Since the Supreme Court decision of January 2006, other states may move forward with legislation similar to Oregon, particularly Vermont and California (Miller & Hedlund, 2005; Okie, 2005). In spring 2008, citizens in the state of Washington collected signatures for a fall ballot measure modeled after Oregon's DWDA. Oregon may be looked to for guidance, direction, and expertise in this end-of-life choice (Task Force to Improve the Care of Terminally Ill Oregonians, 2007). Although the full impact of the act is still debated (Werth & Wineberg, 2005), much has been learned from health professionals as this legal right has become established, particularly for those who work in hospice (Mesler & Miller, 2000; Miller, Hedlund, & Soule, 2006; Miller, Mesler, & Eggman, 2002). The lessons learned in Oregon about assisted death have been many, and the challenges that lie ahead for this end-of-life option will continue to be deliberated and researched.

☐ The Choice to Prolong Life and the Futility Debate

As noted at the beginning of this chapter, the case of Terri Schiavo brought national attention to the differences in values that exist in our society in relation to the question of how life should end. The case of Barbara Howe in Massachusetts was not quite so high profile as the Schiavo case, but nonetheless illustrates some of the struggles of those who choose to prolong life and oppose discontinuing life support under any circumstances.

Over a period of 14 years, Barbara Howe suffered from progressive ALS, or Lou Gehrig's disease. ALS is a neurological disease that gradually paralyzes a person's body while leaving the mind relatively intact. Mrs. Howe eventually entered what is referred to as a *locked-in* state. She could no longer communicate if she was in pain; she needed a ventilator to breathe; and she needed artificial nutrition and hydration to continue to survive. She had appointed her oldest daughter as her healthcare proxy, and she had told her daughter that she wanted aggressive medical care for as long as she could appreciate her family and showed any sign of brain functioning. As her proxy, her daughter insisted on continuing acute medical care. The treatment team at Massachusetts General Hospital (MGH), however, became increasingly uncomfortable with doing so after some of the patient's bones broke during a routine turning and when her right eye had to be removed because of corneal damage that resulted from her inability to blink and lubricate her eyes. The hospital staff believed that she was suffering and might be in great pain (Kowalczyk, 2003).

The patient had only one movement left. Her left eye could be seen to widen when her daughter entered the room. Her family took this as a sign of recognition, and her daughter continued to insist on life-sustaining treatment. The hospital took the case to Probate and Family Court and sought to have the daughter's decision as healthcare proxy overturned. Initially, the judge upheld the daughter's decision but advised her to refocus not on what her mother had said she wanted, but on her best interests given her current circumstances. A year later, MGH went back to court and negotiated with Mrs. Howe's daughter to withdraw life-sustaining treatment in approximately 3.5 months. Barbara Howe died 3 weeks before the date on which treatment was to be withdrawn (Kowalczyk, 2005).

In the case of Barbara Howe, the treatment staff not only thought that further acute treatment was futile but also felt that it was harmful. The family, however, believed that Mrs. Howe's life and death were in God's hands, and that they were observing her autonomous wishes to have her life prolonged for as long as possible (Kowalczyk, 2003). Such differences in end-of-life values and opinions have come to be referred to as the *futility debate.*

Unfortunately, there have been many attempts to define futility of treatment, and none have been particularly successful. Definitions have ranged from treatment that will probably only produce an insignificant outcome, to treatment that is more likely to be more burdensome than beneficial, to treatment that has proved useless in the last 100 similar cases (Beauchamp & Childress, 2001). No consensus has been reached on any of these definitions, in part because in most medical situations near the end of life, nothing is absolute. Rather, there are probable or likely outcomes that can have different degrees of relevance to the various parties involved. Thus, the dying person, his or her surrogate, the treatment staff, and the hospital administration may all have different definitions and thresholds for what, if anything, is considered futile treatment (Truog, Brett, & Frader, 1992).

From the perspective of the patient and his or her family, this situation raises serious concerns about whether decisions about futility of treatment will be unduly influenced by the physician's or hospital's values and biases as opposed to the patient's values and wishes (Werth & Kleespies, 2006). A well-known case in point is that of Baby Ryan (Capron, 1995). Ryan was born 6 weeks premature, asphyxiated, and with barely a heartbeat. His physicians at a hospital in Seattle, Washington, diagnosed him as having brain damage, an intestinal blockage, and kidneys that did not remove toxins from his blood. He was sustained on intravenous feedings and dialysis for several weeks. His doctors thought that the outlook was bleak, but they consulted with a children's hospital in Seattle about the possibility of long-term dialysis for Ryan. The children's hospital, however, refused to accept him for treatment and stated that it would be immoral to treat this child and prolong his agony with no likely positive outcome.

Ryan's parents did not wish to accept the opinion that their son's condition was hopeless and that it would be best if he were allowed to die. Because they feared that the hospital had already decided to remove him from dialysis, they sought and obtained an emergency court order that directed the hospital to take whatever immediate steps were necessary, including renal dialysis, to stabilize and maintain his life. The case drew media attention, and physicians at another children's hospital in Portland, Oregon, offered to accept Ryan for treatment. His parents had him transferred to Portland where the doctors performed surgery to clear his blocked intestines. He recovered from the surgery and gradually was able to switch to nutrition by mouth. In a month and a half, Ryan no longer required dialysis and seemed free of any permanent neurological deficits. A scan showed no structural brain damage, and he went home with his parents.

Ethically, the dispute over futility has been between those who invoke the principle of autonomy or self-determination and those who argue for the integrity of the practice of medicine and distributive justice (Finucane & Harper, 1996; Truog, 2000). As was the case with Baby Ryan, and in the initial court hearing with Barbara Howe's daughter, when futility cases have gone to court, the courts have most often ruled on the side of the patient's or surrogate's autonomous choice (e.g., the case of Helga Wanglie; Miles, 1991). Such legal opinions have, in their turn, left healthcare professionals feeling disenfranchised and as though they have no moral weight in the decision-making process. The demands of medical treatment, however, require the participation of the medical staff and place obligations on them. It would seem that they should have a voice in treatment decisions.

One proposed solution to this dilemma was to abandon definition-based approaches to futility in favor of a case-by-case, fair process approach. This approach was formulated by a task force of the Houston Bioethics Network, a consortium of ethics committees from hospitals in the Houston area (Halevy & Brody, 1996). The Houston policy acknowledges that no policy on futility can be value free and entirely objective. It offers a series of steps for resolving futility dilemmas on an individual case basis. The process gives voice to each of the involved parties (i.e., patient, surrogate, and treatment providers) and requires a thorough institutional review of each case. The physician is not permitted to make unilateral decisions that treatment is futile.

Under the policy, the physician who is of the opinion that treatment is futile must first discuss with the patient or surrogate the nature of the illness or injury, the prognosis, the reasons for considering treatment futile, and the available options, including palliative and hospice care. He or she must clarify that, if the intervention is not provided, the patient will not be abandoned and will be given comfort care and support. The physician is also to present the options of transferring care to another physician or healthcare institution and of obtaining a second, independent opinion.

If agreement cannot be reached and the patient or surrogate does not wish to arrange transfer, the physician must obtain a second medical opinion and present the case to an institutional review committee (e.g., an EAC). The patient or surrogate must be permitted to be present at the case review and encouraged to express his or her views. If the review committee does not concur with the physician's opinion about futility, then orders to limit or end interventions would not be accepted as valid. If, however, the review committee agrees that the treatment is medically inappropriate, the treatment, under this policy, could be discontinued despite the objections of the patient or surrogate.

The state of Texas is now one of two states that have passed statutes (California Probate Code, 2000; Texas Health and Safety Code, 1999) that allow physicians to write do not resuscitate (DNR) orders against the wishes of a patient (or surrogate), provided they follow a fair process approach similar to that mentioned. Texas also has a section of the Texas' Advance Directive Act (1999) that allows an attending physician, with the review and concurrence of a hospital ethics committee, to discontinue life-sustaining treatment against the wishes stated in a patient's advance directive if the treatment is deemed inappropriate in a fair process approach. The Texas statute was tested in court in the case of Sun Hudson, a 6-month-old infant who was on a ventilator and had a form of dwarfism that is usually fatal (NBC5.com, 2005). The hospital did not want to act in a way that the staff believed would prolong the baby's suffering, but the baby's mother believed that he might gain strength and survive. The mother obtained a court injunction blocking the hospital from removing life support; however, the hospital was successful in getting the judge to lift the injunction, and the infant died a short time after treatment was withdrawn.

Despite the statutes in California and Texas, there is as yet no universal agreement in the medical community that this type of approach to futility questions is an acceptable way to proceed. Moreover, with the exception of the case in Texas mentioned here, the legal status of discontinuing life-sustaining treatment against the objections of a dying patient or his or her surrogate remains untested in most jurisdictions. In the case of Barbara Howe in Massachusetts, the treatment staff and the hospital brought a case of perceived futility to court. The court, however, did not render an opinion but rather worked to achieve an agreement between the parties involved.

□ Conclusion: The Struggle to Make a Choice

This chapter has explored the choices available to those terminally ill individuals who wish to bring life to a close and those who wish to prolong life against all odds. These choices do not come easily, and we have explored many cases and examples of difficult end-of-life situations. We must also state that some patients and families fare well while a loved one is dying and find this a precious and meaningful time. Yet, it is inherently a complicated process that is full of emotions and decisions that are mingled into a cultural, legal, political, and social context. Thus, the path that each individual or family takes through the dying process is unique.

The supports available near the end of life range from formal to informal. Who or what will be involved in someone's last days depends on many factors: the disease process; where the person lives; if hospice or palliative care is appropriate; what the terminally ill person sees as important; the choices made; the influence of family, society, and culture. A struggle over making a choice appears to be normative when death is near. We appear to be a society that does not plan well for our last event despite the fact that choices exist. We also tend to be a death-denying culture that has great faith in our ability to conquer illness and disease. The ethical, moral, political, and legal debates will rage on for the foreseeable future. The best that we can do at this point is to continue to debate the choices along with the struggles and, at the end, have hope that all terminally ill patients can be given care that provides comfort and dignity.

References

Battin, M. P. (1994). *The least worst death: Essays in bioethics on the end of life*. New York: Oxford University Press.

Battin, M. P., & Lipman, A. G. (1996). *Drug use in assisted suicide and euthanasia*. New York: Haworth.

Beauchamp, T., & Childress, J. (2001). *The principles of biomedical ethics* (5th ed.). New York: Oxford University Press.

Bodenheimer, T. S., & Grumbach, K. (2005). *Understanding health policy*. New York: McGraw-Hill.

Boisaubin, E. (1993). Legal decisions affecting the limitation of nutritional support. *The Hospice Journal, 9*, 131–147.

California Probate Code, Section 4736 (West 2000).

Callahan, D. (2005). Death: "The distinguished thing." *Hastings Center Report Special Report, 35*(6), S5–S8.

Capron, A. (1995, March–April). Baby Ryan and virtual futility. *Hastings Center Report, 25*, 20–21.

Child Abuse Prevention and Treatment and Adoption Reform Act, Public Law 98-457 (1984).

Christakis, N., & Lamont, E. (2000). Extent and determinants of error in doctors' prognoses in terminally ill patients: Prospective cohort study. *British Medical Journal, 320*, 469–472.

Committee on Bioethics, American Academy of Pediatrics. (1994). Guidelines on forgoing life-sustaining treatment. *Pediatrics, 93*, 532–536.

Cruzan v. Director, Missouri Department of Health, 497 DS 261 (1990).

Finucane, T., & Harper, M. (1996). Ethical decision-making near the end of life. *Clinics in Geriatric Medicine, 12,* 369–377.

Fohr, S. (1998). The double effect of pain medication: Separating myth from reality. *Journal of Palliative Medicine, 1,* 315–328.

Ganzini, L., & Dobscha, S. K. (2004). Clarifying distinctions between contemplating and completing physician-assisted suicide. *Journal of Clinical Ethics, 15,* 119–122.

Ganzini, L., Harvath, T. A., Jackson, A., Goy, E. R., Miller, L. L., & Delorit, B. A. (2002). Experiences of Oregon nurses and social workers with hospice patients who requested assistance with suicide. *New England Journal of Medicine, 347,* 582–588.

Ganzini, L., Nelson, H., Schmidt, T., Kraemer, D., Delorit, M., & Lee, M. (2000). Physicians' experiences with the Oregon Death With Dignity Act. *New England Journal of Medicine, 342,* 557–563.

Grisso, T., & Appelbaum, P. (1998). *Assessing competence to consent to treatment: A guide for physicians and other health professionals.* New York: Oxford University Press.

Halevy, A., & Brody, B. (1996). A multi-institution collaborative policy on medical futility. *Journal of the American Medical Association, 276,* 571–574.

Hendin, H. (1995). *Suicide in America.* New York: Norton.

Hendin, H. (1999). Suicide, assisted suicide, and euthanasia. In D. Jacobs (Ed.), *The Harvard Medical School guide to suicide assessment and intervention* (pp. 540–560). San Francisco: Jossey-Bass.

Hoefler, J. M. (1994). *Deathright: Culture, medicine, politics, and the right to die.* Boulder, CO: Westview Press.

In re Baby K, 16F3d 590 (4th Cir. 1994).

In re Quinlan, 755 A2A 647 (N.J.), cert. denied, 429 U.S. 922 (1976).

Kleespies, P. (2004). *Life and death decisions: Psychological and ethical considerations in end-of-life care.* Washington, DC: American Psychological Association.

Kleespies, P., Hughes, D., & Gallacher, F. (2000). Suicide in the medically ill and terminally ill: Psychological and ethical considerations. *Journal of Clinical Psychology, 56,* 1153–1171.

Kowalczyk, L. (2003, September 28). *Mortal differences divide hospital and patient's family.* Retrieved March 13, 2005, from http://www.boston.com/yourlife/health/children/articles/2003/09/28/mortal_differences_divide_hospital_ and_patient's_family

Kowalczyk, L. (2005, June 8). *Woman dies at MGH after battle over care: Daughter fought for life support.* Retrieved February 26, 2006, from http://www.boston.com/new/local/articles/2005/06/08/woman_dies_at_MGH_after_battle_over_care

Krakauer, E., Penson, R., Truog, R., King, L., Chabner, B., & Lynch, T. (2000). Sedation for intractable distress of a dying patient: Acute palliative care and the principle of double effect. *The Oncologist, 5,* 53–62.

Lynn, J. (2005). Living long in fragile health: The new demographics shape end of life care. *Hastings Center Report Special Report, 35*(6), S14–S18.

McCamish, M., & Crocker, N. (1993). Enteral and parenteral nutrition support of terminally ill patients: Practical and ethical perspectives. *The Hospice Journal, 9,* 107–129.

Meisel, A. (1995). *The right to die* (2nd ed.). New York: Wiley.

Meisel, A., Snyder, L., & Quill, T. (2000). Seven legal barriers to end-of-life care. *Journal of the American Medical Association, 284,* 2495–2501.

Mesler, M. A., & Miller, P. J. (2000). The structure and process of an inherent dilemma. *Death Studies, 24,* 135–155.

Miles, S. (1991). Informed demand for "non-beneficial" medical treatment. *New England Journal of Medicine, 325,* 512–515.

Miller, F., & Meier, D. (1998). Voluntary death: A comparison of terminal dehydration and physician-assisted suicide. *Annals of Internal Medicine, 128,* 559–562.

Miller, F., Quill, T., Brody, H., Fletcher, J., Gostin, L., & Meier, D. (1994). Sounding board: Regulating physician-assisted death. *New England Journal of Medicine, 331,* 119–123.

Miller, P., Hedlund, S., & Soule, A. (2006). Conversations at the end-of-life: The challenge to support patients who consider Death With Dignity in Oregon. *Journal of Social Work in End-of-Life and Palliative Care, 2,* 25–43.

Miller, P. J. (2000). Life after death with dignity: The Oregon experience. *Social Work, 45,* 263–271.

Miller, P. J., & Hedlund, S. C. (2005). "We just happen to live here." Two social workers share their stories about Oregon's Death With Dignity law. *Journal of Social Work in End-of-Life and Palliative Care,* 1, 71–86.

Miller, P. J., Mesler, M. A., & Eggman, S. T. (2002). Take some time to look inside their hearts: Hospice social workers contemplate physician-assisted suicide. *Social Work in Health Care, 35,* 53–64.

Miller, R. B. (1996). Assisted suicide and euthanasia: Arguments for and against practice, legalization and participation. In M. Battin & A. Lipman (Eds.), *Drug use in assisted suicide and euthanasia* (pp. 11–41). New York: Haworth.

Mishara, B. (1999). Synthesis of research and evidence on factors affecting the desire of terminally ill or seriously chronically ill persons to hasten death. *Omega, 39,* 1–70.

Murray, T., & Jennings, B. (2005). The quest to reform end of life care: Rethinking assumptions and setting new directions. *Hastings Center Report Special Report, 35*(6), S52–S57.

NBC5.com. (2005). *Houston mother loses fight to keep baby on life support.* NBC5.com. Retrieved on April 11, 2007, from http://www.nbc5.com/health/4286333/detail.html??z=dp&dpswid=1167317&dppid=65194

Nicholson, B., & Matross, G. (1989, May). Facing reduced decision-making capacity in healthcare: Methods for maintaining client self-determination. *Social Work, 34,* 234–238.

Okie, S. (2005). Physician-assisted suicide—Oregon and beyond. *New England Journal of Medicine, 352,* 1627–1630.

Oregon Death With Dignity Act, Oregon Revised Statutes 127.800–127.995 (1995).

Oregon Department of Human Services, Public Health Division. (2007). *Ninth annual report on Oregon's Death With Dignity Act.* Portland, OR: Author. Retrieved April 12, 2007, from http://egov.oregon.gov/DHS/ph/pas/ar-index.shtml

Orentlicher, D. (1997). The Supreme Court and physician-assisted suicide: Rejecting assisted suicide but embracing euthanasia. *New England Journal of Medicine, 337,* 1236–1239.

President's Commission for the Study of Ethical Problems in Medicine and Behavioral Research. (1983). *Deciding to forego life-sustaining treatment*. Washington, DC: U.S. Government Printing Office.

Preston, T. (1998). The rule of double effect [Letter to the editor]. *New England Journal of Medicine, 338*, 1389.

Quill, T., & Byock, I. (2000). Responding to intractable terminal suffering: The role of terminal sedation and voluntary refusal of food and fluids. *Annals of Internal Medicine, 132*, 408–414.

Quill, T., Dresser, R., & Brock, D. (1997). The rule of double effect—a critique of its role in end-of-life decision making. *New England Journal of Medicine, 337*, 1768–1771.

Quill, T., Lo, B., & Brock, D. (1997). Palliative options of last resort: A comparison of voluntarily stopping eating and drinking, terminal sedation, physician-assisted suicide, and voluntary active euthanasia. *Journal of the American Medical Association, 278*, 2099–2104.

Quill, T., Meier, D. E., Block, S. D., & Billings, J. A. (1998). The debate over physician-assisted suicide: Empirical data and convergent views. *Annals of Internal Medicine, 128*, 552–558.

Schorr, A. (1998). Re: The rule of double effect [Letter to the editor]. *New England Journal of Medicine, 338*, 1389–1390.

Singer, P. (1992). Nephrologists' experience with and attitudes toward decisions to forego dialysis. *Journal of the American Society of Nephrology, 7*, 1235–1240.

Snyder, J., & Swartz, M. (1993). Deciding to terminate treatment: A practical guide for physicians. *Journal of Critical Care, 8*, 177–185.

Statement of Schindler Family. May 17, 2004. Retrieved May 20, 2004, from http://www.terrisfight.org/press/051704statement.html

Task Force to Improve the Care of Terminally Ill Oregonians. (2007). *The Oregon Death With Dignity Act. A guidebook for health care providers*. Portland, OR: Author. Retrieved April 12, 2007, from http://www.ohsu.edu/ethics

Texas Advance Directive Act, Chapter 166, Section 46 (1999).

Texas Health and Safety Code, Section 166 (1999).

Thibault, G. (1997). Prognosis and clinical predictive models for critically ill patients. In M. Field & C. Cassel (Eds.), *Approaching death: Improving care at the end of life* (pp. 358–362). Washington, DC: National Academy Press.

Tolle, S. W., Rosenfeld, A. G., Tilden, V. P., & Park, Y. (1999). Oregon's low in-hospital death rates: What determines where people die and satisfaction with decision on place of death? *Annals of Internal Medicine, 130*, 681–185.

Tolle, S. W., Tilden, V. P., Drach, L. L., Fromme, E. K., Perrin, N. A., & Hedberg, K. (2004). Characteristics and proportion of dying Oregonians who personally consider physician-assisted suicide. *Journal of Clinical Ethics, 15*, 111–118.

Truog, R. (2000). Futility in pediatrics: From case to policy. *Journal of Clinical Ethics, 11*, 136–141.

Truog, R., Brett, A., & Frader, J. (1992). The problem with futility. *New England Journal of Medicine, 326*, 1560–1564.

Vacco v. Quill, 521 U.S. 793 (1997).

Washington v. Glucksberg, 521 U. S. 702 (1997).

Werth, J. L., Jr., and Kleespies, P. (2006). Ethical considerations in providing psychological services in end-of-life care. In J. L. Werth Jr., & D. Blevins (Eds.), *Psychosocial issues near the end of life: A resource for professional care providers* (pp. 57–87). Washington, DC: American Psychological Association.

Werth, J. L., Jr., & Wineberg, H. (2005). A critical analysis of criticisms of the Oregon Death with Dignity Act. *Death Studies, 29,* 1–27.

Wilson, W., Smedira, N., Fink, C., McDowell, J., & Luce, J. (1992). Ordering and administering of sedatives and analgesics during the withholding and withdrawal of life support from critically ill patients. *Journal of the American Medical Association, 267,* 949–953.

III

SECTION

Aspects of End-of-Life Choices and Decision Making

10

CHAPTER

Decision Making in Palliative Care

Victor T. Chang and Nethra Sambamoorthi

Introduction

Decision making can be challenging in palliative care (American Medical Association [AMA] Council, 1999; Back & Arnold, 2005; Gould, Williams, & Arnold, 2000; Karlawish, Quill, & Meier, 1999). In a patient-centered system that values patient autonomy, the patient's and caregiver's genuine participation in, and acceptance of decisions about, the patient's treatment are given high importance. Informed, clear decision making is important for patients, caregivers, and clinicians and may result in better compliance with treatment recommendations (DiMatteo, Giordani, Lepper, & Croghan, 2002) and long-term satisfaction (Jackson, Chamberlin, & Kroenke, 2001). The process of decision making has many components, including definition of a problem and possible solutions (choices), acquisition and communication of information regarding alternative choices, selection of ways to rank choices, acknowledging constraints, and selecting one choice. In palliative care, as in other medical care, patients, caregivers, and healthcare professionals should all participate and interact in making decisions. In this chapter, we review the decision-making process with an emphasis on the perspective of the patient and family/caregiver[1] in different settings. We start with general approaches and then consider specific situations in palliative medicine.

☐ The Process of Preparing for Decision Making

Before making a decision, the decision maker has to first accomplish a number of tasks. In this aspect of decision making, we start with the patient or caregiver's *perspective*, by which we mean the world as seen by the patient or caregiver. We then summarize information on preferences and values, followed by representation of knowledge and information processing. These last two terms are taken from the field of cognitive psychology. *Knowledge representation* refers to how persons conceptualize, organize, and store information. *Information processing* is a broader term and refers to how persons accept and use information and how this process is affected by emotions and the sociocultural context. The following illustrates this process for patients and caregivers.

Patient Decision Making

Patient's Perspective

The patient has to balance the information of a terminal outcome with his or her personal goals and relationships. General goals that may become important include survival, a sense of normalcy (Bottorff et al., 1998), and dignity (Chochinov, 2002). Psychologically, the patient has to cope with successive waves of physical deterioration. One qualitative study exploring patient decision making identified the process to include maintaining control over the disease, creating a system of support and safety, finding meaning, and creating a legacy (Coyle, 2006). Decision making can be affected by medically related issues (e.g., symptom distress, perceptions of staff and of treatment options, financial expenses, physical dependence); social issues (e.g., caregiver burden, support from others, family responsibilities, financial concerns); cultural issues (e.g., role expectations and fulfillment); spiritual issues (e.g., expectations of the afterlife); and emotional issues (e.g., hopelessness, grief, sorrow, anger, anxiety).

Patient's Preferences

Preferences help patients prioritize what they want done and form a first step in defining goals of care. Preferences may be shaped by personal or societal values and may guide choices. Treatment preferences of seriously ill patients revolve around the issues of likelihood of treatment success, treatment burden, and likelihood of cognitive and functional impairments related to treatment (Fried, Bradley, Towle, & Allore, 2002). Large-scale interview studies of patients in North America have identified common themes in patient preferences regarding care at the end of life. These include management of pain and symptoms, strengthening relationships, achieving a sense of control and closure, decision making about advance directives, and minimizing burden to family and society (Singer, Martin, & Kelner, 1999; Steinhauser et al., 2000).

Knowledge Representation

The theory and research related to knowledge representation are vast, and there are many ideas, but across these, there is a general consensus of a few key aspects. Most cognitive scientists consider the structure of one's knowledge as a series of interconnected nodes of information, with each node representing a single concept (e.g., death, life, dignity). How the nodes are interconnected is determined by learning and experience, including socialization into different cultures, religions, and so forth. This structure forms the basis for how information is received or heard by a person and how it is used. For example, a person who has only seen instances of dying in which there was poor symptom management and no support from an interdisciplinary team may associate the concept of death with pain and anguish, resulting in fear and other undesirable emotional reactions. This therefore will form the context within which that person makes decisions.

Biomedical knowledge, and therefore communicative understanding, is often rudimentary among nonmedically trained individuals. In a survey of 102 laypersons, researchers found poor comprehension of medical terms, including such information as where the liver was located (46%). However, the majority of respondents thought they understood the questions (Chapman, Abraham, Jenkins, & Fallowfield, 2003). In a multisite survey of inpatients regarding cardiopulmonary resuscitation (CPR), only 11% could name more than two components of CPR (Heyland et al., 2006). A survey of patients with advanced cancer who were receiving chemotherapy found that 29% thought they were receiving curative therapy (Craft, Burns, Smith, & Broom, 2005). A second consideration in knowledge representation is that the patient may be balancing the biomedical knowledge against other competing systems of knowledge, such as religious, cultural, magical, or family beliefs, that may hold higher validity in the patient's mind.

Information Processing

Patients want information, especially that which is treatment related (Rutten, Arora, Bakos, Aziz, & Rowland, 2005). However, individual patients vary in the amount of information desired and in their comprehension of what they have been told. This reflects the stressful nature of the clinical encounter, the patient's coping mechanisms (Miller, 1995), and how patients interact with their healthcare providers. The ability to process information may be limited because of stress. Recall of information can be impaired, especially of technical information. Research in decision aids and other psychological investigations have shown that how the information is presented, including how it is framed and whether a graphical format is used, can affect perception and processing (Wills & Holmes-Rovner, 2003). Additional factors relevant to patient reasoning include anecdotes (analogy, past experiences, and those of loved ones); fears and other emotions, (Redelmeier, Rozin, & Kahneman, 1993); the use of heuristics (rules of thumb), the presence of biases (e.g., zero risk, aversion to loss, avoidance of regret) (Chapman & Elstein, 2000); concurrent depression with inability to make a decision; and uncertainty about making the decision (decisional conflict) (O'Connor, 1995).

The role of religion in decision making has received increasing attention. Studies suggest that patients who are more religiously oriented may show less concern with prognosis, less interest in living wills, and increased willingness to undergo procedures (Johnson, Elbert-Avila, & Tulsky, 2005; True et al., 2005). Personal religious beliefs in miracles can also affect decisions. Careful exploration of unstated assumptions may be needed to understand a seemingly medically illogical decision (Lo et al., 2002).

Thus, information processing is a very complex process. It is not possible simply to examine the information presented to a person to ensure appropriate decision making; it is also necessary to consider the influence of such factors as existing knowledge about what is being discussed, past experiences, beliefs, biases, culture, religious beliefs, and emotional states.

Both Spannhake (chapter 3, this volume) and Raye (chapter 5, this volume) provide illustrations of this situation in their personal stories. Spannhake's emotional state was severely compromised because of the pain he was experiencing, which influenced the decision he was willing to make regarding treatment. As noted in other chapters in this book (see Hayslip and colleagues, chapter 17; Doka, chapter 16), persons who are less religious tend to support hastened death to avoid anticipated suffering and to maintain control at the end of life; this was precisely the case described by Raye in her family's assistance in her father's death.

Caregiver Decision Making

Caregiver decision making assumes added importance in palliative care, during which most patients will at some point become unable to decide for themselves, often without any written advance directives. This is an area of intense clinical and research interest. Although the cognitive elements of information processing are the same as those outlined for patients, there are additional factors to consider when exploring decision making among caregivers.

Caregiver Perspectives

Caregivers are confronted with the patient's needs and symptoms and, often, shrinking financial resources, limited support, and their own physical and knowledge limitations (Rabow, Hauser, & Adams, 2004; Wolff, Dy, Frick, & Kasper, 2007), which can all influence information processing. In one large survey of primarily female family members providing care at home, nearly 90% required assistance of some kind (Emanuel, Fairclough, & Slutsman, 1999). Supportive care challenges for caregivers generally include one or more of the following barriers: (a) family related, (b) health system, and (c) communication and informational. Specific barriers are also possible and can include impaired concentration of the caregivers, conspiracies of silence, timing of information, and caregiver rejection of support (Hudson, Aranda, & Kristjanson, 2004).

Caregiver Preferences

Whether explicit or not, caregivers must balance their own preferences with that of honoring the patient's preferences, in the context of what a patient needs and the amount of support available. The gap between the amount of support available and caring for the patient's needs is stressful, and much of the information needed by caregivers centers on how to provide and get help for the patient.

Although caregivers want information, less is known about how the information is organized and interpreted by them. The potential lack of comprehension by caregivers is illustrated in a French study: After meeting the medical doctor, half of the representatives of intensive care unit (ICU) patients were unable to understand the diagnosis, prognosis, or treatment plans for the ICU patient (Azoulay et al., 2000). It is unknown to what extent this applies to the United States, but the results would presumably be similar. In a systematic review of articles on family decision making, reasoning about end-of-life decisions was seen by family members as the result of the context of a larger family relationship with the patient, developed over time, including previous family deliberations over his or her clinical course (Meeker & Jezewski, 2005).

One important area for palliative care decision making is discordance—when the patient and caregivers disagree about care (disagreements between patient/caregivers and medical staff also occur but are not discussed here; see Csikai, chapter 11, this volume). Familial conflicts have been reported in patients receiving treatment for lung cancer (Zhang

& Siminoff, 2003) and in deciding on the place of death (Tang, Liu, Lai, & McCorkle, 2005). Although families have been shown to value consensus in decision making as well as the sense of acting as the patient's advocate (Meeker & Jezewski, 2005), almost every area can become conflictual in palliative care, from perception of pain severity and its management, to choosing between disease-oriented treatments designed to provide a small improvement in survival and treatments for comfort only.

Balancing the perspectives of caregivers in the decision-making process requires the involvement of healthcare providers. In an interview study of 461 bereaved family members of older patients, the most common recommendation for healthcare professionals was better communication (44%), followed by more physician time (17%), and symptom control (10%) (Hanson, Danis, & Garrett, 1997). When such issues are addressed, caregiver involvement in the process may be facilitated and improved on, minimizing the influence of stress and other socioemotional and healthcare system barriers.

□ Models of Decision Making

Decision making can be classified as descriptive models (how decisions are actually made), normative models (how best decisions can be made), and prescriptive models (what can be done to improve decision making). Commonly encountered decision-making approaches are summarized under these three groups, although recognize that there is some overlap. As shown in Table 10.1, the models vary by how much relative involvement different stakeholders have throughout the process and at what points in the care process the model may be appropriate.

Descriptive Models

Descriptive models summarize observations of how different participants (e.g., the patient, caregivers, medical staff) in the decision-making process might select a course of action when a decision has to be made.

Physician-Centered Approach

In this approach, the physician makes the decision with the implicit agreement of the patient and the caregiver. Although patient input may be solicited, it is not strongly associated with the decision reached by the provider. This is an example of the paternalistic approach to care that is often

TABLE 10.1 Summary of Decision-Making Models

Model	Defining Feature	Conditions When Likely to Be Important	Applications to Palliative Care
Physician centered	MD makes decisions	When patient would prefer not to be or is unable to be actively involved	Decision making for unconscious patients without health care proxy
Patient centered	Patient makes decisions	When patient has capacity to decide	Discussions regarding goals of care, such as do not resuscitate orders, or designation of health care proxy
Family centered	Family makes decisions	Patients from some cultures, when patient does not have capacity or desire to be involved	Interdependent cultures, especially when patient does not have capacity
Recognition primed	"Gut reaction" based on experience and intuition	Emergency situations, ill-defined situations	Need to make quick decisions, often in uncertain situations and without known existing patient preferences (transfer to intensive care unit)
Rational choice	Explicit listing of choices and preferences	Conflict resolution, need for optimizing a solution	Family conferences
Utility and uncertainty	Measure of patient preferences under uncertainty	Need to mathematically model complex decisions	None at this time
Shared	Patient and MD make decisions	Most decisions when patient has capacity and desire	Many decisions, such as when to pursue or stop disease-modifying therapy
Structured	Similar to rational choice, but no clear decision maker specified	Need for optimizing a solution, especially when decision is responsibility of a team	None at this time

criticized in contemporary literature. Nevertheless, it may be appropriate when the patient, or sometimes the caregiver, is unwilling or unable to participate.

Patient-Centered Decision Making

Patient-centered decision making is a logical consequence of patient-centered care and autonomy, by which the patient makes caregiving decisions for personal care. This approach can cause more anxiety for patients (Gatellari, Voigt, Butow, & Tattersall, 2002) but occurs more frequently as patients become more experienced with an illness (Grunfeld et al., 2006). Patient-centered care is a core tenant of the palliative care movement and feelings of anxiety can be minimized with the appropriate degree and format of communication and support from loved ones and healthcare providers.

Family-Centered Decision Making

The family-centered decision-making style can most commonly be seen in Asian and southern European cultures. The family makes the decision with the physician, and not the patient, often with nondisclosure of diagnosis to the patient, with the intent of protecting the patient. It is more likely to occur when the patient is elderly and the prognosis is poor (Back & Huak, 2005). Accommodation to family-centered decision making for patients from other cultures can be a difficult process for North American practitioners (Lapine et al., 2001). One simple approach is to ask the patient if he or she would like to have the family take over (Freedman, 1993). The willingness of providers to do this emphasizes the importance of flexibility when palliative care physicians see patients who have recently immigrated from other parts of the world. In practice, when the patient is unable to communicate, palliative care teams will employ family-centered approaches (Lan & Quill, 2004; Levine & Zuckerman, 1999).

Normative Models

Normative models address processes through which decisions are made in healthcare settings from a theoretical viewpoint as opposed to research indicating what actually happens. Four common types of processes are presented, along with how they may be executed in actual clinical settings:

Recognition-Primed Decisions

Recognition-primed decisions are based primarily on experience and intuition (Klein, 2001). The decision that results from some piece of information is largely automatic or a "knee-jerk" reaction. An example might be the decision to initiate CPR in a hospital emergency room (ER) setting or medical inpatient ward, where initiation of CPR is rarely questioned and automatically engaged in as a standard of care. In palliative care, this may be seen in an immediate decision by patients or caregivers that an option is not acceptable. For example, personal and cultural beliefs may immediately result in rejecting any decision that involves reducing or stopping curative care.

Rational Choice Strategy Decisions

The rational choice strategy (RCS) decision is usually held as the standard for ideal decision making and lends itself to mathematical analyses, such as with decision trees, in which each choice is given a weight, and an optimal choice can often be determined (Hunink et al., 2001) with sufficient information. Characteristics of this approach include defining the goals to be achieved, defining the goals of the decision to be made, and resolving conflicts through open communication among all participants. It is assumed that decisions are arrived at and accomplished in the absence of extraordinary time pressures. This approach makes explicit the choices and values of all participants. Clinically, this might apply to multidisciplinary or family conferences held to discuss the management of a patient. One example in palliative care is the ethical grid approach, in which the views of the patient, caregivers, and team regarding the medical situation, patient preferences, quality of life, and contextual features are elicited and respected in reaching a decision (Kuhl & Wilensky,1999).

Psychological Models

We include the area of psychological models under normative models because it provides important insights from various psychological theories about decision making. It is a collection of assumptions about how decisions are made that includes theoretical approaches such as contingent decision behavior, dominance structuring theory, and differentiation and consolidation theory. According to several of these theories, the choice of decision rules and strategy depends on the problem, person, and social context. One alternative decision among those possible may eventually dominate over others for various reasons related to information processing. Another way to examine the decision-making process is to consider the interaction of the psychological process before and the anticipated processes after the decision. It is assumed that before a decision is made, alternatives are differentiated from each other by decision rules, attractiveness representations, and potential regret, followed by the defense of a decision against possible threats once it is made (Svenson, 1992). In prospect theory, alternatives are laid out as in rational choice, and psychological cognitive processes are examined to develop preferences. Specifically, decision makers are thought to have a reference level, an aspiration level, and a risk level. Framing effects are recognized—risk taking tends to be minimized when gains are expected and maximized when losses are expected. (Hastie & Dawes, 2000; Tversky & Kahneman, 1981). In practice, patients appear to use a more intuitive, emotionally driven process that incorporates normative data when deciding among options (Weinberger, personal communication, 2006). More research is needed to understand how closely these models reflect actual decision making in palliative care.

Utility- and Uncertainty-Based Decision Making

According to the utility- and uncertainty-based decision-making approach, in the presence of uncertainty, preferences by a person are assigned to different outcomes. Decision trees are constructed by which options are weighted, and optimal choices are determined by both preferences and probabilities assigned to different outcomes. The application of this type of decision making to clinical care has been limited by the inability of patients to provide numerical values for preferences. This model is identified as normative because it contains certain principles and methods that could be part of a prescriptive method.

Prescriptive Models

Prescriptive models reflect current approaches to decision making, with the intent of improving decisions made by patients. We focus primarily on one approach, shared decision making, because it has become the dominant perspective adopted in the literature.

Shared Decision-Making Approach

Shared medical decision making is a process by which all stakeholders jointly agree on a course of treatment given knowledge about patient preferences and the expected results of various decisions (Frosch & Kaplan, 1999). The emphasis on the collaboration between patients and providers reflects an increasing interest on the part of patients to be part of the decision-making process and societal trends for increased patient autonomy (Charles, Gafni, & Whelan, 1997; Deber, Kraetschmer, & Irvine, 1996; McNutt, 2004). This is currently considered the ideal approach to decision making.

In practice, shared decision making can have different meanings. One is that the physician shares the information with the patient, and the patient makes the decision. Another interpretation is that the patient shares his or her values and preferences with the physician, and the physician makes the decision. A recent review identified 418 articles on shared decision making in the context of a patient provider relationship: 161 had a conceptual definition, and 31 separate concepts were identified. The authors presented an integrated model, consisting of essential components (define and explain the problem, present options, discuss risks and benefits, elicit patient values and preferences, discuss patient ability and self-efficacy, present a recommendation, check or clarify understanding, make a decision or agree to delay, arrange for follow-up); ideal components (unbiased information, present evidence, define desire for involvement, mutual agreement); and general qualities (deliberation/negotiation, flexibility/individualized approach, information exchange, involves at least two people, middle ground, mutual respect, patient education, patient participation, process/ stages) (Makoul & Clayman, 2006).

Some theorists have held that not all decisions may call for shared decision making. According to Whitney (2003), for example, decisions are defined by (a) importance of a decision (major or minor) and (b) certainty of an appropriate course of treatment. He held that only decisions that have high importance and low certainty require involvement of the patient. Situations of low importance (minor decisions) and high certainty are unlikely to generate patient preference for collaboration (e.g., choice of intravenous fluids). Situations of high importance and high certainty can lead to an easy consensus of treatment choices under a shared, collaborative approach to decision making but may also result in conflicts if disagreements arise in preferences between the patient and provider. However, such situations also lend themselves well to the shared decision-making process to reach consensus.

Patients, as a group, tend to be ambivalent about shared decision making. In a Canadian survey of 436 patients with newly diagnosed cancer and 482 control patients, 59% of newly diagnosed patients preferred a passive role, whereas 64% of the control participants preferred an active role in decision making (Degner & Sloan, 1992). Age, education, and gender were key predictors of preferences. Neither symptom distress nor extent of disease affected preferences. These results suggest that not all patients want to have an active role in decision making. In a survey of 78 patients with advanced cancer seen at a palliative care clinic, active decision making was chosen by 16 (20%), shared decision making by 49 (63%), and passive decision making by 13 (17%) patients. Full agreement between physicians and patient ratings of the type of decision-making approach was present for 30 (38%) patients (Bruera, Sweeney, Calder, Palmer, & Benisch-Tolley, 2001). Furthermore, interviews with cancer inpatients at a university medical center showed a wide range of meanings assigned to participation in decision making and the importance of specific knowledge about the disease. Both nurses and physicians were considered authoritative sources of information, and barriers to participation included the patient's rating of lack of knowledge about the disease, arrogance of the nursing and medical staff, lack of time to talk, and high rates of staff turnover. For patients, participation included not only medical decisions but also nursing decisions and gathering information (Benbassat, Pilpel, & Tidhar, 1998; Sainio, Lauri, & Eriksson, 2001).

A predictor of the degree of shared decision making with physicians is the level of patient trust of healthcare providers. In a study of 606 patients seen in clinics at a Toronto hospital, blind trust was associated with a passive role and high levels of trust and disease familiarity with shared decision making. Low levels of trust were associated with a more skeptical approach to decision making (Kraetschmer, Sharpe, Urowitz, & Deber, 2004). Other factors include amount of experience with the disease, age, personal attitude toward shared decision making, type of decision, and interactions with healthcare personnel (Say, Murtagh, & Thomson, 2006).

The willingness of family members to participate in decision making also cannot be assumed. The family members may not even be physically present in today's era of modern communications. Studies of family members of ICU patients showed that approximately 40% of family members in Canada (Heyland, Cook, et al., 2003) and 50% of family members in France (Azoulay et al., 2004) would prefer not to be involved. In the French study, predictors for the desire to participate included the desire for more information, and a predictor for decreased desire to participate was the sense of comprehension of the care given. Although similar studies have not been conducted in the United States, these conclusions are likely to be consistent in the United States as well.

The concept of shared decision making has led to the development of decision aids and other tools. A decision aid is a standardized evidence-based tool intended to facilitate the process of arriving at an informed, values-based choice among two or more healthcare alternatives (O'Connor, Graham, & Visser, 2005). The role of decision aids remains an area of investigation, with applications to date in patients with advanced emphysema (Dales et al., 1999; Wilson et al., 2005) and for treatment decisions in patients with advanced cancer (Leighl, Butow, & Tattersall, 2004). One review of the development of decision aids for patients with early prostate cancer found substantial heterogeneity in the types of information providers thought were appropriate, in what patients considered important, and how formats for presenting data affected retention of information (Feldman-Stewart, Brundage, McConnell, & MacKillop, 2000). Decision aids may be more helpful for the integration of information than for clarifying values. Nurse-administered decision aids, such as the Ottawa decision support framework, provide additional ways to help patients with difficult decisions (Murray, Miller, Fiset, O'Connor, & Jacobsen, 2004). Further, questions include how to integrate the decision aid into the decision-making process and how decision aids are to be evaluated (Elwyn et al., 2006; Feldman-Stewart & Brundage, 2000).

Structured Decision Making

In addition to shared decision making, one other predictive model deserves mention because it is reflected in the contemporary literature. Structured decision-making (SDM) models rely on the underlying concept that a decision regarding a problem is really a set of decisions, each of which covers a specific aspect of the problem at hand. For example, in managing an outpatient with advanced cancer, when new symptoms arise that are highly indicative of a medical emergency, a structured decision approach would encompass consideration of factors such as reassessment of treatment options, goals of care, communication with the patient, negotiating family conflicts, and affirmation of patient choices (Weissman, 2004). This involves a detailed, step-by-step walk-through of each decision that needed to be made in a case. This approach is especially relevant when a chief decision maker is lacking, but a decision is relegated to a team, requiring skills in conferences and managing multiple objectives.

Summary and Comparison

Table 10.1 summarizes and compares the models. These decision models are not mutually exclusive in that all may be applicable at different points in a patient's trajectory in advanced illness. There is substantial heterogeneity in how patients and their caregivers approach a decision, with the preferences of decision makers influencing which model, and when a given model, is appropriate and adopted.

□ Decision Making in Palliative Care

In this section, we review special concerns that arise in palliative care and decision-making issues specific to various diseases and sites of care common at the end of life.

Special Features of Decisions in Palliative Care

A number of features in palliative care lend poignancy and desperation to the decision-making process. For most illnesses, the outcome is not known at the time of decision making. Here, one outcome, death, is known, as well as the anticipation that it will occur soon. However, the length of survival is unknown. The limitations of physicians' ability to estimate a prognosis is well known. Furthermore, patients have to reconcile different estimates by different providers (Davey, Butow, & Armstrong, 2003). Patients and caregivers often receive different opinions from different subspecialists (Penson, Kyriakou, Zuckerman, Chabner, & Lynch, 2006), which may be couched in euphemisms. The potential for misunderstanding is illustrated by the following findings.

The SUPPORT (Study to Understand Prognoses and Preferences for Outcomes and Risks of Treatment) study found that patients with metastatic lung or colon cancer greatly overestimated their probabilities of surviving greater than 6 months, and this perception led them to seek more aggressive treatments (Weeks et al., 1998). The extent to which patients wish to know their prognosis is highly individual, and the means by which it is communicated may have to be tailored to the patient's communication preferences (Butow, Dowsett, Hagerty, & Tattersall, 2002; Clayton, Butow, & Tattersall, 2005). In one survey of 206 primary family caregivers regarding physician caregiver communication at the time of hospice referral, 20% stated they had not been told the patient's disease was incurable, 40% never received a prognosis, and 33% had not discussed hospice with the caregiver. Physician discussions influenced caregivers' perceptions of illness, but only 25% of caregivers agreed with the medical doctor's prognosis (Cherlin et al., 2005). This uncertainty by patients and caregivers regarding expected survival affects willingness to take risks when making decisions.

Cancer patients seen in consultation at an Australian tertiary care cancer center were informed about treatments and side effects, but only 57% were told about survival, 30% were given a management choice, and a mere 10% were asked if they comprehended what they had heard (Gatellari et al., 2002). In another study of Dutch patients who were seeing an oncologist to decide between palliative chemotherapy and watchful waiting, the incurability of disease was mentioned 84% of the time, the procedure of chemotherapy in 77%, effect of chemotherapy on survival in 55%, and watchful waiting was mentioned as a single sentence in 23% and explained in 27% (Koedoot et al., 2004). No such studies have been performed in the United States. These kinds of data suggest that changes in communication patterns and sources of information have the potential to alter patient decisions (Matsuyama, Reddy, & Smith, 2006).

Crow (chapter 4, this volume) demonstrated her frustration with poor communication from the medical provider caring for her brother. The lack of information and open discussion created frustration and anger and likely was partially the impetus for the arguments that subsequently resulted with her father in trying to adapt to the situation. Further, decision making on the part of the family would likely have been more constructive and appropriate to respect the wishes of her brother had the physicians described the nature and extent of the injuries incurred in the accident, something that did not occur until an outside provider was brought in to assist.

The second feature of decision making near the end of life that is unlike other fields of medicine is that discussions often center on perceived withdrawal of care, rather than interventions, although there are large cultural variations in desire for care. The burden of medical diagnostic tests is weighed more heavily, the value of simple medical treatments (oxygen, blood transfusions, intravenous lines, gastrostomy tubes) is questioned, and placement decisions (e.g., in a nursing home, with or without hospice care) become paramount. For many people, although not all, information often becomes more important as a way to cope with uncertainty (see Csikai, chapter 11, this volume).

A third feature is that the context or clinical setting frequently changes, often shifting from acute medical care to end-of-life care to medical crisis, and decisions have to be revisited and revised. Each of these settings has different traditions in approaching illness, and the underlying assumptions of the setting and healthcare personnel may be confusing to patients and family members.

A fourth feature is ambivalence. Ambivalence to death can arise from deep fear of the unknown. Decisions regarding end-of-life care are not embraced the same way as are decisions about curative treatment. Patients may prefer to receive treatments and to remain partially ignorant to avoid confronting death, even at the risk of worsened health (De Haes & Koedoot, 2003). This ambivalence is not only personal but also rooted in social and cultural norms (Burt, 2003) and may be more pronounced in younger patients. From a decision-making standpoint, this means that a decision may always be subject to last-minute changes unless consolidation of the decision is effective.

A fifth feature is the potential for misunderstanding when the physicians and patients come from different backgrounds. As noted, this can arise in family-centered models of decision making. In the United States, differences between European Americans and African Americans have been the main area of research interest, with some additional studies on patients from Asian decent and different socioeconomic backgrounds. These studies suggest a universality in perspectives of the most important elements of family involvement in decision making that can cross cultural barriers (Born, Greiner, Sylvia, Butler, & Ahluwahlia, 2004; Koffman & Higginson, 2001; see Hayslip, Hansson, Starkweather, & Dolan, chapter 17, this volume).

A sixth feature is *conflict*, defined as a "clash, competition, or mutual interference of opposing or incompatible forces or qualities (as ideas, interests, wills)" characterized by antagonism (*Websters*, 1976, p. 585). The presence of conflict in palliative care often generates headlines, and the topic has been recently reviewed (Mpinga, Chastonay, & Rapin, 2006; see

Cerminara, chapter 8, this volume). Methods to solve these conflicts constitute another aspect of decision making and may include consultation with ethics committees, pragmatic ethics (Fins & Miller, 2000), mediation (Dubler & Liebman, 2004), and sometimes litigation (Meisel, 2005). Two situations that commonly lead to such conflicts are when the patient does not have the capacity to make decisions (see Volicer, chapter 18, this volume) and when there is a request for hastened death (see Raye, chapter 5, this volume).

□ Decision Making Across Diseases and Sites of Care

Although there are many commonalities across different terminal diseases, some conditions may have unique influences on decision making. The same is true when considering different sites where care can occur. The unique characteristics interact in complex ways with psychosocial and spiritual factors discussed throughout this book. There are two related factors, however, that often differentiate the decision-making processes across disease states and sites of care: prognostication and communication. These variables are illustrated for some of the common terminal diseases in the United States.

As noted, prognostication is difficult, and many providers are hesitant to offer survival estimates for fear of being wrong; however, some diseases have more predictable trajectories than others. For example, most forms of cancer have a fairly predictable course, and prognosis is somewhat more certain, yet it can be difficult to know when to stop curative treatment because of the increasing range of treatments available (see Field, chapter 6, this volume).

Most of the other leading causes of death (e.g., congestive heart failure, chronic obstructive pulmonary disease, dementia; see Field, chapter 5, this volume) have a more uncertain trajectory, making prognosticating, and hence decision making, very difficult. In addition, patients with dementia and other severe central nervous system disorders pose unique challenges because their mental capacity to participate in decision making is limited or absent; thus, decisions fall almost exclusively to the medical team and the family. Such situations necessitate choosing certain decision-making models over others. For example, in one study of decision making for hospice placement, patients receiving hospice care were older, more likely to have accepted their prognosis, and to know about hospice at the time of the decision, however, the majority of decisions to enter hospice were made by families (Chen, Haley, Robinson, & Schonwetter,

2003). These types of family-based decisions are influenced by numerous factors, such as communication needs and unmet needs of patients, and interact with caregiver characteristics.

The interaction of these factors can be seen in a survey of 65 Dutch caregivers, who were asked to rate the relative importance of several factors they viewed as supportive. Communication was rated as the most important, followed by information about nursing skills, their own health, their social network, bereavement, and a support program (Jansma, Schure, & de Jong, 2005). In a study of caregivers for veterans with cancer, caregiver needs were related to information and symptom management. Unmet needs and caregiver depression led to increased caregiver burden (Hwang et al., 2003). A study of Australian caregivers also identified a relationship between unmet patient needs, increased caregiver burden, and worsened caregiver health (Sharpe, Butow, Smith, McConnell, & Clarke, 2005). Thus, communication and information are critical to decision making, interacting with the social and emotional characteristics of the decision maker.

A similar illustration of such an interaction can be seen in a British survey of caregivers regarding treatment decisions for patients with advanced dementia; approximately half of the caregivers wanted all four of the available treatments suggested on the survey: CPR, intravenous fluids, intravenous antibiotics, and oral antibiotics. Information about quality of life and severity of dementia did not affect the choices (Potkins et al., 2000). This type of evidence points to the need to understand the motivations and reasons for the care choices elected by family members to determine the reasons one decision is chosen over another.

Regardless of the terminal illness one may confront, there seem to be several common themes across caregiving situations of patients, and these include symptom control, diverse attitudes regarding what end-of-life care should look like in terms of prolonging life, and problematic communications. However, certain disease states have unique characteristics that should be considered. Further, the site within which decision making occurs similarly influences the perspectives of patients, family, and providers (Jansma et al., 2005; Sharpe et al., 2005).

As noted by Field (chapter 5, this volume) and Prevost and Wallace (chapter 12, this volume), institutions are the most common site of end-of-life care. Communication and access to accurate information to inform decision making continue to be crucial in such settings, but it is also important to consider the influence and circumstances that will be present while decisions are made.

For example, decision making in the ICU presents patients and family with the entire spectrum of medical interventions within a compressed time frame, but the burden is usually experienced most by families because patients frequently do not have capacity to participate in the process. The need for family support is increasingly recognized in such situations (Davidson et al., 2007). Caregivers deal with high levels of stress and uncertainty and rely heavily on staff interactions while making decisions in the ICU. A high prevalence of anxiety (69%) and depression (34%) among family members was found in a survey of 920 family members of French ICU patients (Pochard et al., 2001). The following communication needs were identified: for information, for honesty, for clear communication, for informed clinicians, and for clinicians to listen (Norton, Tilden, Tolle, Nelson, & Eggman, 2003).

Medical ICU nurses at one hospital suggested that barriers to a decision for transition to palliative care included family misunderstandings, family discord, younger patient age, and shifting medical decisions (Badger, 2005). Families often identify staff as a source of stress. In an interview study of 48 family members 1 year after the ICU stay of a loved one at a major American medical center, 22 (46%) perceived conflict with staff and perceived unprofessionalism as a frequent source of stress. Discussions regarding end-of-life care did not upset these respondents (Abbot, Sago, Breen, Abernethy, & Tulsky, 2001). Conversely, adequate information, good decision making, and respect and compassion for the patient were predictors of satisfaction in postmortem surveys of Canadian ICU family members (Heyland, Rocker, O'Callaghan, Dodek, & Cook, 2003). Thus, the interaction of healthcare providers and family members is critical to the decision-making process, directly influencing perceived levels of stress and burden and indirectly having the potential to affect the caregiving choices.

Another common site of death is in nursing homes (see Prevost and Wallace, chapter 12, this volume). Although end-of-life preferences and experiences of nursing home residents and family members have received significant attention in the literature, decision making has not. Common decisions include when to transfer patients to an acute care facility and when to start a palliative care approach, which could include specific treatment decisions, in addition to electing hospice care.

Although 25% of all deaths occur in nursing homes (Centers for Disease Control and Prevention [CDC], 2003), these facilities have a reputation of providing poor end-of-life care, with both physical and psychosocial issues neglected (Blevins & Deason-Howell, 2003; Harrington, 2001; Kayser-Jones, 2002). In a national sample of family members of patients who had died 9–15 months prior, respondents expressed concerns over untreated physical symptoms, poor communications with physicians, lack of respect for patients, and inadequate emotional support. Although home hospice fared better than nursing homes or hospitals, all sites showed significant deficiencies (Teno et al., 2004). All of these factors have the potential to impact the decision-making process and the eventual decisions made by patients and family members near the end of life.

Summary and Conclusions

This chapter summarized various decision-making approaches commonly employed in medical settings and their relevance to palliative care. We also highlighted various issues that are unique to persons near the end of life across and within particular disease states and different settings. What emerges from this review of patient and caregiver perspectives is the great breadth of individual, group, and cultural variations in approaches to decisions, concepts of autonomy, the need for different types of information at different depths of description, and styles of communicating. The complex interaction of all of these factors needs to be considered in the understanding of the decision-making process.

Also illustrated throughout this chapter was the need for additional research on many aspects of the decision-making process for patients, caregivers, and providers near the end of life. Future advances may lie in more flexible interpretation of autonomy by physicians for different groups (Wenzelberg, Hanson, & Tulsky, 2005), improved communication, and a better understanding of interactions among the various participants and issues important to decision-making processes.

Acknowledgment

We thank Samer Nasr, M.D., Brooke Sorger, Ph.D., and Lawrence Weinberger, Ph.D., for their comments. Authors' time was partially supported by funding by the Department of Veterans Affairs (grant VA HSRD IIR 02-103).

Note

1. *Family* in this chapter is used in the broadest sense, to include biological relatives and spouses or friends and other loved ones.

References

Abbot, K. H., Sago, J. G., Breen, C. M., Abernethy, A. P., & Tulsky, J. (2001). Families looking back: One year after discussion of withdrawal or withholding of life support. *Critical Care Medicine, 29*, 197–201.

American Medical Association (AMA) Council on Ethical and Judicial Affairs. (1999). Medical futility in end of life care. *Journal of the American Medical Association, 281*, 937–941.

Azoulay, E., Chevret, S., Leleu, G., Pochard, F., Barboteu, M., Adrie, C., et al. (2000). Half the families of intensive care unit physicians experience inadequate communication with physicians. *Critical Care Medicine, 28*, 3044–3049.

Azoulay, E., Pochard, F., Chevret, S., Adrie, C., Annane, D., Bleichner, G., et al. (2004). Half the family members of intensive care unit patients do not want to share in the decision-making process: A study in 78 French intensive care units. *Critical Care Medicine, 32*, 1832–1838.

Back, A., & Arnold R. (2005). Dealing with conflict in caring for the seriously ill. "It was just out of the question." *Journal of the American Medical Association, 293*, 374–381.

Back, M. F., & Huak, C. Y. (2005). Family centered decision-making and non-disclosure of diagnosis in a southeast Asian oncology practice. *Psycho-Oncology, 14*, 1052–1059.

Badger, J. M. (2005). Factors that enable or complicate end-of-life transitions in critical care. *American Journal of Critical Care, 14*, 513–522.

Benbassat, J., Pilpel, D., & Tidhar, M. (1998). Patients' preferences for participation in clinical decision-making: A review of published surveys. *Behavioral Medicine, 24*, 81–88.

Blevins, D., & Deason-Howell, L. M. (2002). End-of-life care in nursing homes: The interface of policy, research, and practice. *Behavioral Sciences and the Law, 20*, 271–286.

Born, W., Greiner, K. A., Sylvia, E., Butler, J., & Ahluwahlia, J. (2004). Knowledge, attitudes, and beliefs about end-of-life care among inner-city African Americans and Latinos. *Journal of Palliative Medicine, 7*, 247–256.

Bottorff, J. L., Steele, R., Davies, B., Garossino, C., Porterfield, P., & Shaw, M. (1998). Striving for balance: Palliative care patients' experiences of making everyday choices. *Journal of Palliative Care, 14*, 7–17.

Bruera, E., Sweeney, C., Calder, K., Palmer, L., & Benisch-Tolley, S. (2001). Patient preferences versus physician perceptions of treatment decisions in cancer care. *Journal of Clinical Oncology, 19*, 2883–2885.

Burt, R. A. (2003). *Death is that man taking names. Intersections of American medicine, law, and culture.* Berkeley: University of California Press.

Butow, P. N., Dowsett, S., Hagerty, R., & Tattersall, M. H. N. (2002). Communicating prognosis to patients with metastatic disease: What do they really want to know? *Supportive Care in Cancer, 10*, 161–168.

Centers for Disease Control and Prevention (CDC). (2003). *Characteristics of hospice care discharges and their length of service, United States, 2003*. Retrieved January 10, 2003, from http://www.cdc.gov/nchs/pressroom/03facts/hospicecare.htm

Chapman, G. B., & Elstein, A. S. (2000). Cognitive processes and biases in medical decision-making. In G. B. Chapman & F. A. Sonnenberg (Eds.), *Decision-making in health care. Theory, psychology, and applications* (pp. 183–210). New York: Cambridge University Press.

Chapman, K., Abraham, C., Jenkins, V., & Fallowfield, L. (2003). Lay understanding of terms used in cancer consultations. *Psycho-Oncology, 12*, 557–566.

Charles, C., Gafni, A., & Whelan, T. (1997). Shared decision-making in the medical encounter: What does it mean? (or it takes at least two to tango). *Social Sciences and Medicine, 44*, 681–692.
Chen, H., Haley, E., Robinson, B. E., & Schonwetter, R. S. (2003). Decisions for hospice care in patients with advanced cancer. *Journal of the American Geriatrics Society, 51*, 789–797.
Cherlin, E., Fried, T., Prigerson, H., Schulman-Green, D., Johnson-Hurzeler, R., & Bradley, E. H. (2005). Communication between physicians and family caregivers about care at the end of life: When do discussions occur and what is said? *Journal of Palliative Medicine, 8*, 1176–1185.
Chochinov, H. (2002). Dignity conserving care. A new model for palliative care. Helping the patient to feel valued. *Journal of the American Medical Association, 287*, 2253–2260.
Clayton, J. N., Butow, P. N., & Tattersall, M. H. (2005). When and how to initiate discussion about prognosis and end of life issues with terminally ill patients. *Journal of Pain and Symptom Management, 30*, 132–144.
Coyle, N. (2006). The hard work of living in the face of death. *Journal of Pain and Symptom Management, 32*, 266–274.
Craft, P. S., Burns, C. M., Smith, W. T., & Broom, D. H. (2005). Knowledge of treatment intent among patients with advanced cancer: A longitudinal study. *European Journal of Cancer Care, 14*, 417–425.
Dales, R. E., O'Connor, A., Hebert, P., Sullivan, K., McKim, D., & Llewellyn-Thomas, H. (1999). Intubation and mechanical ventilation for COPD: Development of an instrument to elicit patient preferences. *Chest, 116*, 792–800.
Davey, H. M., Butow, P. N., & Armstrong, B. K. (2003). Cancer patients' preferences for written prognostic information provided outside the clinical context. *British Journal on Cancer, 89*, 1450–1456.
Davidson, J. E., Powers, K., Hedayat, K. M., Tieszen, M., Kon, A. A., Shepard, E., et al. (2007). Clinical practice guidelines for support of the family in the patient-centered intensive care unit: American College of Critical Medicine Task Force 2004–2005. *Critical Care Medicine, 35*, 605–622.
Deber, R. B., Kraetschmer, N., & Irvine, J. (1996). What role do patients wish to play in treatment decision-making? *Archives of Internal Medicine, 156*, 1414–1420.
Degner, L. F., & Sloan, J. A. (1992). Decision-making during serious illness: What role do patients really want to play? *Journal of Clinical Epidemiology, 45*, 941–950.
De Haes, H., & Koedoot, N. (2003). Patient centered decision-making in palliative cancer treatment: A world of paradoxes. *Patient Education Counsel, 50*, 43–49.
DiMatteo, M. R., Giordani, P. J., Lepper, H. S., & Croghan, T. W. (2002). Patient adherence and medical treatment outcomes: A meta-analysis. *Medical Care, 40*, 794–811.
Dubler, N. N., & Liebman, C. B. (2004). *Bioethics mediation. A guide to shaping shared solutions.* New York: United Hospital Fund of New York.
Elwyn, G., O'Connor, A., Stacey, D., Volk, R., Edwards, A., Coulter, A., et al. (2006). Developing a quality criteria framework for patient decision aids: Online international Delphi consensus process. *British Medical Journal, 333*, 417–422.

Emanuel, E. J., Fairclough, D. L., & Slutsman, J. (1999). Assistance from family members, friends, paid care givers, and volunteers in the care of terminally ill patients. *New England Journal of Medicine, 341,* 956–963.

Feldman-Stewart, D., & Brundage, M. D. (2000). Challenges for designing and implementing decision aids. *Patient Education Counsel, 54,* 265–273.

Feldman-Stewart, D., Brundage, M. D., McConnell, B. A., & MacKillop, W. J. (2000). Practical issues in assisting shared decision-making. *Health Expectations, 3,* 46–54.

Fins, J. J., & Miller, F. G. (2000). Clinical pragmatism, ethics consultation, and the elderly patient. *Clinical Geriatric Medicine, 16,* 71–81.

Freedman, B. (1993). Offering truth. One ethical approach to the uninformed cancer patient. *Archives of Internal Medicine, 153,* 572–576.

Fried, T. R., Bradley, E. H., Towle, V. R., & Allore, H. (2002). Understanding the treatment preferences of seriously ill patients. *New England Journal of Medicine, 346,* 1061–1066.

Frosch, D. L., & Kaplan, R. M. (1999). Shared decision-making in clinical medicine: Past research and future directions. *American Journal of Preventive Medicine, 17,* 285–294.

Gatellari, M., Voigt, K. J., Butow, P. N., & Tattersall, M. (2002). When the treatment goal is not cure? Are cancer patients equipped to make informed decisions? *Journal of Clinical Oncology, 20,* 503–513.

Gould, S. D., Williams, W., & Arnold, R. (2000). Conflicts regarding decisions to limit treatment. A differential diagnosis. *Journal of the American Medical Association, 283,* 909–914.

Grunfeld, E. A., Maher, J., Browne, S., Ward, P., Young, T., Vivat, B., et al. (2006). Advanced breast cancer patients' perceptions of decision-making for palliative chemotherapy. *Journal of Clinical Oncology, 24,* 1090–1098.

Hanson, L. C., Danis, M., & Garrett, J. (1997). What's wrong with end-of-life care? Opinions of bereaved family members. *Journal of the American Geriatrics Society, 45,* 1339–1344.

Harrington, C. (2001). Residential nursing facilities in the United States. *British Medical Journal, 323,* 507–510.

Hastie, R., & Dawes, R. M. (2000). *Rational choice in an uncertain world. The psychology of judgment and decision making.* Thousand Oaks, CA: Sage.

Heyland, D. K., Cook, D. J., Rocker, G. M., Dodek, P. M., Kutsogiannis, D. J., Peters, S., et al. (2003). Decision-making in the ICU: Perspectives of the substitute decision maker. *Intensive Care Medicine, 29,* 75–82.

Heyland, D. K., Frank, C., Groll, D., Pichora, D., Dodek, P., Rocker, G., et al. (2006). Understanding cardiopulmonary resuscitation decision-making. Perspectives of seriously ill hospitalized patients and family members. *Chest, 130,* 419–428.

Heyland, D. K., Rocker, G. M., O'Callaghan, C. J., Dodek, P. M, & Cook, D. J. (2003). Dying in the ICU: Perspectives of family members. *Chest, 124,* 392–397.

Hudson, P. L., Aranda, S., & Kristjanson, L. J. (2004). Meeting the supportive needs of family caregivers in palliative care. Challenges for health professionals. *Journal of Palliative Medicine, 7,* 19–25.

Hunink, M., Glasziou, P., Siegel, J., Weeks, J., Pliskin, J., Elstein, A., et al. (2001). Valuing outcomes. In M. Hunink, P. Glasziou, J. Siegel, J. Weeks, J. Pliskin, A. Elstein, et al. (Eds.), *Decision-making in health and medicine* (pp. 88–125). New York: Cambridge University Press.

Hwang, S. S., Chang, V. T., Alejandro, Y., Osenenko, P., Davis, C., Cogswell, J., et al. (2003). Caregiver unmet needs, burden, and satisfaction in symptomatic advanced cancer patients at a Veterans Affairs (VA) medical center. *Palliative Supportive Care, 1*, 319–329.

Jackson, J. L., Chamberlin, J., & Kroenke, K. (2001). Predictors of patient satisfaction. *Social Sciences and Medicine*, 52, 609–620.

Jansma, F. F. I., Schure, L. M., & de Jong, B. M. (2005). Support requirements for caregivers of patients with palliative cancer. *Patient Education Counsel, 58*, 182–186.

Johnson, K. S., Elbert-Avila, K. I., & Tulsky, J. A. (2005). The influence of spiritual beliefs and practices on the treatment preferences of African Americans: A review of the literature. *Journal of the American Geriatrics Society, 53*, 711–719.

Karlawish, J. H., Quill, T., & Meier, D. (1999). A consensus-based approach to providing palliative care to patients who lack decision-making capacity. *Annals of Internal Medicine, 130*, 835–840.

Kayser-Jones, J. (2002). The experience of dying: An ethnographic nursing home study. *The Gerontologist, 42* (Special Issue III), 11–19.

Klein, G. (2001). *Sources of power. How people make decisions*. Cambridge, MA: MIT Press.

Koedoot, C. G., Oort, F. J., de Haan, R. J., Bakker, P. J., de Graeff, A., & de Haes, J. C. (2004). The content and information given by medical oncologists when telling patients with advanced cancer what their treatment options are: Palliative chemotherapy or watchful waiting. *European Journal on Cancer, 40*, 225–235.

Koffman, J., & Higginson, I. J. (2001). Accounts of carers' satisfaction with health care at the end of life: A comparison of first generation black Caribbeans and white patients with advanced disease. *Palliative Medicine, 15*, 337–345.

Kraetschmer, N., Sharpe, N., Urowitz, N., & Deber, R. B. (2004). How does trust affect patient preferences for shared decision-making? *Health Expectations, 7*, 317–326.

Kuhl, D. R., & Wilensky, P. (1999). Decision-making at the end of life: A model using an ethical grid and the principles of group process. *Journal of Palliative Medicine, 2*, 75–86.

Lan, F., & Quill, T. (2004). Making decisions with families at the end of life. *American Family Physician, 70*, 719–723, 725–726.

Lapine, A., Wang-Cheng, R., Goldstein, M., Nooney, A., Lamb, G., & Dersey, A. R. (2001). When cultures clash. Physician, patient and family wishes in truth disclosure for dying patients. *Journal of Palliative Medicine, 4*, 475–480.

Leighl, N. B., Butow, P. N., & Tattersall, M. H. N. (2004). Treatment decision aids in advanced cancer: When the goal is not cure and the answer is not clear. *Journal of Clinical Oncology, 32*, 1759–1762.

Levine, C., & Zuckerman, C. (1999). The trouble with families: Toward an ethic of accommodation. *Annals of Internal Medicine, 130*, 148–152.

Lo, B., Ruston, D., Kates, L. W., Arnold, R. M., Cohen, C. B., Faber-Langendoen, D., et al. (2002). Discussing religious and spiritual issues at the end of life. A practical guide for physicians. *Journal of the American Medical Association, 287,* 749–754.

Makoul, G., & Clayman, M. L. (2006). An integrative model of shared decision-making in medical encounters. *Patient Education Counsel, 60,* 301–312.

Matsuyama, R., Reddy, S., & Smith, T. J. (2006). Why do patients choose chemotherapy near the end of life? A review of the perspective of those facing death from cancer. *Journal of Clinical Oncology, 24,* 3490–3496.

McNutt, R. A. (2004). Shared decision-making. Problems, process, progress. *Journal of the American Medical Association, 292,* 2516–2518.

Meeker, M. A., & Jezewski, M. A. (2005). Family decision-making at end of life. *Palliative Supportive Care, 3,* 131–142.

Meisel, A. (2005). The role of litigation in end of life care. A reappraisal. *Improving End of Life Care: Why Has It Been So Difficult? Hastings Center Report Special Report, 35*(6), S47–S51.

Miller, S. M. (1995). Monitoring versus blunting styles of coping with cancer influence the information patients want and need about their disease. *Cancer, 76,* 167–177.

Mpinga, E. K., Chastonay, P., & Rapin, C. (2006). Conflits en fin de vie. [End of life conflicts in palliative care.] *Recherche en soins infirmiers, 86,* 68–96.

Murray, M., Miller, T., Fiset, V., O'Connor, A., & Jacobsen, M. (2004). Decision support: Helping patients and families to find a balance at the end of life. *International Journal of Palliative Nursing, 10,* 270–277.

Norton, S. A., Tilden, V. P., Tolle, S. W., Nelson, C. A., & Eggman, S. T. (2003). Life support withdrawal: Communication and conflict. *American Journal of Critical Care, 12,* 548–555.

O'Connor, A. M. (1995). Validation of a decisional conflict scale. *Medical Decision-Making, 5,* 25–30.

O'Connor, A. M., Graham, I. D., & Visser, A. (2005). Implementing shared decision-making in diverse health care systems. The role of decision aids. *Patient Education Counsel, 57,* 247–249.

Penson, R. T., Kyriakou, H., Zuckerman, D., Chabner, B. A., & Lynch, T. J., Jr. (2006). Teams: Communication in multidisciplinary care. *Oncologist, 11,* 520–526.

Pochard, F., Azoulay, E., Chevret, S., LeMaire, F., Hubert, P., Canoui, P., et al. (2001). Symptoms of anxiety and depression in family members of intensive care unit patients. Ethical hypothesis regarding decision-making capacity. *Critical Care Medicine, 29,* 1893–1898.

Potkins, D., Bradley, S., Shrimanker, J., O'Brien J., Swann, A., & Ballard, C. (2000). End of life treatment decisions in patients with advanced dementia: Carer's views and the factors which influence them. *International Journal of Geriatric Psychiatry, 15,* 1005–1008.

Rabow, M. W., Hauser, J. M., & Adams, J. (2004). Supporting family caregivers at the end of life. They don't know what they don't know. *Journal of the American Medical Association, 291,* 483–491.

Redelmeier, D. A., Rozin, P., & Kahneman, D. (1993). Understanding patients' decisions: Cognitive and emotional perspectives. *Journal of the American Medical Association, 270,* 72–76.

Rutten, L. J. F., Arora, N. K., Bakos, A. D., Aziz, N., & Rowland, J. (2005). Information needs and sources of information among cancer patients: A systematic review of research (1980–2003). *Patient Education Counsel, 57,* 250–261.

Sainio, C., Luri, S., & Eriksson, E. (2001). Cancer patients' views and experiences of participation in care and decision-making. *Nursing Ethics, 8,* 97–113.

Say, R., Murtagh, M., & Thomson, R. (2006). Patients' preference for involvement in medical decision-making: A narrative review. *Patient Education Counsel, 60,* 102–114.

Sharpe, L., Butow, P., Smith, C., McConnell, D., & Clarke, S. (2005). The relationship between available support, unmet needs and caregiver burden in patients with advanced cancer and their carers. *Psycho-oncology, 14,* 102–114.

Singer, P. A., Martin, D. K., & Kelner, M. (1999). Quality end of life care: Patient's perspectives. *Journal of the American Medical Association, 281,* 163–168.

Steinhauser, K. E., Christakis, N. A., Clipp, E. C., McNeilly, M., Grambow, S., McIntyre L., et al. (2000). Factors considered important at the end of life by patients, family, physicians and other care providers. *Journal of the American Medical Association, 284,* 2476–2482.

Svenson, O. (1992). Differentiation and consolidation theory of human decision-making: A frame of reference for the study of pre and post-decision processes. *Acta Psychologica, 80,* 143–168.

Tang, S. T., Liu, T. W., Lai, M. S., & McCorkle, R. (2005). Discrepancy in the preferences of place of death between terminally ill cancer patients and their primary family caregivers in Taiwan. *Social Sciences and Medicine, 61,* 1560–1566.

Teno, J. M., Clarridge, B. R., Casey, V., Welch, L. C., Wetle, T., Shield, R., et al. (2004). Family perspectives on end of life care at the last place of care. *Journal of the American Medical Association, 291,* 88–93.

True, G., Phipps, E. J., Braitman, L. E., Harralson, T., Harris, D., & Tester, W. (2005). Treatment preferences and advance care preferences at the end of life: The role of ethnicity and spiritual coping in cancer patients. *Annals of Behavioral Medicine, 30,* 174–179.

Tversky, A., & Kahneman, D. (1981). The framing of decisions and the psychology of choice. *Science, 211,* 453–458.

Websters Third New International Dictionary. (1976). Springfield, MA: Merriam.

Weeks, J. C., Cook, F., O'Day, S. J., Peterson, L. M., Wenger, N., Reding, D., et al. (1998). Relationship between cancer patients' predictions of prognosis and their treatment preferences. *Journal of the American Medical Association, 279,* 1709–1714.

Weissman, D. E. (2004). Decision-making at a time of crisis near the end of life. *Journal of the American Medical Association, 292,* 1738–1743.

Wenzelberg, G. S., Hanson, L. C., & Tulsky, J. C. (2005). Beyond autonomy: Diversifying end of life decision-making approaches to serve patients and families. *Journal of the American Geriatrics Society, 53,* 1046–1050.

Whitney, S. N. (2003). A new model of medical decisions: Exploring the limits of shared decision-making. *Medical Decision-Making, 23,* 275–280.

Wills, C. E., & Holmes-Rovner, M. (2003). Patient comprehension of information for shared treatment decision-making. *Patient Education Counsel, 50,* 285–290.

Wilson, K. G., Aaron, S. D., Vandemheen, K. L., Hebert, P. C., McKim, D. A., Fiset, V., et al. (2005). Evaluation of a decision aid for making choices about intubation and mechanical ventilation in chronic obstructive pulmonary disease. *Patient Education Counsel, 57,* 88–95.

Wolff, J. L., Dy, S. M., Frick, K. D., & Kasper, J. D. (2007). End-of-life care. Findings from a national survey of informal caregivers. *Archives of Internal Medicine, 167,* 40–46.

Zhang, A. Y., & Siminoff, L. A. (2003). The role of the family in treatment decision-making by patients with cancer. *Oncology Nursing Forum, 30,* 1022–1028.

11

CHAPTER

Communication Related to End-of-Life Care and Decisions

Ellen L. Csikai

□ Introduction

Communication and decision making about end-of-life care may occur in various settings such as homes, physicians' offices, or hospitals and with the input of various participants. The need for end-of-life care communication may result from sudden illness or injury or deterioration because of a chronic health condition. Individuals may also wish to plan for end-of-life care with their families in advance of becoming ill through various forms of advance directives. Regardless of the setting or immediate need for end-of-life care communication, it is often a difficult undertaking for all involved.

Many factors contribute to making communication about end-of-life care among the most dreaded discussions one can have during a time of illness or injury. In Western society, we tend not to talk about death or to accept it as a part of life. We often do not even say the word "death" or that someone "died." Instead they "passed away," "went home," or are "gone."

Relatedly, scientists/researchers are continually searching for and "discovering" new medical treatments to cure disease and prolong life. Many people go through life believing that "it" (death) will not happen to them. If a new or experimental treatment to prolong life is developed and used to treat their disease long enough, perhaps a cure will be discovered for that particular disease at some point in the future. The reality is that everyone will die, and communication about the care individuals wish to have near the end of life is necessary. However, it does not occur for many because of fears associated with the process of death or unrealistic expectations for a cure. Thus, many may die without meaningful connections either spiritually (with whomever they deem as a higher power) or practically, leaving unfinished family business (emotional or concrete).

□ Communication About Dying and Death

Typically, a series of conversations takes place between patients and families with their physicians and other healthcare providers when patients are facing an advanced illness. Options for end-of-life care may and should be discussed during many of these conversations, not just when death appears to be imminent (Larson & Tobin, 2000; Wenrich et al., 2001). Advance care planning, "the process by which patients, together with their families and health care practitioners, consider values and goals and articulate preferences for future care" (Tulsky, 2005, p. 360) may take place. With each change in medical status, the goals of care need to be reexamined, and patients and families need to be given the opportunity to express how they wish care to be carried out in accordance with their definition of quality of life (e.g., how aggressively to treat a deteriorating condition or what care to give if the patient is in an irreversible coma). Particularly when the medical team is recommending a change from curative care to palliative care, clear communication of options leading to decisions must occur. An example of such a process was described by Lyon (Richard & Lyon, chapter 2, this volume) with her family-centered advance care planning model.

Reluctance to Talk About Death

In today's society, talking about death is a taboo. "Everyone is ambivalent about death" (Dubler, 2005, p. S19). Some people fear that there is a connection between talking and action and believe that talking about death will make it happen, even if it is not remotely possible. Although no scientific evidence exists that open, honest, and thoughtful communication about dying has detrimental effects on either patients or families (Corr, 1998), some cultural and spiritual belief systems do include this perception, and this is an important determinant of the type and content of communication desired from healthcare professionals by individuals who hold these beliefs (see Hayslip, Hansson, Starkweather, & Dolan, chapter 17, this volume).

Often, patients and families are reluctant to initiate discussion about death, dying, and end of life, so it is incumbent on physicians and other healthcare professionals to do so. A number of factors have been found to inhibit this discussion by patients and families. Patients may conceal important indicators that a disease is progressing, such as pain or other debilitating symptoms, feelings of loss, or fears about prognosis and death. Patients also may perceive a stigma associated with end-of-life discussions and being labeled as "terminal." Cultural prohibition and deferment of such discussion to family members may also occur. In a parallel fashion, families may be reluctant to accept the advanced nature of a patient's illness or his or her expressed preferences for care. They may also overestimate the patient's chance for cure and not permit discussion of end-of-life care options but instead demand the medical team "do everything" (Larson & Tobin, 2000; see Chang & Sambamoorthi, chapter 10, this volume).

Numerous reasons why physicians may avoid end-of-life care discussions have been cited in the literature and discussed among healthcare professionals anecdotally from their experiences. These reasons include fear of causing pain and relating bad news; lack of knowledge about advance directive laws; lack of training in delivering "bad news"; anticipation of disagreement with patients or families; and legal-medical concerns (Morrison, 1998). In addition, the very culture of medicine and socialization to the discipline discourages discussion about death. Physicians are trained to cure disease. When this is not possible and the "enemy" is not defeated, physicians may believe they have failed. Few want to admit that the enemy has won and thus avoid talking about the dying patient.

Although changing slowly, educational preparation to handle end-of-life care discussions is minimal in all professions. Unacknowledged fears about loss and death may inhibit discussion as well and create a barrier to emotional engagement that may unintentionally result in projection of the professionals' feelings onto patients and families (Kvale, Berg, Groff, & Lange, 1999). Finally, physicians and other healthcare professionals are less likely to initiate end-of-life care discussions when they believe they lack the interpersonal skills needed (Larson & Tobin, 2000). As noted, communication skills particularly regarding end-of-life care receive little focus in medical school and residency training programs (Lunney, Foley, Smith, & Gelband, 2003).

The healthcare system is often a culprit in discouraging end-of-life conversations. Currently, these discussions are not a part of routine care for most physicians and healthcare professionals. This communication is perceived to be inherently difficult and emotional for patients and families, which may lead clinicians to decide that they do not have the time or inclination to conduct them. The healthcare system also does not value psychosocial conversations about end-of-life care, as evidenced by the lack of adequate compensation to physicians for their time to conduct conversations about advance care planning or end-of-life care. Contact time with individual patients also appears to be steadily decreasing, and there seem to exist fewer long-term patient-physician relationships today. Patients and families may be meeting providers with whom they have not developed a rapport or a sense or trust. In addition to these factors, medical care is often provided by multiple providers, so that it may be unclear who has the primary responsibility for initiating and continuing end-of-life care conversations and who should coordinate care among the various providers through the progression of an illness.

□ Communication About Diagnosis and Prognosis

Although true for the diagnosis of a serious illness, uncertainty regarding prognosis or course of progression of an illness causes considerable anxiety in the medical and lay communities. If a physician says that you will die within 3 months, what is the soonest that you might die, and what are the chances that you will live longer? "Uncertainty characterizes all medical decision-making" (Tulsky, 2005, p. 362).

How much information to disclose to seriously ill patients is another source of debate. Although some argue that precise information is needed so that patients and families can make informed decisions, others believe that maintaining an optimistic outlook can lead to better medical outcomes (Ubel, 2001). Concerns about maintaining hope in patients with serious illness not only can have very real consequences in terms of outcomes but also can determine how much about the patient's condition and prognosis is disclosed. Physicians may struggle to promote hope in patients with advanced illness and to support a positive outlook (Butow, Dowsett, Hagerty, & Tattersall, 2002). They frequently convey a more optimistic prognosis than is medically indicated, or the physician may avoid giving a prediction about prognosis. This may be the result of a belief that talking about death will distress patients (Christakis, 2000; Wenrich et al., 2001) or bring out emotions that the physician is not prepared to address.

Another factor to consider in communicating prognosis is the readiness of the patient and caregiver to hear the information. Because there exists a high level of prognostic uncertainty, patients and families may not be willing to acknowledge or accept a poor prognosis and opt for more aggressive treatment than is recommended. Also, it becomes more threatening to acknowledge a poor prognosis as the disease progresses; thus, maintaining what may be unrealistic hope is more palatable (Fried,

Bradley, & O'Leary, 2006). Even when kept informed about changes in prognosis throughout the last year of patients' lives, one study found both patients' and family caregivers' life-expectancy predictions remained or became more uncertain or became only slightly less optimistic over time. In this study, even in the month prior to patients' deaths (from cancer, chronic obstructive pulmonary disease, or congestive heart failure), only a small proportion of patients believed their life expectancy was less than 1 year (Fried et al.). The finding that few patients and caregivers corrected their prognostic misunderstandings as the patients' illnesses progressed was likely because of the small numbers of patients and caregivers who indicated that their physician discussed prognosis with them. It also could be the result of other previously documented reasons, such as physicians' inaccurate prognostication skills and lack of training in communication skills (Fried et al.).

Some may interpret overly optimistic views on life expectancy as "unrealistic" hope, but an important question to consider is whether the patient's beliefs are interfering with the ability to plan for current and future care. Rather than trying to take away patients' hopes that might be helping them cope with the illness, the discussion can be approached in a way that preserves hope for the "best" but prepares for the "worst" (Tulsky, 2005). The conversation can be directed toward managing resources in terms of what can still be done to help the patient and family through the end stage of the illness.

The language of medicine is often confusing to patients and families and complicates understanding of diagnosis and prognosis. Because this language is part of everyday medical communication, healthcare professionals sometimes fail to recognize when there has been a misunderstanding regarding the meaning of medical terms used during a discussion of the patient's illness. The following is an extreme example of this phenomenon that came to light during a hospice admission visit by a nurse and a social worker with a middle-aged man with pancreatic cancer and his wife.

> The nurse and I arrived at the home and were greeted by his wife. The patient was in a back bedroom. As is often the case, the wife asked to speak with us first before seeing the patient, who was very ill. We asked her what she understood about her husband's diagnosis and prognosis, and what she said was astonishing. She understood from the doctor that her husband was "terminal," and asked us what his illness had to do with the bus station. (Walters, 2005, p. 30)

Another problem with medical terminology is that it often blames, isolates, or seems to ridicule the patient. A frequently used phrase in oncology is that a patient "failed" a particular treatment regimen, which implies the patient is to blame for the treatment that failed her or him.

Perhaps if the person would have tried harder, the treatment would have been successful. It also may imply that the patient has also failed his or her physician by not having a better response and thus might no longer be of interest and therefore be abandoned by the physician. In another twist of word meanings, when test results reveal little or no evidence of cancer, the doctor is "not impressed" with the findings. A layperson would likely believe that being unimpressed could mean bad news, but in this context it has a positive meaning. Also the phrase, "the tumor is progressing" seems like it should be good news, but it is distinctly not good news. These everyday medical phrases are not everyday language to patients and families and can lead to misinterpretation and misunderstanding of diagnosis and prognosis (Walters, 2005).

Along with factual information given in clear and understandable language (not jargon), most patients and families want to know the physician's recommendation regarding options offered to them. Helping patients and families understand each option, including risks and benefits, can facilitate making the decision that is right for them at that time. Physicians may wish to ask social workers or other mental health professionals to join them in helping patients with these decisions.

Attending to the feelings associated with the content of the conversations about diagnosis and prognosis is important because emotions can have an impact on decision making. After hearing "bad news," patients and families are often not able to comprehend much about the details that follow in the discussion about end-of-life care options (Sell et al., 1993; Tulsky, 2005). This is compounded by the frequently missed opportunities by physicians to enter the realm of patients' and families' emotions (Curtis et al., 2002, 2005). Tulsky (2005) offered the following guidance to physicians regarding attending to patients' affect: "Acknowledge the emotion; identify loss; legitimize the feelings; offer support; explore" (p. 363). It is important that physicians and other care providers receive training in these areas because these conversations may occur without access to a social worker or other mental health professional who is perhaps more skilled at recognizing and working through intense emotions.

□ The Communication Process

Communication is a basic process that all living things experience. To meet our basic human needs (e.g., food, shelter, safety, belonging), we must make our needs and wishes known to others through some form of communication, either verbal or nonverbal. Not doing so places people at risk of physical and emotional discomfort. Communication can be seen as a process that cannot be conducted by oneself. The process includes the involvement of at least one communicator and one listener. These roles necessarily are interchangeable throughout the process. So when one is talking, the other party is listening, and both respond according to the verbal and nonverbal cues given. Information exchange is important in meeting the needs of both parties.

Effective communication begins with a relationship between the two (or more) parties involved in the situation. Social workers and other mental health professionals learn early in their educational programs how to form therapeutic relationships through which communication leading to facilitation of problem solving occurs. These relationships must be based on rapport and trust and can be enhanced through displaying unconditional positive regard for individuals' dignity and well-being, warmth (conveying a feeling of interest, concern in an individual), empathy (acknowledging that you understand an individual's situation), and genuineness (relating to an individual in a natural, sincere, spontaneous, open, and genuine manner) (Hepworth, Rooney, Rooney, Strom-Gottfried, & Larsen, 2006).

Effective communication in a helping relationship also involves understanding the issues and problems faced by patients and their families. Through communication, the intent or meaning of information conveyed can be made clear to others. Words need to be used in a way that others can understand. Verbal and nonverbal cues must match so that the intended message is delivered. Listening skills are also important so that what others are literally saying, as well as what they mean or intend to say with their words, is heard. Barriers to communication regarding the intent of the message include lack of clarity, vagueness, and cultural differences, while barriers to the message's impact include divided attention, other concerns, and biases (Kirst-Ashman & Hull, 2009).

Family-Team Conferences

One useful communication strategy that promotes coordination among team members and families' understanding of patients' medical conditions and treatment options is a family-team conference. The purpose of a family-team conference is to provide an opportunity for the healthcare providers to meet the family, inform them of the patient's condition, discuss the treatment plan, answer questions, and include the family (or surrogates) in the decision-making process. Such a meeting is appropriate particularly when there is a change in the patient's medical status, when a conflict is present between patient and family or between family and healthcare providers, when there is a belief that the goals of care should be transitioned to palliative care, or when the family requests a conference or healthcare providers believe that a meeting would be helpful (Csikai & Chaitin, 2005).

Curtis (2000) provided suggestions to physicians about how to approach end-of-life care discussions in family conferences that can also be useful to other health professionals participating in the discussions: (a) put time and thought into preparing for the discussion; (b) plan where the discussion should take place; (c) talk with patient or family about who they would like present at the meeting and what will be covered during the meeting; and (d) anticipate what is likely to happen after the meeting. Physicians are not expected to possess all of the skills necessary for effective communication about end-of-life care, just as mental health professionals are not expected to know the intricacies of medical treatments. Discussions about end-of-life care need to draw on the expertise of several disciplines to be able to adequately address patients' and families' concerns (Larson & Tobin, 2000).

Further outlined by Curtis (2000) were some steps that may facilitate good communication during family meetings (see Table 11.1). As noted, it will be important to keep cultural considerations in mind as one decides how to talk about issues during these meetings.

In one study (Curtis et al., 2002), audiotapes of family conferences were analyzed to discern the content of what was discussed regarding withdrawal of life-sustaining treatments and end-of-life care options. The researchers were able to identify a framework for this content that was believed to be representative of effective end-of-life discussions with families. In essence, there needs to be preparation for each meeting, including discussion with the team members regarding what information will be presented, about potential reactions from family members that may occur, and planning a strategy for providing recommendations and ending the meetings. These are all elements that serve to facilitate good communication during a family-team conference (see Table 11.2).

□ Communication in Health Care

Informed Consent

Communication in health care hinges on the concept of informed consent. Informed consent is a basic process by which patients or their surrogates are "informed" about their situation and give "consent" before any medical treatment takes place (except in emergencies). The patient's consent is needed across the spectrum of decision-making situations—from the most basic of procedures, such as routine lab work that may be drawn in

TABLE 11.1 Steps to Facilitate Good Communication During Family Meetings

1. Make preparations prior to a discussion about end-of-life care
    - Review previous knowledge of the patient or family
    - Review previous knowledge of the patient's attitudes and reactions
    - Review your knowledge of the disease: prognosis, treatment options
    - Examine your personal feelings, attitudes, biases, and grieving
    - Plan the specifics of location and setting: a quiet, private place
    - Have advance discussions with the patient and family about who will be present
2. Holding a discussion about end-of-life care
    - Introduce everyone present
    - If appropriate, set the tone in a nonthreatening way: "This is a conversation I have with all of my patients."
    - Find out what the patient or family understands
    - Find out how much the patient or family wants to know
    - Be aware that some patients do not want to discuss end-of-life care
    - Discuss prognosis frankly in a way that is meaningful to the patient
    - Do not discourage all hope
    - Avoid temptation to give too much medical detail
    - Make it clear that withholding life-sustaining treatment is not withholding caring
    - Use repetition to show that you understand what the patient or family is saying
    - Acknowledge strong emotions and use reflection to encourage patients or families to talk about these emotions
    - Tolerate silence
3. Finishing a discussion of end-of-life care
    - Achieve common understanding of the disease and treatment issues
    - Make a recommendation about treatment
    - Ask if there are any questions
    - Ensure basic follow-up plan and make sure the patient or family know how to reach you for questions

Source: From "Communicating With Patients and Their Families About Advance Care Planning and End-of-Life Care," by J. R. Curtis, 2000, *Respiratory Care, 45*, p. 1388.

the physician's office to check a cholesterol level, to withdrawing life-sustaining ventilator support that will allow a patient to die. Consent may be implied, verbal, or written, depending on the situation. Medical treatment

TABLE 11.2 Summary of Content of Family Discussions About End-of-Life Options

1. Introductions and openings
    - Introductions
    - Purpose
    - Elicit agenda
2. Information exchange
    - Review patient's condition
    - Discuss patient's baseline
    - Values history
    - Clarification of terms
    - Significance of information
    - Symptoms
    - Affirming experiences
3. Discussions of what the future might hold
    - Prognosis for survival
    - Prognosis regarding future quality of life
    - Uncertainty
4. Decisions
    - Surrogate decision making
    - Discussions of existing advance directives
    - Options
    - Choices
    - Code
    - Transitions from curative to palliative care
    - Burden and benefit
    - Withdraw life-sustaining treatments
5. Discussions of death and dying
    - Dying
    - Death
6. Closings
    - Summary of conference
    - Family control of timing
    - Assure patient comfort
    - Further discussions
    - Continuity issues
    - Contact information

TABLE 11.2 Summary of Content of Family Discussions About End-of-Life Options (Continued)

• Gratitude
• Next steps

Source: "Studying Communication About End-of-Life Care During the ICU Family Conference: Development of a Framework, by J. R. Curtis, R. A. Engelberg, M. D. Wenrich, E. L. Nielsen, S. E. Shannon, P. D. Treece, P. D., et al., 2002, *Journal of Critical Care, 17*, p. 151.

may also be legally refused (consent not given), even if that refusal could result in death (Meisel & Cerminara, 2004; see Cerminara, chapter 8, this volume).

The informed consent process is a conversation that is normally initiated by the physician or other healthcare provider who has specialized knowledge of the patient's illness and the treatment options available. "The goal [in informed consent] is to create the best environment for the patient to execute an informed, self-determined choice" (Csikai & Chaitin, 2005, p. 127). The physician's role is to reveal knowledge about the condition, concerns, and advice, and the participant's role is to ask questions and state concerns and preferences. Thus, in the best situation, both patients and physicians/providers are giving and obtaining information needed about proposed medical treatments for the patient's illness (Csikai & Chaitin). In end-of-life care discussions, physicians are to address the goals of care and provide information about the treatment options themselves, including risks, benefits, and potential outcomes for the patient's quality of life. Patients and families need to provide information about their expectations and hopes for the outcome. Together, perhaps with other health professionals present, such as a nurse or a social worker, deliberation of the options will take place. After the information is exchanged and weighed, an informed decision can be made and then carried out. Informed consent should also be a continuous process—not a one-time event. As the patient's condition changes, recommendations and preferences for treatment options may change, so periodic updates are needed.

Informed consent presumes that a patient has the capacity to make decisions. To determine capacity, four criteria may be used: (a) evidence of a choice; (b) evidence of an understanding of the relevant information; (c) rational manipulation of relevant information provided; and (d) appreciation of the consequences of the situation (Roth, Applebaum, Sellee, Reynolds, & Huber, 1982). If a patient lacks the capacity to give informed consent, then treatment decisions should be discussed with the patient's surrogate. This person, normally a family member, is someone identified either by the patient or by law to "speak" for the patient. When the patient has no family, a court-appointed guardian is needed. Ideally, according to the principle of autonomy that provides the foundation for informed consent laws, patients are able to make their own decisions. When surrogates are involved in the decisions, there is a much greater likelihood of conflict among family members who have differing opinions about the appropriate course or aggressiveness of treatment and between surrogates and the healthcare team.

Facilitating Effective Communication

Trust in healthcare providers is fundamental for good medical care. This belief that providers are acting in the best interests of the patients must be shared by patients, families, and the other members of the healthcare team. The nature of medical care as it currently exists necessitates that physicians and others develop relationships and trust with patients and their families quickly. Tulsky (2005) gives the following suggestions to physicians that may facilitate trust: "Encourage patients and families to talk; do not contradict or put down other health care providers, yet recognize patient concerns; acknowledge errors; be humble; demonstrate respect; and do not force decisions" (p. 362).

Patients and families often form relationships with multiple providers, including physicians, nurses, social workers, and others who will help guide their medical care. Individuals may literally be "thrown" into a relationship with providers through an emergency situation, or they may have been able to choose a provider who will provide care long term, such as their family physician. Often as an illness progresses, the number of providers increases as specialists in the disease may be consulted (e.g., oncologists, nephrologists). The more providers there are, the more complex communication becomes and the greater the chance of conflict among providers and between the patients and families and the providers.

In recent years, the patient-physician relationship has become "crowded," particularly in the acute care setting involving many other "nonmedical" personnel, such as discharge planners, financial officers, length-of-stay managers, and reimbursement specialists, who do not necessarily have medical best interests foremost on their agenda. Cost-containment issues may thrust these individuals into the treatment decisions of patients, families, and healthcare professionals. Many more and diverse individuals are thus involved in medical decisions, creating a greater risk of "misunderstanding, misinformation, disagreement, and dispute" (Dubler, 2005, p. S22).

In addition to verbal communication, physicians and other healthcare professionals can communicate with each other through written documentation in a patient's medical record and outpatient consultation reports sent in a timely manner to the primary care physician. The recent move toward electronic medical records has made information immediately available to the healthcare team and has helped in the coordination of medical care.

Communication in Different Healthcare Settings

Communication about end-of-life care can be conceptualized as a series of overlapping continua: setting for the discussion, participants in the discussion, and the information shared in the discussion. The acuity of the patient's illness at the time that an end-of-life care discussion is held may dictate the setting or environment for the discussion. It may also indicate who needs to be involved in the discussion. In addition, if the situation is such that the condition is immediately life threatening, then much more detailed information may need to be shared with the patient and family.

Meetings in which a terminal prognosis and end-of-life care options are discussed may be held in the physician's office, with the patient and physician as the only participants, or in the intensive care unit (ICU), where there may be a family-team conference. Such a conference would include the patient, family members, physicians (primary care and specialists), primary nurse, social worker, and others as determined by their level of involvement and input needed in the conference, such as physical therapist, respiratory therapist, or nutritionist.

The content of these discussions may also range from minimal information, options discussed, but no recommendations made to patients (with also little or no interpretation of technical information, making decision making difficult) to full disclosure of information and options, including all risks and benefits (also making decision making difficult because too much information is given without interpretation or recommendation). The recommendations of the healthcare professionals involved in the patient's care are important in helping patients and families make needed decisions. Social workers and other mental health professionals can assist with interpreting what various medical treatments may mean for the patient's quality of life and regarding care that families may need to provide for the patient during the end stage of a disease.

An additional aspect to add to these three considerations is the timing of the discussions. At one end of the continuum, discussions about care options may be unplanned and occur spontaneously, for example, while the physician is on patient rounds in the hospital. At the other end, meetings may be planned (on a medical unit or ICU) when all family and professionals who need and want to attend and provide input are available.

Primary Care or Specialist Physician's Office

The two settings that most of us are likely familiar with and where much communication about medical diagnosis, prognosis, and even end-of-life care occurs are the primary care physician's office or specialist's office (or clinic). Because of the increasing fiscal concerns in the healthcare system, many medical tests and procedures that were once done while in the hospital are now administered on an outpatient basis. Primary care or specialty physicians then receive the results and discuss them with patients in the office or clinic setting. Treatment options are offered (with recommendations), and decisions are made. Advance care planning also ideally occurs in this setting. Patients and physicians can have a conversation about patients' end-of-life care wishes when the situation is not emergent and document these in their medical records to be prepared if such a situation arises. A formal advance directive document may not be completed but having this conversation will greatly ease the burden of decision making at the end of life for the physician and the patients' family. The following is an example of a case that could be considered uncomplicated, with continuous communication through end-of-life care.

> Mrs. A, a 98-year-old woman, has been Dr. W's patient for the past 30 years. She lives with her daughter (75 years old). She has been fairly independent and able to be left alone at home while her daughter goes out to volunteer at the local library. Mrs. A was diagnosed with congestive heart failure (CHF) 10 years ago. In the past 2 years, she has been hospitalized three times for exacerbations of the CHF. Her lung capacity is deteriorating, and she has been losing weight steadily over the last 6 months. Mrs. A and her daughter are now meeting with Dr. W in his office to discuss the progression of illness and treatment options, including risks and benefits. Hospice care was the recommended option for care as Dr. W believes that her condition will continue to deteriorate fairly rapidly. Mrs. A agrees to have no further treatment as some procedures, such as draining her lungs, have become increasingly painful to her. This recommendation was not a surprise to either the patient or daughter because they have had frank discussions with the physician about the patient's diagnosis and what it would mean for her quality of life over the past several years. They reviewed the situation periodically and went over options. An advance directive, specifying the daughter as a healthcare proxy, was formulated about 5 years ago; however, it was not in effect now because the patient was still capable of making her own decisions. Although saddened, the daughter agrees with the recommendation and will continue to care for her mother. Mrs. A's wishes are that she be comfortable and not in pain at the end of

life. After the meeting, Dr. W made a referral to hospice and will continue to follow her medical care through the hospice agency.

In other cases, specialists may be consulted by primary care physicians when the medical condition faced is complicated or requires more than routine or general medical care. This is often done to discover or confirm a new diagnosis of an illness. This physician may then become a primary source of information and communication about this new illness. The following case illustrates such a situation:

> Mr. D, a 54-year-old man, has been feeling generally fatigued over a 6-month period and noticed his voice becoming "raspy." His primary care physician, Dr. M, ordered a chest x-ray, which revealed a large tumor on his left lung. Dr. M discussed the results with Mr. D and his wife and recommended that they see Dr. S, an oncologist, for confirmation of the diagnosis of lung cancer. Dr. S explained that a biopsy would determine the cell type, which would be an indication of how effective various treatments might be in curing the cancer. The biopsy revealed that the cancer was aggressive, and the oncologist prepared to engage in a discussion in his office with Mr. D, his wife, and one of his two daughters about prognosis and potential treatment options. Dr. S discussed options but was not optimistic about the chance for cure. His recommendation was for the patient to be evaluated by the hospital's palliative care team and for possible referral to hospice. Mr. D and family were all tearful on hearing this news. Mr. D's wife did not want him to give up and talked him into trying chemotherapy. Because this conversation occurred in the oncologist's office, it was not possible to involve the primary physician directly. However, the specialist had forwarded the test results to the primary care physician and had a conversation with him about which treatment options and recommendations would be presented to Mr. D. The primary care physician concurred with the specialist that hospice enrollment should be recommended; however, because of the knowledge he had about this family as a result of the relationship that he formed with the D's during the past 10 years, he cautioned the specialist that the conversation could be very emotional, and that Mrs. D, who was a dominant figure in the family, may not want to stop the "fight."

The process of family decision making described by Lyon (Richard & Lyon, chapter 2, this volume) is an example of how healthcare professionals can engage the family unit to ensure that the patient's wishes come to the forefront of a care-planning conference. It was clear that Richard had different preferences for care than his grandparents, and ensuring an open dialogue that is facilitated by the provider can reduce the likelihood of conflict when a critical event occurs and forces a family to make difficult decisions.

The Intensive Care Unit

Family members with loved ones in the ICU have rated communication with healthcare providers as one of the most important skills for those providers and rated communication skills as equally or more important than clinical (medical/technical) skill (Curtis, 2000). Through focus groups with patients, family members, physicians, and other healthcare professionals, aspects important in the communication process between dying patients and physicians were identified as follows (Wenrich et al., 2001, p. 868):

1. Talking with patients in an honest and straightforward way
2. Being willing to talk about dying
3. Giving bad news in a sensitive way
4. Listening to patients
5. Encouraging questions from patients
6. Being sensitive to when patients are ready to talk about death

The following case provides a demonstration of these elements carried out by members of the healthcare team in the ICU with family members:

> An 82-year-old woman living alone suffered a massive stroke at home. Her son lived nearby and found her lying on the floor of her bathroom when he stopped by to take her grocery shopping. She was breathing but had an extremely weak pulse. He immediately called 911, and paramedics transported her to the local emergency room (ER). Her medical condition was now stable with support from medications to regulate her blood pressure. She awakened occasionally but was not coherent during these times and became easily agitated. After 2 days of treatment and observation in the ICU, the health care team believed a family-team conference was necessary to discuss the patient's prognosis and treatment options. The patient's son, daughter-in-law, and two granddaughters were present as well as the attending physician (critical care), neurologist, primary nurse, and the social worker. The meeting was held in the social worker's private office outside the unit. The physicians relayed that the patient's prognosis was for little meaningful recovery, and that they believed the most likely scenario is that the patient would have another massive stroke within days or weeks, causing death, because controlling

her blood pressure has been difficult. The team recommended withdrawing the life-sustaining treatment (medications) and allowing her to die. The team encouraged the son and family to think about the patient's quality of life and what decisions she might have made if she were able to say so right now. While the son was considering options overnight, the patient suffered another stroke and was now declared brain dead. A follow-up family meeting was held that morning with only the attending physician and the son as now the choice may be different because of the changed circumstances.

Although this situation illustrates how communication can be effective and facilitative in an ICU, a very different process was described by Crow (chapter 4, this volume) in her experience when her brother became hospitalized. Withholding of information by medical providers and failing to consider the stressful nature of unexpected situations increases the likelihood of indecision and conflict among family members making decisions on behalf of a loved one. Further, as Crow describes, second-guessing the quality of decisions made as a result of poor information through hindsight can result in added distress, guilt, and dissatisfaction with the healthcare system.

Emergency Room

The ER is another setting in which families may meet with more than one healthcare professional regarding medical situations that require immediate and often critical "life-and-death" decisions. The time-sensitive and critical nature of a patient's injuries complicates decision making for family members as they struggle to deal with the emotional impact of the situation.

Mr. G was a 35-year-old pedestrian crossing the street on the way to his car after work, around 6:00 p.m. He was hit by a drunk driver who did not stop at a red light at that intersection. Mr. G sustained severe head and spinal cord injuries and was in a coma. He was also diagnosed with a ruptured spleen, and the surgeon recommended emergency surgery to stop internal bleeding. Mr. G's wife and father arrived at the ER, were greeted by the social worker, and were escorted to the "family room." The G's have two small children, who are at home with the grandmother. The social worker acts as a liaison with the medical team and relays as much information to them as possible until the physicians are free to speak with the family about the patient's medical condition. The surgeon meets with the family to attempt to gain informed consent for the needed surgery, without which Mr. G will die from internal bleeding. He explains the many risks of the surgery, especially given the extent of Mr. G's other injuries. The ER physician is brought to the family room by the social worker and discusses the overall situation and tells them that a neurosurgeon is currently evaluating Mr. G's head and neck injuries. Although the ER physician believes that the patient will likely not survive his head injuries, he will defer to the neurosurgeon's evaluation. They begin to discuss options and the goals of care. The family is in shock and can only focus on the information that Mr. G may die without the surgery to repair damage to his spleen. They do not hear that Mr. G. will likely not recover or if he does he will remain ventilator dependent because of the severity and placement of the spinal cord injury. The physicians leave the room, and the social worker continues to talk with the family about the situation. She first asks them to repeat what they heard the ER physician and surgeon tell them. She then works with them to clarify information that they do not appear to have heard or understood. She also encourages them to talk about Mr. G and how he lived his life, his values, and what treatment he would want in this situation as they await the evaluation of the neurosurgeon.

Social workers and other mental health professionals working with families in the ER must engage in crisis intervention to enable the families to focus on the immediacy of the medical treatment they may be asked to consent to on behalf of the seriously ill or injured individual. Professionals must be cognizant that because of the unplanned nature of the situations, families often are not prepared at that moment for decisions about which life-sustaining procedures or treatments are desirable. Remaining in close contact with the family and coordinating access to information from the medical team are paramount to building trust with families and allaying fears about what is happening throughout the crisis in the ER.

□ Conclusion

As a foundation to understanding the importance of communication, the chapter discussed the reluctance to talk about death and dying in U.S. society. This hesitation extends from laypersons to medical professionals. Given this, it is not surprising that the communication process and elements that promote good communication in situations involving end-of-life decisions are not easy and do not come naturally to many people. Therefore, of particular importance are building positive relationships with individuals and families and utilizing family-team conferences for relaying information about medical care/treatment options and presenting recommendations and decisions that must be made. To provide examples of real-life situations, the chapter's final sections described typical cases that may occur in primary care physicians' offices, specialists' offices, ICUs, and ERs and provided information about how good communication may be fostered in those settings.

Ideally, good communication will lead to medical care that achieves the patient's and family's goals, consistent with their conceptualization of a quality of life and cultural values. In approaching the end of life, many complex emotions may be experienced in anticipation of loss, and although conflict may occur during the process, this does not always indicate or lead to a poor outcome. As long as relationships among dying individuals, families, and healthcare providers are built on trust and communication continues, difficult decisions can be made and good outcomes are possible at the end of life.

☐ References

Butow, P. N., Dowsett, E., Hagerty, R., Tattersall, M. H. (2002). Communicating prognosis to patients with metastatic disease: What do they really want to know. *Supportive Care Cancer, 10*, 161–168.

Christakis, N. A. (2000). *Death foretold: Prophecy and prognosis in medical care*. Chicago: University of Chicago Press.

Corr, C. (1998). Death in modern society. In G. H. D. Doyle & N. MacDonald (Eds.), *Oxford textbook of palliative medicine* (pp. 31–39). Oxford, England: Oxford University Press.

Csikai, E. L., & Chaitin, E. (2005). *Ethics in end-of-life decisions in social work practice*. Chicago: Lyceum Books.

Curtis, J. R. (2000). Communicating with patients and their families about advance care planning and end-of-life care. *Respiratory Care, 45*, 1385–1394.

Curtis, J. R., Engelberg, R. A., Wenrich, M. D., Nielsen, E. L., Shannon, S. E., Treece, P. D., et al. (2002). Studying communication about end-of-life care during the ICU family conference: Development of a framework. *Journal of Critical Care, 17*, 147–160.

Curtis, J. R., Engelberg, R. A., Wenrich, M. D., Shannon, S. E., Treece, P. D., & Rubenfeld, G. D. (2005). Missed opportunities during family conferences about end-of-life care in the intensive care unit. *American Journal of Respiratory and Critical Care Medicine, 171*, 844–880.

Dubler, N. N. (2005). Conflict and consensus at the end of life. *Hastings Center Special Report, 35*(6), S19–S25.

Fried, T. R., Bradley, E. H., & O'Leary, J. (2006). Changes in prognostic awareness among seriously ill older persons and their caregivers. *Journal of Palliative Medicine, 9*, 61–69.

Hepworth, D. H., Rooney, R. H., Rooney, G. D., Strom-Gottfried, K., & Larsen, J. A. (2006). *Direct social work practice: Theory and skills* (7th ed.). Belmont, CA: Wadsworth.

Kurst-Ashman, K. K., & Hull, G. H., Jr. (2009). *Understanding generalist practice* (5th ed.). Belmont, CA: Wadsworth.

Kvale, J., Berg, L., Groff, J. Y., & Lange, G. (1999). Factors associated with residents' attitudes toward dying patients. *Family Medicine, 31,* 691.

Larson, D. G., & Tobin, D. R. (2000). End-of-life conversations: Evolving practice and theory. *Journal of the American Medical Association, 284,* 1573–1578.

Lunney, J. R., Foley, K. M., Smith, T. J., & Gelband, H. (2003). *Describing death in America: What we need to know executive summary.* Washington, DC: Institute of Medicine.

Meisel, A., & Cerminara, K. L. (2004 and annual supplements). *The right to die: The law of end-of-life decision-making* (3rd ed.). New York: Aspen.

Morrison, M. F. (1998). Obstacles to doctor-patient communication at the end of life. In M. D. Steinberg & S. J. Youngner (Eds.), *End-of-life decisions: A psychosocial perspective* (pp. 109–136). Washington, DC: American Psychiatric Press.

Roth, L. R., Applebaum, P. S., Sellee, R., Reynolds, C. F., & Huber, G. (1982). The dilemma of denial in the assessment of competency to consent to treatment. *Journal of Psychiatry, 139,* 910–913.

Sell, L., Devlin, B., Bourke, S. J., Munro, N. C., Corris, P. A., & Gibson, G. J. (1993). Communicating the diagnosis of lung cancer. *Respiratory Medicine, 87,* 61–63.

Tulsky, J. A. (2005). Beyond advance directives: Importance of communication skills at the end of life. *Journal of the American Medical Association, 294,* 359–365.

Ubel, P. A. (2001). Truth in the most optimistic way. *Annals of Internal Medicine, 134,* 1142–1143.

Walters, W. (2005). Words matter: Looking at medical language. *Hematology and Oncology News and Issues, 4*(9), 30–35.

Wenrich, M. D., Curtis, J. R., Shannon, S. E., Carline, J. D., Ambrozy, D. M., & Ramsey, P. G. (2001). Communicating with dying patients within the spectrum of medical care from terminal diagnosis to death. *Archives of Internal Medicine, 161,* 868–874.

12

CHAPTER

Dying in Institutions

Suzanne S. Prevost and J. Brandon Wallace

☐ Introduction

A hundred years ago, most Americans died at home. Disease and death were common throughout life. Young and old alike fell ill and often died from infectious diseases such as pneumonia, tuberculosis, or diarrhea and enteritis. Early death kept the average life expectancy low (47 years in 1900) (National Center for Health Statistics [NCHS], 2006). When death did occur, it was often sudden, following only a few days or, at most, a few weeks of illness. There were few physicians and even fewer hospitals or nursing homes. Most care was provided at home by female family members—mothers, wives, sisters, and daughters. Thus, people typically lived their final days at home in the care of family members (Lynn & Adamson, 2003).

Beginning in the 1930s and accelerating rapidly following World War II, the healthcare industry expanded dramatically in the United States. The emergence of third-party payers (private and public health insurance) made health care a lucrative business. By the 1960s and 1970s, most American communities had several medical doctors, one or more hospitals, and various other medical institutions, such as nursing homes and rehabilitation centers. Advances in health care, especially in the prevention and treatment of infectious disease, reduced death rates among the young and dramatically increased life expectancy. Even death in old age changed as abrupt death from acute illness gave way to gradual decline and death brought on by chronic conditions such as heart disease, cancer, stroke, respiratory disease, and diabetes. Further, the management and treatment of chronic ailments improved as new technological and pharmacological advances continued to extend life and increasingly postponed death to extreme old age.

By the 1980s, these changes had radically altered the experience of death in America. Although most Americans could expect to live well into old age, with life expectancy at birth approaching 75 years (NCHS, 2006), they could also expect an extended period of decline in which chronic disease gradually reduced their health and increased their dependency on others. Further, it was likely that their last few days, perhaps even weeks or months, would be spent in a hospital or nursing home under the care of paid medical professionals (Lynn & Adamson, 2003). In fact, by 1989, 62.3% of all deaths occurred in hospitals, while another 19.2% occurred in nursing homes, with only 15.9% of deaths occurring at home (Center for Gerontology and Health Care Research, 2004).

However, increasing concerns about the institutionalization of death, the cost and efficacy of some life-sustaining technologies, and growing public perceptions of death in hospitals as somewhat inhumane led to a rethinking of end-of-life care by both policy makers and the medical community (Last Acts, 2002). Influenced by the hospice movement, many healthcare providers began to focus on palliative (comfort-oriented) care rather than curative or rehabilitative care for the terminally ill. Further, the implementation of the prospective payment system in which hospitals are paid a predetermined rate for each Medicare admission based on the patient's Diagnosis Related Group (DRG), encouraged hospitals to discharge patients earlier. Also influential was federal legislation passed in the late 1980s and 1990s that added and gradually increased a hospice benefit to Medicare and gave states the option of adding hospice benefits to their Medicaid programs (McMillan, Mentnech, Lubitz, McBean, & Russell, 1990). These changes led to a reduction in the percentage of deaths occurring in hospitals. By 1997, 51.7% of deaths occurred in hospitals, and in 2001 this percentage dropped to 49.5%. These declines were accompanied by increases in the percentage of deaths occurring in nursing homes (23.0% in 1997 and 23.2% in 2001) and at home (22.5% in 1997 and 23.4% in 2001) (Center for Gerontology and Health Care Research, 2004).

In spite of these national trends, there are appreciable regional differences in the location of death. For example, in 2001 most southern and many eastern states had a higher proportion of deaths occurring in hospitals than did most northern and western states. At the same time, states in the upper Midwest had the highest proportion of deaths in nursing homes, while states in the south and east had the lowest. These differences are likely the result of variations in the availability of healthcare resources, such as the number of hospital and nursing home beds and access to home health services; divergent state policies and programs, including Medicaid reimbursements for hospice or home health care; and regional differences in racial composition, income, and cultural values (Flory et al., 2004; Mitchell, Teno, Miller, & Mor, 2005; Tolle, Rosenfeld, Tilden, & Park, 1999).

Other factors are associated with where a person dies as well. Studies have shown that minorities, individuals with less education, and those enrolled in health maintenance organizations (HMOs) are more likely to die in hospitals, while the very old, people with long-term functional limitations, and those with cognitive limitations are more likely to die in nursing homes (Flory et al., 2004; Iwashyna & Chang, 2002; Johnson et al., 2005; Levy, Fish, & Kramer, 2004; Weitzen, Teno, Fennell, & Mor, 2003). Specific medical conditions also affect the location of death. Patients with dementia, for example, are more likely to die in nursing homes, while those with cancer are more likely to die at home (Flory et al.; Mitchell et al., 2005). Not surprisingly, the number of in-hospital deaths decreases and at home or nursing home deaths increase as the availability and utilization of hospice services increases. Hospital deaths also are less likely if patients have a living will or if do not resuscitate (DNR), do not hospitalize, or other advance directives are in place (Degenholtz, Rhee, & Arnold, 2004; Pekmezaris et al., 2004). Continuity of care provided by a family physician, the availability of informal care networks in the home and community, and access to formal home health providers also reduce the likelihood of death in a hospital (Brazil, Howell, Bedard, Krueger, & Heidebrecht, 2005; Burge, Lawson, Johnston, & Cummings, 2003; Klinkenberg et al., 2005; McWhinney, Bass, & Orr, 1995). In sum, numerous factors determine where a person dies. However, the general trend over the last decade and a half has been a declining rate of death in hospitals and increasing rates of death in nursing homes or private residences.

It is important to note that research addressing preferences for place of death has typically found most terminal patients and their families (50–90%) prefer death in private residences (Koffman & Higginson, 2004; Tang, Liu, Lai, & McCorkle, 2005; Tiernan, O'Connor, O'Siorain, & Kearney, 2002). Although some suggest that family members are more likely than patients to express preferences for institutional settings, by far the majority would prefer to have their loved one die at home (Brazil et al., 2005). Yet, in spite of these preferences, most deaths still occur in hospitals and nursing homes, suggesting that such preferences are often being ignored or, more often, are not communicated effectively to healthcare providers. Others point out that what patients and their families prefer and what is best for the patient are not always the same. For example, if a patient's pain and suffering cannot easily be managed outside the hospital or if the available informal care networks are inadequate, it is not in the patient's best interest to be discharged home. Thus, although terminal patients might prefer to die at home, it is not always feasible for them to do so. The situation confronted by Crow (chapter 4, this volume) is an example for which it was not feasible for her brother to die outside an institution; however, he was able to be transferred to a home-like setting (i.e., a residential hospice) on the removal of artificial life support. Further, initial preferences for place of death often change as patients' conditions worsen and stresses on family caregivers increase (McCall & Rice, 2005).

□ Dying in Hospitals

The primary philosophy of care in most hospitals is the rapid restoration of health from acute illness. Physicians, nurses, and other healthcare providers are trained to restore health to the sick. The business model of the hospital, especially since the implementation of the prospective payment system, also focuses on quickly treating and discharging patients. Hence, the current trend is to move patients rapidly through hospital systems, often meaning that patients are discharged "sicker and quicker." This scenario tends to create a sense of loss or failure on the part of healthcare providers in hospitals, specifically physicians, but also nurses, social workers, and other professionals, when a patient is determined to be terminal or dying. In many hospital settings, there is great hesitancy to give up the cause and allow a patient to die.

In spite of the philosophical incongruence of dying in an acute care facility, more Americans die in hospitals than anywhere else, and hospitals can offer some unique services and advantages for dying patients and their families. First, in comparison to other types of institutions, hospitals provide more immediate and constant access to professional-level providers, including physicians, nurses, social workers, pharmacists, dieticians, psychologists, and clergy. The skill mix and educational preparation of direct care providers tends to be higher than what is available in other settings, such as nursing homes. With greater educational preparation, there is greater potential that providers have had some type of specific educational preparation in the care of the dying. Unfortunately, even with the recently increased emphasis on enhancing end-of-life care, a 2005 survey by Ogle, Mavis, and Thomason found that only 46% of 275 medical residency programs were providing formal training in end-of-life care.

Hospitals also offer more immediate access to specific therapeutic interventions that may be helpful in the dying process, including a wider range of medications, nutritional supplements, supportive devices such as ventilators and feeding tubes, and mechanical comfort measures such as therapeutic beds and mattresses or heating and cooling blankets. Acute care reimbursement policies also tend to allow for more liberal access to such interventions while patients are in these facilities.

More immediate access to resuscitation providers and interventions is available in the hospital setting. However, this is a double-edged sword for the dying because these interventions are more likely to be used in hospitals, regardless of patient and family preferences related to such interventions. For example, in a study of 270 hospitalized cancer patients, the wishes expressed in advance directives often did not affect whether they received resuscitative interventions (Kish, Martin, & Price, 2000).

Most hospitals offer easy access to supportive personnel such as social workers, counselors, or clergy. The availability of different types of clergy varies depending on the type of facility. Hospitals with a formal religious affiliation tend to have more individuals to provide clerical support, but they tend to be aligned with a limited number of religious denominations.

The provision of palliative care consultants and palliative care teams is a popular, recent trend in hospitals. The number of palliative care programs in hospitals increased from 15% of hospitals in 2000 to 25% of hospitals in 2003 (Morrison, Maroney-Galin, Kralovec, & Meier, 2005). Larger hospitals, veterans' hospitals, and academic medical centers are more likely to have palliative care programs. Hospitals operated by the Catholic church are also more likely to have such programs than hospitals owned by other religious groups (Morrison et al.).

Common Decisional Conflicts Related to Dying in Hospitals

Numerous ethical dilemmas and challenging decisions typify the dying experience in hospitals. Four of the most common decisions are addressed here. In each of these situations, optimal outcomes are achieved when the patient and family have discussed these questions and scenarios and have achieved consensus on their preferences prior to the patient's last few days of life.

When and By What Criteria Should Dying Patients Be Admitted and Discharged From Acute Care Hospitals?

Most people want to die at home, but fewer than 25% actually die there. A common dilemma for informal caregivers is the decision of whether, and when, to admit a dying family member to a hospital, particularly if the patient has previously stated a preference for dying at home. Usually, a decision to admit is prompted by a significant increase in symptoms or an acknowledged inability of home-based caregivers to provide sufficient physical care or symptom management. A related challenge is determining the right time to discharge a dying patient from hospital to home. The critical factor in both scenarios is the amount and type of support available to the home-based care provider. Teno and colleagues (2004) found that families of patients who died at home with hospice support were much more likely (70.7%) to rate the overall quality of end-of-life care as excellent compared to those who died in hospitals (46.8%) and those who died at home with standard home care nursing support (46.5%).

What Are the Best Strategies for Managing Symptoms of the Dying Process, Specifically Pain?

Pain control is a common challenge for dying patients and their family members in hospitals. The lack of effective pain management in hospitals is well documented. Among the 9,105 hospitalized adults in the SUPPORT (Study to Understand Prognoses and Preferences for Outcomes and Risks of Treatment) (1995) trial, 50% of the conscious patients who died were reported to have experienced moderate-to-severe pain in their last days of life.

One of the most common obstacles to effective pain management in hospitals is the fear of complications related to the use of strong analgesics, specifically opioid narcotics (Portenoy et al. 2006). Providers, patients, and family members often fear the potential side effects of addiction, excessive drowsiness, depressed respirations, and constipation; yet, opioids remain the most powerful and effective drugs for the relief of severe terminal pain. Research demonstrates that these fears are largely unsubstantiated, and there is ample justification for the use of these drugs to control pain in dying patients (American Pain Society, 1995). Again, advanced conversations and planning can help to clarify patient and family preferences, priorities, and fears or misunderstandings. For example, do the patient and family agree that it would be acceptable for the patient to be drowsy as long as his or her pain is controlled? Family members and other caregivers should be prepared to continually assess the patient's pain status and advocate for aggressive pain management interventions as needed.

Untreated or undertreated pain can compromise, if not drive, decision making near the end of life. Spannhake (chapter 3, this volume) recounts his experiences with a life-threatening illness, noting an overwhelming desire to be medicated to the point of unconsciousness, regardless of the risks, because of the excruciating pain he experienced. It is imperative that family members and providers understand how undertreated pain can have an impact on medical decision making and how to be supportive when pain is untreatable.

When and By What Criteria Should Lifesaving Interventions Be Used? And, When Should They Be Withdrawn?

One of the most common dilemmas in hospitals is the challenge of withdrawing treatment when the patient has not signed an advance directive, when the directive lacks clarity or specificity, or when there is conflict between providers and family members or conflict among family members. A frequent undercurrent in the acute care environment is the fear of liability for not taking the preferred action, particularly when the preference has not been documented in advance. In a study of 274 patients who died in hospitals, 84% had some intervention discontinued prior to death, but only 35% of those patients were able to participate in those decisions when they occurred (Faber-Langendoen, 1996). This study points to the urgency of not only initiating an advanced directive prior to hospitalization, but also carefully considering the pros and cons of the degree of specificity used (see Ditto, chapter 13, this volume). Ideally, families will discuss issues such as the following: What should be done if a patient experiences a cardiac or respiratory arrest while in the hospital? Should resuscitation be attempted? Should emergency medications be administered? Should chest compressions be performed? Should the patient be intubated and placed on a mechanical ventilator? Further, if a patient is determined to be terminal after aggressive interventions are initiated, questions concern such things as how long, or by what criteria, should mechanical ventilation, tube feedings, medications such as antibiotics, or intravenous fluids be continued.

The family-centered model Lyon describes using with Richard and his grandparents is an example of how families can work to come to consensus on advance directives prior to a point at which a critical decision is necessary (Richard & Lyon, chapter 2, this volume). As noted, this is a process that takes time, negotiation, and sometimes professional counseling to ensure decisions are well reasoned and respect the wishes of the dying individual and family members.

Patient autonomy and family preferences are critical issues in relation to these questions. However, patients and families should be advised of the growing trend among hospitals to establish policies that help to define cases of futility, for which aggressive life-saving interventions are not likely to be effective. If a case is determined to be futile, providers may legally elect to avoid or discontinue the use of such interventions regardless of patient or family preferences for aggressive action.

What Is the Optimal Level of Care for Dying Patients in Hospitals (e.g., Intensive Care, Standard Medical-Surgical Care, or Hospice Care)?

Many people dread the possibility of dying in an intensive care unit (ICU) with tubes and monitors attached to every body part. Yet, each year this scenario is a reality for approximately 500,000 people who die in U.S. ICUs (Birkmeyer, Birkmeyer, Wennberg, & Young, 2000). In spite of the common distaste for this scenario, transferring to a lower level of care (e.g., if a DNR decision is made after a patient has spent several days in the ICU) can be traumatic for patients and family members who have established relationships and trust in the ICU providers. Some important factors to consider in this situation are the potential for futility associated with aggressive and expensive critical care interventions as well as the potential for increased family presence and interaction in less-aggressive and more peaceful care delivery environments. In hospitals, like other care delivery settings, dying patients and families who receive hospice care or other specialized palliative care have the greatest level of satisfaction with the end-of-life experience (Baker et al., 2000; Higginson et al., 2002; see Crow, chapter 4, this volume).

Communication in Hospitals

An overriding issue of concern related to end-of-life decision making in hospitals is the need for open, honest, and effective communication among providers, patients, and families (see Csikai, chapter 11, this volume). In a study by Russ and Kaufman (2005), family members interviewed after a death reported multiple problems with communication, including providers who avoided them and did not answer questions or return calls until the patient was close to death and then demanded rapid decisions about withholding or removing life support measures.

Enhanced communication can potentially ease the burden of end-of-life decision making for each of the scenarios described. Elements of effective end-of-life communication include provider accessibility, timeliness, honesty, and full disclosure of information—particularly related to prognosis and the potential for success of interventions. Families also need realistic projections related to the potential investment of time and financial resources for life support measures. Crow (chapter 4, this volume) provides a dramatic example of how poor medical communication not only increases the stress on families but also can compromise decision making.

☐ Dying in Nursing Homes

In 2000, 25% of all U.S. deaths occurred in nursing homes (National Hospice and Palliative Care Organization, 2002). As our elderly population expands, a projected 40% of deaths may occur in nursing homes by the year 2040 (Brock & Foley, 1998). Nursing homes have always been in the business of end-of-life care; yet, the desire and need for focused improvements in the quality of end-of-life nursing home care has been emphasized in recent literature. For example, in a survey of 461 family members regarding recent end-of-life experiences in various settings, nursing home settings had the most opportunities for improvements (Hanson, Danis, & Garrett, 1997).

Most residents who die in nursing homes receive no palliative interventions or specific end-of-life care, and those who do often receive it only during the last few days of their lives (Travis, Loving, McClanahan, & Barnard, 2001). Although the use of hospice care in nursing homes is on the rise, recent studies have documented rates of dying nursing home residents receiving hospice care between 6% and 8.5% (Hanson, Reynolds, Henderson, & Pickard, 2005; Miller & Mor, 2001; Prevost & Wallace, 2004). The few nursing home residents who do receive hospice care have superior pain assessments, less-invasive procedures, and enhanced quality of life, all at lower overall costs (Gage & Dao, 2000).

Dying nursing home residents require intense and highly specialized assessments and interventions, including focused attention to their physical needs (e.g., nutrition, hydration, and pain management); emotional care and counseling; spiritual care; family care; advance planning; and ethical decision making. Nursing home staff members face challenges in providing these intense interventions for a variety of reasons, including lack of education and knowledge, minimum staffing, and high turnover rates.

Several investigators have studied obstacles to effective end-of-life care in nursing homes (Blevins & Deason-Howell, 2002; Ersek, Kraybill, & Hansberry, 2000; Ersek & Wilson, 2003; Stillman, Strumpf, Capezuti, & Tuch, 2005). In 2000, the Health Care Financing Administration (now called the Centers for Medicare and Medicaid Services) concluded that more than 90% of U.S. nursing homes failed to meet the minimum staffing standard of 2 hours of certified nursing assistant (CNA) time per resident per day (Shankroff, Miller, Feuerberg, & Mortimore, 2000). Since CNAs provide the overwhelming majority of nursing home care with limited educational preparation, it is not surprising that they often feel unprepared to address the challenging and controversial issues that arise at the end of life.

In addition to the minimal staffing patterns and the limited educational preparation of the caregivers, nursing homes struggle with some of the highest rates of staff turnover in the healthcare industry. The mean annual turnover rate among the long-term care workforce is 45% (Edwards, 2005). Nursing home caregivers who receive targeted educational interventions to expand their knowledge of end-of-life care are unlikely to work in these settings very long.

Both staff and family members have identified lack of effective communication as a problem (Ersek et al., 2000). In a study of family members interviewed after a death, 23% of them could not recall any discussions with providers about end-of-life decisions (Hanson et al., 1997). This indicates that either the discussions did not happen or family members did not remember them, which is common when communication is ineffective or poorly timed, as is often the case during periods of intense emotional stress.

Common Decisional Conflicts Related to Dying in Nursing Homes

When and By What Criteria Should a Dying Patient Be Admitted to a Nursing Home?

One of the first and most common dilemmas associated with the trajectory of nursing home death is the decision to move a dying family member into a nursing home facility. This decision is generally prompted by one of two scenarios: either the family caregiver becomes physically and emotionally overwhelmed with the demands of providing terminal care at home or the dying patient experiences an episode that ultimately results in a decision to transition from acute, restorative care to terminal, long-term care.

In this placement process, patients and families are challenged by several significant questions and decisions. First, is there bed space available in a desirable facility? If space is available in more than one facility, which one is best suited to meet the needs of this patient and the patient's family? Second, what resources or support systems are available to pay for nursing home expenses? Third, does the facility have a hospice service or other specific palliative care resource readily available?

Which Nursing Home Residents Should Be Classified as Near the End of Life?

Sometimes, nursing home caregivers have conflicting opinions about which residents need end-of-life care and who is responsible for initiating end-of-life care planning and interventions with residents and their families. Physicians and nurse practitioners, the primary providers for nursing home residents, also struggle with diagnosis and assignment of terminal status. Prognostication based on a clinical assessment is particularly challenging when residents suffer from a variety of chronic illnesses and cognitive impairments (Miller et al., 1998). Further, it is difficult to make an accurate prognosis when the individual has conflicting physical phenomena, difficulty communicating, or memory lapses or experiences gradual decline over extended periods of time.

In recent years, several researchers have used the nursing home Minimum Data Set (MDS) as a source of predictors of mortality, or terminal status, among nursing home residents (Flacker & Kiely, 2003; Mitchell et al., 2004; Porock et al., 2005; Wallace & Prevost, 2006). Many of these investigators concluded their studies by publishing lists of risk factors, or models for mortality prediction, but no published studies have reported evaluation or use of any of these models in actual clinical facilities. A research-based clinical tool that simplifies and increases the accuracy of terminal prognostication among nursing home residents could help facilitate end-of-life care planning and hospice interventions for dying residents.

To What Extent Should Restorative Versus Palliative Interventions Be Used?

Although hospitals emphasize restoring health to acute patients as quickly as possible, nursing homes typically focus on rehabilitative care and the management of chronic disease. Nevertheless, shifting focus to palliative care can be problematic for nursing home care planners and staff, especially because, as discussed, identifying terminal patients can be difficult. However, because many nursing home residents will eventually die, it is important that nursing home staff be willing and able to make this shift to ensure dying patients receive optimal end-of-life care.

Once a patient has been identified as terminal, nursing home care planners must decide whether to discontinue rehabilitative services such as physical therapy and occupational therapy, withdraw life-sustaining interventions like respirators or tube feeding, and shift the focus to pain management and comfort care. These choices should reflect patient and family preferences, especially those communicated in living wills and advance directives. Hence, it is important for patients and families to discuss these issues in advance and to communicate their desires to care providers. Care providers in turn must know which advance directives are in place and be willing to solicit family input when decisions are being made.

A particularly difficult decision that providers often have to make involves whether to hospitalize a terminal patient experiencing an acute event. Again, physicians and nurses are trained to treat acute conditions in an effort to relieve suffering and extend life, and patients and their families are socialized to seek medical attention for treatable acute conditions. However, it may be in the best interest of terminal patients not to treat life-threatening acute conditions and to focus instead on making their last few days or hours as comfortable as possible. Nevertheless, choosing not to hospitalize and not to treat acute events can be difficult (see Volicer, chapter 18, this volume). As before, patients, families, and providers should consider what to do in such situations in advance rather than waiting for a crisis to make such decisions (see Ditto, chapter 13, this volume).

Which Palliative Measures Should Be Available, Who Should Provide Them, and Who Will Pay for Them?

Palliative care involves comfort care and pain management as well as measures designed to address the psychological, social, and spiritual concerns of dying patients and their families. Nursing homes are often ill-equipped to provide such care. Staff are seldom adequately trained in palliative care, and limited resources may make it impossible to ensure that pain is adequately monitored or that a variety of pain remediation therapies are available. In addition, few facilities can afford to keep full-time counselors, psychologists, or chaplains on staff.

Increasingly, nursing homes have turned to external palliative care specialists or contracted with outside hospice organizations to provide palliative care to their patients. Although the latter arrangement can improve the end-of-life care provided by nursing homes, access to hospice in nursing homes is often driven by the ability to make a definitive 6-month terminal prognosis rather than by the needs of the individual residents (Miller et al., 1998). To receive the Medicare hospice benefit in a nursing home, the attending physician and the medical director of the affiliated hospice must certify that the resident is terminally ill with less than 6 months to live. Plus, residents or their surrogates must give the hospice full responsibility for their care and waive the right to receive standard Medicare benefits, including curative treatments related to their terminal diagnosis. These decisions can be very difficult for providers, residents, and families, particularly if the terminal prognosis is uncertain. Some physicians fear the accusation of fraud if residents happen to live beyond the 6-month projection (Martin, 1999).

Among medical providers, the overriding goal to cure can create challenges and competing interests in documenting prognoses and planning related end-of-life interventions. Plans directed toward curing or rehabilitating may not be in the best interest of the dying resident. Also, nursing home regulations and reimbursement structures that emphasize restorative and rehabilitative care rather than terminal or palliative care can interfere with the process of classifying a patient as terminal (Miller, Teno,

& Mor, 2004). This cure-oriented philosophy and the related goals of care can conflict with end-of-life care directed toward a peaceful death.

Opportunities for Improvement in Nursing Homes

Limited staff knowledge is frequently assumed to be a major cause of end-of-life care deficits in nursing homes. Therefore, targeted education on end-of-life care is recommended (Last Acts, 2002). Consequently, investigators recently have tested educational interventions for enhancing end-of-life care in nursing homes. Ersek (2003) edited a core curriculum specifically for palliative care nursing assistants. Later, Ersek, Grant, and Kraybill (2005) used this and other nationally recognized end-of-life curricula to develop and implement a program called the Palliative Care Educational Resource Team (PERT). Evaluation of the PERT program revealed increases in end-of-life knowledge, self-evaluation of end-of-life skills, and supervisor's evaluations of staff participation in end-of-life care. Hanson and colleagues (2005) conducted a quality improvement project using hospice providers to educate staff in seven nursing homes. The researchers also met monthly with nursing home staff to provide performance data and plan organizational change strategies. Their program was effective in increasing baseline pain assessments from 18% to 60% of residents and increasing end-of-life discussions from 4% to 17% of residents, but hospice enrollment only increased from 4% to 6.8%.

As stated, end-of-life care in nursing homes could also be enhanced by improving the identification of dying patients. Early identification of potentially terminal patients would allow nursing home staff to begin making the shift from curative and rehabilitative care and possibly to seek a terminal diagnosis from attending physicians, thus allowing the patient to be moved to hospice care. At the policy level, changes in Medicare that would extend nursing home hospice benefits to all patients deemed by their care plan team to need them, whether or not they have a formal terminal diagnosis, could greatly increase the use of hospice services and improve end-of-life care.

☐ Dying in Residential Hospices

Residential hospices or hospice homes are places where terminal patients may live while receiving hospice care. The care is similar to that provided to terminal individuals living in their own residences; the difference is that it is provided in a facility or home operated by the hospice organization rather than in a private home. Federal and state policies have limited the development and use of residential hospices in the United States. For example, although Medicare will pay a residential hospice for the end-of-life care it provides, it does not cover the costs of rooming and boarding hospice patients. These costs must be paid by the patients themselves, their families, or the hospice organization. Some residential hospices rely on charitable contributions to defray these costs (National Hospice and Palliative Care Organization, 2004). The Centers for Medicare and Medicaid Services (2003) is currently investigating the feasibility of using residential hospices to provide hospice care to terminal patients in rural areas who do not have caregivers available in the home.

There is little research on dying in residential hospices other than that which discusses dying with hospice in general. There are studies that describe the development and operations of individual residential hospices (Carter, 1998; Neubecker, 1994; Woodall & Dennis, 2003) and the training and educational needs of residential hospice staff (Evans, Bibeau, & Conley, 2001; Jacques & Hasselkus, 2004; Murray, Fiset, & O'Connor, 2004), but more research is needed on how the experience of dying in a residential hospice differs from dying in a private home with hospice care.

☐ Conclusion

Although a sizable majority of Americans indicate a preference for dying at home, most deaths today occur in institutional settings, with roughly half occurring in hospitals and just under a quarter occurring in skilled nursing facilities. Table 12.1 provides a comparison of the three most common locations and scenarios for dying. The type and quality of end-of-life care provided by these settings can vary tremendously. Hospitals, with their focus on acute conditions and curative care, tend to emphasize keeping patients alive rather than making their deaths as easy and comfortable as possible. Licensed, professional care providers have access to the latest health-monitoring and life-sustaining technologies and eagerly employ them to extend their patients' lives, often with little attention to quality of life in the final days. Although the resources to provide palliative care are obviously available in hospitals, physicians and nurses are trained to preserve life and see that as their primary function. To them, death is sometimes perceived as failure. Thus, they tend to be reluctant to admit that patients are dying, and when they do so, they are often ill-equipped psychologically and emotionally to provide optimal palliative care. In light of this scenario, two of the most important decisions for hospitalized patients and their families are whether they concur that death is imminent and whether they are ready to relinquish the fight to prolong life. Once the patient and family reach the point of acceptance that death

TABLE 12.1 Differences in End-of-Life Care by Location

Location of Care	Primary Treatment Focus	Availability and Use of Life-Sustaining Technologies	Available Care Providers	Availability and Use of Palliative Care and Hospice
Acute hospital	Acute and curative	Readily available and frequently used	Paid professional staff, most are licensed	Palliative care available but treatment focus limits use; hospice availability limited
Skilled nursing facility	Chronic and rehabilitative	Moderate availability and use	Paid professional staff, most are unlicensed	Palliative care available; use of palliative care increasing; hospice availability also increasing
Residential hospice/ home-based hospice	Palliative	Not typically available	Informal care providers with some paid professional support	Hospice and palliative care available by definition; quality depends on training and expertise of care providers

is imminent, a strong patient advocate such as a nurse case manager or social worker can assist them in redirecting the life-saving efforts of the healthcare team.

By design, skilled nursing facilities are not acute care facilities. Rather, their focus is on the treatment and control of chronic conditions and the maintenance or improvement of functional ability. Nursing home patients are typically too sick to be cared for at home but not sick enough to require hospitalization. Although some will recover sufficiently to be discharged home, many will experience a gradual decline in health and functional ability that will ultimately end in death. Because a larger proportion of nursing home patients die, nursing home staff are more accustomed to and accepting of death. It is more likely to be seen as a normal, even welcomed, end to a lengthy period of sickness and decline. Thus, nursing homes are less likely to employ extraordinary means to keep patients alive, especially because many nursing home patients have advance directives in place to indicate that they do not want such interventions. Concomitantly, they are also more likely to provide palliative care and in recent years have increased the role of hospice in the provision of palliative care. However, nursing homes may have difficulty determining when a gradually declining patient is near death and thus in need of end-of-life care. Further, the limited training received by many nursing home staff often leaves them ill-equipped for dealing with dying patients and their families. Hence, although nursing homes are often more accommodating with regard to palliative care, they may not always possess the resources or have those with the knowledge and skills necessary to provide the highest-quality end-of-life care. Again, in the nursing home setting, one of the first major decisions is achieving consensus that the resident has indeed entered into a terminal or dying trajectory. Once this phase is recognized, consultation with a palliative care specialist or hospice provider should be pursued. These experts can guide the patient and family through the subsequent and more specific decision-making processes, including documenting preferences for advance directives, resuscitative interventions, and terminal symptom control.

Although the focus of this chapter is dying in institutions, a brief word about dying in a residential hospice or with home-based hospice care is in order. Clearly, such settings are the most accommodating to palliative care. After all, that is in fact the focus of care. However, they are also least accommodating to life-sustaining medical technologies. Patients and families choosing noninstitutional hospice care must make certain that this is the right decision for them. In addition, community-based hospice care presupposes an active, well-trained hospice organization and capable and competent informal caregivers. If hospice services are not available in a given area or if there are too few staff and volunteers, hospice care may not be an option. Further, if the education and training of hospice staff and volunteers is inadequate, the provision of quality end-of-life care is compromised. Most important, without a network of committed, capable, and caring informal care providers, home-based hospice care is likely to be inadequate. Thus, home- and community-based hospice care is only an option if there are sufficiently committed and skilled care providers available in the community.

Most American deaths occur in institutional settings, and the type of institution can have a tremendous impact on caregiver attitudes and expertise related to dying as well as the resources available to support the dying process. The key to achieving the optimal scenario lies in anticipating the questions and choices that will arise, discussing them in advance, and documenting patient and family preferences before a time of crisis occurs.

☐ References

American Pain Society Quality of Care Committee. (1995). Quality improvement guidelines for the treatment of acute pain and cancer pain. *Journal of the American Medical Association, 274*, 1874–1880.

Baker, R., Hyg, M., Wu, A., Teno, J., Kreling, B., Damiano, A., et al. (2000). Family satisfaction with end-of-life care in seriously ill hospitalized adults. *Journal of the American Geriatrics Society, 48,* S61–S69.

Birkmeyer, J. D., Birkmeyer, C. M., Wennberg, D. E., & Young, M. P. (2000). *Leapfrog safety standards: Potential benefits of universal adoption.* Washington, DC: Leapfrog Group.

Blevins, D., & Deason-Howell, L. M. (2002). End-of-life care in nursing homes: The interface of policy, research, and practice. *Behavioral Sciences and the Law, 20,* 271–286.

Brazil, K., Howell, D., Bedard, M., Krueger, P., & Heidebrecht, C. (2005). Preferences for place of care and place of death among informal caregivers of the terminally ill. *Palliative Medicine, 19,* 492–499.

Brock, D., & Foley, D. (1998). Demography and epidemiology of dying in the U.S. with emphasis on deaths of older persons. *Hospitals, 13,* 49–60.

Burge, F., Lawson, B., Johnston, G., & Cummings, I. (2003). Primary care continuity and location of death for those with cancer. *Journal of Palliative Medicine, 6,* 911–918.

Carter, C. (1998). Hospice: Residential care center. The first year. *The Kansas Nurse, 73*(3), 2–3.

Center for Gerontology and Health Care Research. (2004). *Facts on dying 2004.* Retrieved April 6, 2007, from http://www.chcr.brown.edu/dying/factsondying.htm

Centers for Medicare and Medicaid Services. (2003). *Rural Hospice Demonstration Project.* Retrieved April 6, 2007, from http://www.cms.hhs.gov/demoprojectsevalrpts/md/itemdetail.asp?filterType=none&filterByDID=0&sortByDID=3&sortOrder=ascending&itemID=CMS024393

Degenholtz, H. B., Rhee, Y., & Arnold, R. M. (2004). Brief communication: The relationship between having a living will and dying in place. *Annals of Internal Medicine, 141,* 113–117.

Edwards, D. (2005). LTC employee turnover costs the nation billions each year. *Nursing Homes and Long Term Care Management, 54*(2), 16.

Ersek, M. (2003). *Core curriculum for the hospice and palliative nursing assistant.* Dubuque, IA: Kendall-Hunt.

Ersek, M., Grant, M., & Kraybill, B. (2005). Enhancing end-of-life care in nursing homes: Palliative care educational resource team (PERT). *Journal of Palliative Medicine, 8,* 556–566.

Ersek, M., Kraybill, B., & Hansberry, J. (2000). Assessing the educational needs and concerns of nursing home staff regarding end-of-life care. *Journal of Gerontological Nursing, 27,* 16–26.

Ersek, M., & Wilson, S. (2003). The challenges and opportunities in proving end-of-life care in nursing homes. *Journal of Palliative Medicine, 6,* 45–57.

Evans, W. M., Bibeau, D. L., & Conley, K. M. (2001). Coping strategies used in residential hospice settings: Findings from a national study. *American Journal of Hospice & Palliative Care, 18,* 102–110.

Faber-Langendoen, K. (1996). A multi-institutional study of care given to patients dying in hospitals. *Archives of Internal Medicine, 156,* 2130–2136.

Flacker, J. M., & Kiely, K. (2003). Mortality-related factors and 1-year survival in nursing home residents. *Journal of American Geriatrics Society, 51,* 213–221.

Flory, J., Young-Xu, Y., Gurol, I., Levinsky, N., Ash, A., & Emanuel, E. (2004). Place of death: U.S. trends since 1980. *Health Affairs, 23,* 194–200.

Gage, B., & Dao, T. (2000). *Medicare's hospice benefit: Use and expenditures, 1996 cohort.* Washington, DC: U.S. Department of Health and Human Services.

Hanson, L., Danis, M., & Garrett, J. (1997). What is wrong with end-of-life care? Opinions of bereaved family members. *Journal of American Geriatric Society, 45,* 1339–1344.

Hanson, L., Reynolds, K., Henderson, M., & Pickard, C. (2005). A quality improvement intervention to increase palliative care in nursing homes. *Journal of Palliative Medicine, 8,* 576–586.

Higginson, I., Finlay, I., Goodwin, D., Cook, A., Hood, K., Edwards, A., et al. (2002). Do hospital-based palliative teams improve care for patients or families at end of life. *Journal of Pain Management, 23,* 96–106.

Iwashyna, T. J., & Chang, V. W. (2002). Racial and ethnic differences in place of death: United States, 1993. *Journal of the American Geriatrics Society, 50,* 1113–1117.

Jacques, N. D., & Hasselkus, B. R. (2004). The nature of occupation surrounding dying and death. *Occupation, Participation and Health, 24*(2), 44–53.

Johnson, K. S., Kuchibhatala, M., Sloane, R. J., Tanis, D., Galanos, A. N., & Tulsky, J. A. (2005). Ethnic differences in the place of death of elderly hospice enrollees. *Journal of the American Geriatrics Society, 53,* 2209–2215.

Kish, S., Martin, C., & Price, K. (2000). Advance directives in critically ill cancer patients. *Critical Care Nursing Clinics of North America, 12,* 373–383.

Klinkenberg, M., Visser, G., van Groenou, M., van der Wal, G., Deeg, D., & Willems, D. L. (2005). The last 3 months of life: care, transition and the place of death of older people. *Health and Social Care in the Community, 13,* 420–430.

Koffman, J., & Higginson, I. J. (2004). Dying to be home? Preferred location of death of first-generation black Caribbean and native-born white patients in the United Kingdom. *Journal of Palliative Medicine, 7,* 628–636.

Last Acts. (2002). *Means to a better end: A report on dying in America today.* Princeton, NJ: Robert Wood Johnson Foundation.

Levy, C. R., Fish, R., & Kramer, A. M. (2004). Site of death in the hospital versus nursing home of Medicare skilled nursing facility residents admitted under Medicare's Part A benefit. *Journal of the American Geriatrics Society, 52,* 1247–1254.

Lynn, J., & Adamson, D. M. (2003). *Living well at the end of life: Adapting health care to serious chronic illness in old age,* Santa Monica, CA: Rand.

Martin, E. (1999). Helping patients find their way to "good death" [Electronic version]. *American College of Physicians Observer.* Retrieved May 10, 2007, from http://www.acponline.org/journals/news/jun99/gooddeath.htm

McCall, K., & Rice, A. M. (2005). What influences decisions around the place of care for terminally ill cancer patients? *International Journal of Palliative Nursing, 11,* 541–547.

McMillan, A., Mentnech, R. M., Lubitz, J., McBean, A. M., & Russell, D. (1990). Trends and patterns in place of death for Medicare enrollees. *Health Care Financing Review, 12,* 1–7.

McWhinney, I. R., Bass, M. J., & Orr, V. (1995). Factors associated with location of death (home or hospital) of patients referred to a palliative care team. *Canadian Medical Association Journal, 152,* 361–367.

Miller, S., & Mor, V. (2001). The emergence of Medicare hospice care in U.S. nursing homes. *Palliative Medicine, 15,* 471–480.

Miller, S., Mor, V., Coppola, K., Teno, J., Laliberte, L., & Petrisek, A. (1998). The Medicare hospice benefit's influence on dying in nursing homes. *Journal of Palliative Medicine, 1,* 367–376.

Miller, S., Teno, J., & Mor, V. (2004). Hospice and palliative care in nursing homes. *Clinics in Geriatric Medicine, 20,* 717–734.

Mitchell, S., Kiely, D., Hamel, M., Park, S., Morris, N., & Fries, B. (2004). Estimating prognosis for nursing home residents with advanced dementia. *Journal of the American Medical Association, 291,* 2734–2740.

Mitchell, S. L., Teno, J. M., Miller, S. C., & Mor, V. (2005). A national study of the location of death for older persons with dementia. *Journal of the American Geriatrics Society, 53,* 299–305.

Morrison, R. S., Maroney-Galin, C., Kralovec, P. D., & Meier, D. E. (2005). The growth of palliative care programs in the United States. *Journal of Palliative Medicine, 8,* 1127–34.

Murray, M. A., Fiset, V., & O'Connor, B. (2004). Learning needs of nurses at a residential hospice. *Journal of Hospice & Palliative Nursing, 6,* 108–116.

National Center for Health Statistics. (2006). *Health, United States, 2006, with chartbook on trends in the health of Americans.* Hyattsville, MD: Author.

National Hospice and Palliative Care Organization. (2002). *NHPCO facts and figures.* Alexandria, VA: Author.

National Hospice and Palliative Care Organization. (2004). *2004 national data set.* Retrieved February 22, 2006, from http://www.nhpco.org/i4a/pages/index.cfm?pageid=3367

Neubecker, J. (1994). Hospice: A comprehensive program. *Health Progress, 75*(9), 28–31, 40.

Ogle, K. S., Mavis, B., & Thomason, C. (2005). Learning to provide end-of-life care: Postgraduate medical training programs in Michigan. *Journal of Palliative Medicine, 8,* 987–997.

Pekmezaris, R., Breuer, L., Zaballero, A., Wolf-Klein, G., Jadoon, E., D'Olimpio, J. T., et al. (2004). Predictors of site of death of end-of-life patients: The importance of specificity in advance directives. *Journal of Palliative Medicine, 7,* 9–17.

Portenoy, R., Sibirceva, U., Smout, R., Horn, S., Connor, S., Blum, R., et al. (2006). Opioid use and survival at the end of life: A survey of a hospice population. *Journal of Pain and Symptom Management, 32,* 532–540.

Prevost, S., & Wallace, J. (2004). Predicting limited life expectancy in long term care. In *Proceedings: Sigma Theta Tau's 15th International Nursing Research Congress.* Retrieved May 10, 2007, from http://www.nursinglibrary.org/Portal/main.aspx?pageid=4024&pid=4305

Porock, D., Oliver, D., Zweig, S., Rantz, M., Mehr, D., Madsen, R., et al. (2005). Predicting death in the nursing home: Development and validation of the 6-month Minimum Data Set mortality risk index. *Journal of Gerontology, 60,* 491–498.

Russ, A., & Kaufman, S. (2005). Family perceptions of prognosis, silence, and the "suddenness" of death. *Culture, Medicine, and Psychiatry, 20,* 103–123.

Shankroff, J., Miller, P., Feuerberg, M., & Mortimore, E. (2000). Nursing home initiative. *Health Care Financing Review, 22,* 113–115.

Stillman, D., Strumpf, N., Capezuti, E., & Tuch, H. (2005). Staff perceptions concerning barriers and facilitators to end-of-life care in the nursing home. *Geriatric Nursing, 26,* 259–264.

SUPPORT Principal Investigators. (1995). A controlled trial to improve care for seriously ill hospitalized patients: The Study to Understand Prognoses and Preferences for Outcomes and Risks of Treatment (SUPPORT). *Journal of the American Medical Association, 274,* 1591–1598.

Tang, S. T., Liu, T. W., Lai, M. S., & McCorkle, R. (2005). Discrepancy in the preferences of place of death between terminally ill cancer patients and their primary family caregivers in Taiwan. *Social Science and Medicine, 61,* 1560–1566.

Teno, J., Clarridge, B., Casey, V., Welch, L., Wetle, T., Shield, R., et al. (2004). Family perspectives on end-of-life care and the last place of care. *Journal of the American Medical Association, 291,* 88–93.

Tiernan, E., O'Connor, M., O'Siorain, L., & Kearney, M. (2002). A prospective study of preferred versus actual place of death among patients referred to a palliative care home-care service. *Irish Medical Journal, 95*(8), 232–235.

Tolle, S. W., Rosenfeld, A. G., Tilden, V. P., & Park, Y. (1999). Oregon's low in-hospital death rates: What determines where people die and satisfaction with decisions of place of death? *Annals of Internal Medicine, 130,* 681–685.

Travis, S., Loving, G., McClanahan, L., & Barnard, M. (2001). Hospitalization patterns and palliation in the last year of life among residents in long-term care. *The Gerontologist, 41,* 153–160.

Wallace, J., & Prevost, S. (2006). Two methods for predicting limited life expectancy in nursing homes. *Journal of Nursing Scholarship, 37,* 148–153.

Weitzen, S., Teno, J. M., Fennell, M., & Mor, V. (2003). Factors associated with site of death: A national study of where people die. *Medical Care, 41,* 323–335.

Woodall, H. E., & Dennis, W. (2003). Comfort always. The Rainey Hospice House: South Carolina's first inpatient hospice. *Journal of the South Carolina Medical Association, 99*(8), 224–226.

13

CHAPTER

What Would Terri Want?

Advance Directives and the Psychological Challenges of Surrogate Decision Making

Peter H. Ditto

☐ Introduction

The tragic final chapter of Terri Schiavo's life story was unique in many ways (see Cerminara, chapter 8, this volume). Even in an era saturated with celebrity trials and confessional television talk shows, seldom has such an exquisitely personal decision been elevated to the level of full-blown, 21st century style public spectacle. Discussions normally held in reverent tones within the dimly lit corridors of hospitals and hospices were magnified by a 24-hour news cycle and an ongoing culture war into a national conversation—a national shouting match at times—with individuals, interest groups, and even the U.S. Congress aligning themselves with one or the other side of a horribly fractured family to engage in an agonizingly difficult debate over the relative value of a human life versus the essentially human right to decide how one's life should be lived (and therefore ended). The situation seemed uniquely cursed with every difficulty that might befall a family striving to make the right decisions for an incapacitated loved one. Irreconcilable differences between family members about the appropriate course of action, the lack of any written documentation of Terri's wishes about the use of life-sustaining technology, and ambiguity about her level of disability and prognosis for recovery all created a confluence of uncertainty that seemed only to fuel the moral outrage among active partisans and to make simple, comfortable resolutions difficult for almost any thoughtful observer.

In many other ways, however, the issues faced by Terri Schiavo's family were not at all unusual. Every day, thousands of families in the United States and around the world must make decisions about whether to prolong a loved one's life "artificially" with medical treatment.[1] Every day families disagree about how such decisions should be made, are uncertain about what their loved one would have really wanted, and wrestle with doubts about giving up the fight for their loved one's life too early or too late. The end of Terri Schiavo's life may have been unique in the number of different factors that conspired to complicate decision making on her behalf, but taken individually the challenges faced by the Schiavo and Schindler families were all too common ones, and thus an analysis of them can help generate insights that are applicable to the difficulties inherent in end-of-life medical decision making more generally.

In this chapter, I use the Terri Schiavo case as a springboard to review psychological research on end-of-life medical decision making generally and the use of instructional advance directives (i.e., "living wills") in particular. I identify three points of uncertainty and disagreement that were brought into sharp relief in the Schiavo case, which represent general categories of problems faced in almost all instances when decisions about the use of life-sustaining treatment must be made for incapacitated individuals. I conclude with a discussion of some lessons we might learn from the Schiavo case about how to better approach such decisions in the future, but with a disclaimer: There is no easy fix that will make end-of-life decision making simple and conflict free. The line between life and death will nearly always be blurry, and there likely will never be a sure way of knowing the wishes of an individual left wishless by ravages of injury or disease. Despite many commentators' quick leap to endorse living wills as the sure path to avoiding Terri and her family's sad fate, resolving the uncertainty and conflict inherent in end-of-life medical decisions will not be as easy as just filling out a form.

☐ Self-Determination, Surrogate Decision Making, and Substituted Judgment

The fundamental right of individuals to control the important decisions in their lives, especially regarding their own health and bodily integrity, is well founded in U.S. law and embodied by traditional American values of personal liberty and privacy. When medical decisions must be made near the end of life, however, this basic right to self-determination becomes complicated in two important ways.

First, although ethicists often argue that there is no morally relevant distinction between identical outcomes brought about by acts of commission (doing something) versus acts of omission (not doing something), laypeople, legislators, and judges often do see an important difference (Baron & Ritov, 2004; Spranca, Minsk, & Baron, 1991). A good example of this point is that although the right of seriously ill individuals to choose not to avail themselves of life-sustaining medical treatment is relatively noncontroversial as a matter of both law and public opinion, whether these same individuals have the right to take *active* steps to end their own lives remains extremely contentious (Dresser, 2003; Pew Research Center, 2006). This is most obviously true when medication is used to hasten death, as in the classic physician-assisted suicide scenario or in the physician-condoned-but-unassisted death described in Nicola Raye's touching story of her father's passing (see chapter 5 in this volume). But, the same psychological distinction also underlies the ethical difference many people sense between choosing not to initiate life-sustaining treatment in the first place (an act of omission) and stopping life-sustaining treatment that has already begun (an act of commission). In this chapter, I focus only on decisions about whether to begin or continue life-sustaining treatment and do not deal with the important set of psychological issues revolving around the most active forms of hastened death like physician-assisted suicide. In particular, my focus is on situations like those faced by Terri Schiavo's family as well as Laura Crow and her father (see Crow's chapter 4, this volume), in which decisions about the use of life-sustaining medical treatment must be made for individuals who can no longer speak for themselves.

This brings us to the second complication that often faces the exercise of patient self-determination near the end of life. Exercising one's right to choose for oneself is a straightforward affair as long as that self is conscious and competent to make decisions. Unfortunately, in many cases when decisions have to be made about the use of life-sustaining medical treatment, these decisions must be made after the individual is already too sick to speak for himself or herself (e.g., Bradley, Walker, Blecher, & Wettle, 1997). As a legal matter, it is well established that current incompetence does not diminish a formerly competent individual's fundamental right to self-determination (*Cruzan v. Director, Missouri Department of Health*, 1990; Dresser, 2003; see also Cerminara, chapter 8, this volume). As such, Terri Schiavo retained her legal rights to make her own medical decisions despite the fact that near the end of her life she had been unable to speak for herself for more than a decade. The problem of course is a logistical one. How can people like Terri Schiavo or Laura Crow's brain-injured brother exercise their fundamental right to make their own medical decisions?

The key is that someone else must make the decision for them but do so in a way that faithfully represents the decisions they would have made for themselves if they were able. This process is referred to as *substituted judgment* (Baergen, 1995; President's Commission, 1983), and it is generally accepted as the most desirable method of making decisions for incapacitated patients precisely because of the ethical priority accorded to self-determination in medical decision making (Buchanan & Brock, 1990; President's Commission). That is, rather than representing a surrogate decision maker's beliefs about what is best for the patient, the substituted judgment standard requires surrogates to remove their own wishes from the decision-making process and strive only to represent the *patient's* preferences regarding the use of life-sustaining medical treatment. In this way, the interpersonal judgment can be *substituted* for the personal one, and the incapacitated individual can maintain, through a surrogate decision maker, the ability to express choices even though he or she currently lacks decision-making capacity.

From a legal and ethical standpoint then, the decision about whether to terminate the provision of nutrition and hydration to Terri Schiavo was her decision to make. Because Terri was no longer able to make that decision for herself, however, the task facing her loved ones was to ask themselves the essential substituted judgment question, "What would Terri want?"

It is my contention in the following sections that when faced with the prospect of a seriously ill loved one, people have difficulty both asking and answering this important question. Honoring the wishes of an incapacitated individual is no simple psychological feat. Not only must the surrogate remain focused on the task of predicting *the patient's* wishes in the face of other competing standards that might be used to make decisions on the patient's behalf, but prior indications of the patient's wishes (even formal ones recorded in advance directive documents) are seldom as helpful as most people imagine when it comes to predicting how the patient would make a specific decision about the use of a particular medical therapy in a specific set of clinical circumstances. To be sure, it took a unique convergence of medical uncertainty, family dynamics, and historic and cultural forces to catapult Terri Schiavo into the national spotlight. Still, an analysis of the points of conflict in the Schiavo case can be instructive about the problems surrounding end-of-life decision making more generally in that the very intensity of the conflict that surrounded that case serves to highlight issues that are actually quite common but normally struggled with in less-dramatic fashion.

The three central points of uncertainty, and therefore conflict, in the Schiavo case concerned (a) the appropriate standard by which to make decisions on Terri's behalf, (b) the specific nature of Terri's wishes about the use of life-sustaining treatment, and (c) the true nature of Terri's level of disability and prognosis for recovery. These points are discussed in turn, first in terms of how each played out in the Schiavo case specifically and second with an emphasis on identifying issues of general concern in end-of-life medical decision making.

☐ Conflicting Values for End-of-Life Decision Making

Based on the precedent set by *Cruzan v. Director, Missouri Department of Health* (1990) and supported by Florida State law, the legal decision regarding the removal of Terri Schiavo from artificial nutrition and hydration hinged on the provision of "clear and convincing" evidence that this act was consistent with Terri's wishes. The legal arguments presented by the two sides were thus primarily framed in terms of honoring Terri's wishes and therefore her right to self-determination. In fact, the ability of Terri's husband, Michael, to so consistently prevail in the numerous judicial proceedings was likely because of the discipline shown by his legal team in terms of characterizing their case solely as an issue of carrying out Terri's own desire to be removed from artificial life support.

The arguments presented by the Schindler family's legal team, and those presented in the media by the Schindlers and their various supporters, were much less disciplined. At times, the argument was made that Terri would not have wanted her feeding tube removed. This was asserted variously on the basis of either statements she supposedly had made as a adolescent watching television reports about the Karen Ann Quinlan case or her Catholic faith, which according to the position of Pope John Paul II, excludes the provision of food and water from the types of "artificial" life-prolonging treatments (such as mechanical respiration) that individuals have an ethical right to refuse.

At other times, however, the argument for maintaining Terri's nutrition and hydration revealed an ethical stance directly opposed to arguments based on her right to self-determination. For example, in a detailed report on the case written for Florida Governor Jeb Bush, the court-appointed guardian ad litem noted that the Schindler family members explicitly stated during court testimony that "even if Theresa had told them of her intention to have artificial nutrition withdrawn, they would not do it" (Wolfson, 2003, p. 14). The report gives this additional description of the Schindler family's stance toward Terri's medical treatment:

> Throughout the course of the litigation, deposition and trial testimony by members of the Schindler family voiced the disturbing belief that they would keep Theresa alive at any and all costs. Nearly

> gruesome examples were given, eliciting agreement by the family members that in the event Theresa should contract diabetes and subsequent gangrene in each of her limbs, they would agree to amputate each limb, and would then, were she to be diagnosed with heart disease, perform open heart surgery. (p. 14)

The sentiments of the Schindler family are of course understandable and may best be attributed to a purely emotional desire to keep their loved one alive rather than any explicit consideration of abstract ethical principles. Other participants in the legal and media debates, however, made statements quite explicitly based on a "right to life," suggesting that Terri should continue to receive nutrition and hydration, not because she would have wanted to, but because of an ethical obligation to maintain life if the means to do so are within reach. A softer version of this argument was revealed in repeated assertions by President George W. Bush and others that end-of-life medical decisions should "err on the side of life."

At least three other distinct ethical arguments can be identified that were made in support of maintaining Terri's treatment. Closely related to the right-to-life argument, disability rights advocates argued that Terri's nutrition and hydration should be maintained because its discontinuation would reflect a devaluation of the lives of the cognitively disabled. Another argument heard frequently in the media coverage was one based on parental rights. According to this argument, Terri's mother and father had a fundamental right to maintain her life if they so desired (e.g., "If her parents are willing to take care of her, why not let them?"). Finally, a number of statements made about the case revealed an implicit reliance on the "best interest standard" that is generally considered an important principle in surrogate decision making, but only if the substituted judgment standard cannot be applied (Buchanan & Brock, 1990). Examples of this range from the oft-cited concern that removal of artificial nutrition and hydration would cause Terri pain and suffering (and thus was not in her best interest), to the assertion made by Schindler attorney David Gibbs in his argument to federal judge James Whittemore (and recounted in the motion later submitted to the U.S. Supreme Court) that because of its conflict with Terri's Roman Catholic faith, terminating her nutrition and hydration could "jeopardize her eternal soul."

The sheer volume of commentary on the Schiavo case ensured that a wide range of different perspectives would be applied to understand and argue it. But, the more general point should not be missed. In any case when family members must make medical decisions for an incapacitated loved one, there is bound to be emotional anguish and, quite often, interpersonal conflict regarding the appropriate standard by which decisions should be made. The desire to relieve a loved one's suffering or honor his or her wishes to terminate treatment invariably conflict with the sadness and potential guilt that are the unavoidable emotional toll of finally deciding that the battle for a loved one's life is lost. It is likely, therefore, that many surrogate decision makers fully understand and acknowledge their obligation to do what their incapacitated loved one would have wanted but still feel deeply ambivalent about (or even emotionally incapable of) carrying out those wishes.

End-of-life decision making is also ripe for interpersonal conflict. Although the right to self-determination holds a preeminent place in U.S. case law guiding end-of-life decision making, this value hierarchy is hardly universal. Individuals differ in their personal desire to control their own end-of-life medical care (Hawkins, Ditto, Danks, & Smucker, 2005), and sharp individual, cultural, and religious differences exist in the value ascribed to patient autonomy relative to other decision-making standards such as the right to life or family-based decision making (e.g., Blackhall, Murphy, Frank, Michel, & Azen, 1995). Family members inevitably bring unique sets of values to the decision-making process, and thus clashes between these values seem likely. These value conflicts may often be difficult to resolve because people seldom hold explicit ethical positions that they can readily articulate. Rather, individuals tend to respond to ethical dilemmas based on intuitive, emotion-based moral rules (Haidt, 2001), and thus it may be hard for family members to identify the sources of their disagreement and address them.

The conflict seen in the Schiavo case regarding the appropriate values by which to guide decisions about Terri's care, although unusually intense, was hardly unusual. It would seem the exceptional case when family members experience no emotional ambivalence or value conflicts when faced with a decision about whether to discontinue life-prolonging medical treatment for an incapacitated loved one.

□ Conflicting Views of Terri's Wishes

A common refrain in the coverage of the Schiavo case was that the entire conflict would have been avoided if only Terri had expressed her wishes in a living will prior to her collapse. More formally known as *instructional advance directives*, living wills are often presented, by the media and the medical establishment alike, as a cure for all that ails end-of-life medical decision making. If the problem is that people are often too sick to tell others what treatments they want near the end of life, then the solution is to have people write down their wishes when they are still healthy enough to do so. Support for living wills also flows directly from the ethical priority we give to the principle of self-determination. Theoretically, living wills allow people to control their own end-of-life care by communicating their wishes to the surrogate decision makers, who can then carry out those wishes on the patient's behalf (Ditto et al., 2001).

This point is crucial because, despite the fact that Terri Schiavo left no written record of her wishes regarding her end-of-life care, it was the court's conclusions about the nature of Terri's wishes that played a central role in the ultimate decision that her nutrition and hydration could be terminated. Testimony by Michael Schiavo and two members of his family indicated that Terri had expressed her wish to be removed from artificial nutrition and hydration based on statements she had made indicating a general desire not to become a "burden" and not to have her life prolonged artificially with "machines" and "tubes." These statements were vague, and their veracity was questioned by the Schindler family, but ultimately the court accepted this testimony as "clear and convincing" evidence of Terri's wishes.[2] It was thus on the power of these general verbal statements that the courts ultimately decided that it would be honoring Terri's wishes to remove her from the machines and tubes that were maintaining her life.

Among people who approached the Schiavo case without deep value-based convictions, it was likely the fact that such a momentous decision was based on such less-than-definitive evidence that was the source of their greatest discomfort. For some, concern about the lack of any written record of Terri's wishes was compounded by suspicions about the potential conflict of interest represented by her husband's romantic involvement with another woman. If only there had been greater certainty about what Terri would have wanted. If only Terri had completed a living will—so goes the lament—all the controversy, bitterness, and heartache that surrounded her final days could have been avoided.

Again, it is tempting to view the Schiavo case as unique in the extent of uncertainty that surrounded Terri's wishes about the use of life-sustaining medical treatment. In reality, however, uncertainty about the wishes of incapacitated patients is the rule rather than the exception in end-of-life medical care.

First, like Terri, most people die without an advance directive. Despite years of enthusiastic advocacy by major healthcare organizations and the widespread passage of state and federal law encouraging their use, fewer than 25% of Americans (pre-Schiavo) were estimated to have any kind of advance directive (Eiser & Weiss, 2001). There is some evidence that media attention on the Schiavo case has generated some increased interest in advance directives (Pew Research Center, 2006), but the longevity of this interest and whether it will manifest itself in the actual completion of advance directives is still in question. Rates of advance directive completion are particularly low for some ethnic groups (Caralis, Davis, Wright, & Marcial, 1993; Morrison, Zayas, Mulvihill, Baskin, & Meier, 1998; Murphy et al., 1996), and although high-quality data are hard to find regarding the prevalence of advance directive completion among adults in their mid-20s (as Terri was as the time of her collapse), it would seem safe to assume that it also is quite low. Even seriously ill individuals have been found to complete living wills at rates only slightly higher than those found in nonpatient populations (Holley, Stackiewicz, Dacko, & Rault, 1997; Kish, Martin, & Price, 2000). Thus, rather than being the atypical case, most families, like Terri Schiavo's, face the task of end-of-life decision making without written documentation of their loved one's wishes.

Second, even when individuals complete advance directives, these directives seldom provide clear instructions that can be used to guide actual medical decisions. One study, for example, found that only 5% of directives completed by a sample of seriously ill patients contained any specific instructions about the use of life-sustaining treatment (Teno et al., 1997). The majority of the directives were either durable powers of attorney (simply naming the individual they wanted to make decisions for them) or contained only vague instructions with unclear implications for the patient's actual medical condition (e.g., "no heroic measures").

Finally, even when individuals complete directives containing relatively specific treatment instructions, these directives may still do little to improve surrogates' understanding of the patients' treatment wishes. In a study conducted by my research group, we found that allowing a surrogate to review a quite specific advance directive completed by a loved one did not improve the surrogate's ability to predict the treatment preferences that loved one stated in response to a series of hypothetical end-of-life scenarios (Ditto et al., 2001). Moreover, this was true even when surrogates were allowed to discuss the content of the directive with their loved one immediately prior to the prediction task.

There are at least two different reasons why even specific directives may be less helpful than most people might imagine when it comes to clarifying a loved one's end-of-life wishes. First, no directive, no matter how detailed, can possibly anticipate all the medical decisions that might await us (e.g., Brett, 1991). Even specific directives often require that surrogates infer, from that patient's statements about similar but not identical treatments or conditions, a patient's preference for a particular medical treatment in a particular medical condition.

Second, when family members act as surrogate decision makers, they have been found to show at least two types of prediction biases that may compound problems caused by the imperfect mapping of directive statements onto experienced clinical conditions. The first of these is an overtreatment bias such that family members consistently predict that their loved ones will want life-sustaining treatment more often than they really do (Ditto et al., 2001; Fagerlin, Ditto, Danks, Houts, & Smucker, 2001). One way to characterize this bias is that family members tend to "err on the side of life" even when they are trying their best to honor a loved one's wishes. Another bias that has been documented in both family surrogates and physicians is a projection bias (Fagerlin et al.; Schneiderman, Kaplan, Pearlman, & Teetzel, 1993). That is, when trying to predict another person's desire for life-sustaining medical treatment, we often err by assuming that that individual will have wishes similar to our own. Although using one's own wishes to predict another's is not inherently irrational (many people likely approached the Schiavo case by imagining what *they* would want if *they* were in Terri's condition), projection has been found to be a common source of misprediction in studies examining the accuracy of surrogate substituted judgment (Fagerlin et al.; Pruchno, Lemay, Feild, & Levinksy, 2005). It is not hard to imagine that the beliefs of the various members of Terri Schiavo's family might have been influenced by this tendency to believe that Terri's wishes about end-of-life medical treatment were likely to be the same as their own.

☐ Conflicting Views of Terri's Medical Condition

So far, I have argued that family members often bring differing moral standards to bear on difficult decisions about how to treat an incapacitated loved one, and there is often uncertainty and disagreement regarding just what that loved one would want if he or she could only say. The Schiavo case, however, was plagued with one additional source of uncertainty that might seem less typical than these others: the uncertainty that surrounded the actual nature of her medical condition.

Space considerations preclude a full description of the intricacy of the two factions' beliefs about Terri's actual medical history, but the opposing positions boiled down to this: According to Michael Schiavo, his wife, Terri, was in a persistent vegetative state with no chance of improvement or recovery and was responsive to environmental stimulation only at a rudimentary, reflex level. According to Terri's parents and siblings, Terri was in a condition that is generally referred to as a "minimally conscious state," with the potential for some substantial degree of recovery if aggressive treatment was applied, and was aware of and emotionally responsive to their presence (and perhaps even capable of expressing her wishes and intentions). These dramatically different portrayals of Terri's medical condition added another level of decision-making complexity to an already challenging situation. If one accepted Michael's assessment of Terri's medical condition, two things reasonably followed: (a) There was little of "Terri" left to save even if saving her was possible, and thus terminating the treatment that prolonged her marginal existence was morally justifiable; and (b) Terri likely would not have wanted to have her life prolonged if she had no significant cognitive function and no chance of ever recovering it. Conversely, if one accepted the Schindler's assessment of Terri's condition, two quite different things could be reasonably concluded: (a) It was morally wrong to deny treatment to a person with some ability to think and reason and a substantial likelihood of recovery, and (b) Terri would likely have wanted her nutrition and hydration continued if she knew that she might be able to recover and regain some reasonable quality of life. Thus, true knowledge of Terri's actual medical condition had dramatic implications for what could be perceived as the "right" decision to make on her behalf, both in terms of the direct moral implications of the act of withdrawing treatment and in what the nature of her condition would imply about honoring Terri's own treatment wishes.

It is tempting to see the uncertainty and conflict surrounding Terri Schiavo's medical condition as uniquely a function of our limited understanding of vegetative states and the nature of consciousness itself. The issues that seemed so central in the Schiavo case are relatively rare, but the general problem of medical uncertainty is not. In particular, uncertainty about patients' prognoses for recovery often accompanies, and complicates, end-of-life decision making.

Perhaps the single piece of information that people find most helpful in making end-of-life decisions is a clear sense of whether the patient is likely to regain an acceptable quality of life (Fried & Bradley, 2003; Fried, Bradley, Towle, & Allore, 2002). End-of-life decisions involving older adults with multiple medical problems often generate relatively little conflict because it is clear to all that medical treatment can only prolong an imminent and inevitable dying process. Similarly, hypothetical statements about end-of-life wishes are often stated confidently because they assume an unambiguous prognosis (e.g., "I would *definitely* not want to be kept alive if there was *no* chance that I would recover.").

In reality, however, prognostic certainty is a rare commodity. Medical prognoses, by their very nature, are statements of probability. Moreover, rather than involving just a single probability of full recovery given one particular treatment approach, the uncertainties involved in real clinical situations are often complex and multiple, involving numerous probabilities representing various degrees of partial recovery and various likelihoods of different types of unfavorable outcomes associated with multiple possible treatment approaches.

As was well illustrated by the Schiavo case, uncertainty about a loved one's prognosis for recovery creates uncertainty and often conflict about the appropriate course of action. No one wants to give up the fight for their loved one's life prematurely, but how can one know for certain that a decision to terminate treatment is premature? If a physician tells a patient's family that the patient has only a very slight chance of recovery, how does the family know for sure that their loved one is not that rare case that will pull through? If family members disagree about their loved one's future likelihood of recovery, how can the issue ever be resolved in the present? Real end-of-life decision making taking place in real time almost always occurs in a mist of irreducible uncertainty regarding the patient's likelihood of (full or partial) recovery.

The problems caused by prognostic uncertainty can be compounded by the fact that family members typically have a powerful emotional desire to maintain the belief that their loved one will recover. Psychological research provides clear evidence that motivation can bias assessments of the likelihood of wanted and unwanted outcomes (Ditto, Munro, Apanovitch, Scepansky, & Lockhart, 2003; Weinstein, 1980). Thus, family members who want desperately for their loved ones to recover may often be reluctant to end treatment, maintaining their belief in the possibility of recovery even when the medical probabilities seem clear to more dispassionate observers. Consistent with this speculation, it seems likely that in addition to differences in values and disagreements about Terri's wishes about the use of life-sustaining treatment, another clear source of the intense conflict seen in the Schiavo case was the difficulty Terri's parents and siblings seemed to have had accepting the prevailing medical opinion (confirmed by a subsequent autopsy report) that Terri's brain damage left her with no significant cognitive function and no reasonable chance for recovery.

□ The Legacy of the Schiavo Case

The public attention generated by the final weeks of Terri Schiavo's life will almost certainly spawn well-intentioned efforts to address the difficult issues that surround end-of-life medical decision making for incapacitated patients. It is crucial, however, that these efforts be more than just well intentioned.

The Schiavo case was most certainly a compelling family drama, with a story line that mapped seamlessly onto the broader cultural drama playing out in contemporary red state (Republican Party controlled) versus blue state (Democratic Party controlled) America. It will be tempting for lawmakers to view the case in this most superficial light and try to fix it with equally superficial measures. In the previous sections, however, my goal was to illustrate that the decision-making challenges that made the Schiavo case so vexing were neither simple nor uncommon. As such, law and policy makers must approach end-of-life decision making with a full appreciation of both the scope and complexity of the challenges involved. In this final section, I venture a few suggestions about the general form attempts to address these challenges should and should not take.

Clearly, the most problematic form legislation could take would be to attempt to require in some way that under conditions of uncertainty, surrogate medical decisions err on the side of life. Such a provision might seem reasonable at first blush, but it is important to recognize that the impetus for the advance directive movement was widespread public concern about the aggressive use of advanced medical technology to prolong the dying process (President's Commission, 1983). Given the ubiquity of uncertainty in end-of-life situations, a requirement to err on the side of life would institutionalize this fear of pointless medical treatment and repudiate several decades worth of state and federal legislation designed to address this very problem.

Moreover, although such a requirement seems to maintain the ethical priority of self-determination (by suggesting treatment only when the individual's wishes are not clear), the end result of the requirement would almost certainly undermine self-determination in many instances. With reference to the Schiavo case, for example, public opinion polls suggest that a clear majority of the American people would have wanted treatment terminated if they were in a medical situation similar to Terri Schiavo's (Blendon, Benson, & Herrman, 2005; Pew Research Center, 2006). My own research has found that only about 10% of older adults say they would want to receive artificial feeding and fluid if they were in a "coma" with "no chance of recovery" (Coppola et al., 1999; Ditto et al., 2001). The number increases to near 40% if the condition is said to have a "very slight chance of recovery," but this still leaves a substantial majority of individuals in a case similar to Terri Schiavo's for whom a requirement to err on the side of life would result in treatment that opposed their wishes.

Finally, perhaps the clearest result from the public opinion polls conducted in the wake of the Schiavo case is that a substantial majority of the American public, cutting across virtually all religious and political lines, have a distinctly negative reaction to governmental interference in an individual's end-of-life care (Blendon et al., 2005). Although individual Americans clearly differ on the specific values that they believe should guide decisions about the use of life-sustaining medical treatment, most agree that these decisions are a personal matter to be resolved by individuals and their families according to their own moral sensibilities, rather than dictated from outside by judges or, perhaps worst of all, politicians. Based on these data, I suspect that any attempt to use policy or law to impose a value standard on end-of-life decisions (like erring on the side of life) would be responded to poorly by the American public.

This brings us to the opposite approach. One way to address the inherent uncertainty of surrogate decision making is to impose decision standards on individuals from the outside. A quite different way to address the problem is to maximize individual control over end-of-life decisions by developing policy and law to encourage the completion of more and more specific instructional advance directives.

From a strict self-determination perspective, the push toward greater specificity in living wills makes perfect sense. Theoretically, the more clearly and precisely an individual can document his or her wishes prior to incapacitation, the more clearly and precisely those wishes can be followed afterward. Specific instructional directives are also appealing from the perspective of both physicians and attorneys. To the extent that advance medical decision making can mimic the specificity of real-time medical decision making (e.g., "The patient is in medical condition X, and his living will clearly states that if he were to experience condition X he does not want medical treatment Y"), then physicians have not only clear medical instructions by which they can honor patients' wishes but also clear legal protection to enact those wishes in the guise of honoring the patient's right to self-determination.

The problem with this strategy when taken to its logical extreme, however, is that it is unlikely that even a very specific instructional directive will provide the clarity surrogates, physicians, and attorneys seek regarding the wishes of an incapacitated loved one. Suppose Terri Schiavo had documented in her living will: "I do not want life-prolonging medical treatment if I am in a persistent vegetative state with no chance of recovery." Would this statement, which is more specific than the kind of statements found in most living wills (Teno et al., 1997), have resolved the uncertainty and conflict surrounding this case? By "life-prolonging medical treatment," did Terri mean artificial feeding and fluids? Some people would; others would not. Was Terri in a persistent vegetative state? Her husband says she was, but her parents and siblings disagreed. Did she have a chance of recovery? How big a chance? How big a chance of recovery is big enough that we could all agree that Terri would have wanted to take the risk of spending the remaining years or decades of her life unable to communicate, dependent on others for every need, a shell of the vivacious young woman she once was?

One might argue, of course, that these ambiguities could be addressed with even greater specification of wishes. But, there are two other important problems with a push toward hyperspecificity in advance directives.

First, there is considerable evidence to suggest that people are not capable of making detailed predictions about the specific medical treatments they would want to have used on them in specific medical conditions. A quite extensive body of research from both the medical and psychological literature reveals that people's predictions about their behavioral and emotional reactions to future situations are often inaccurate (see Ditto, Hawkins, & Pizarro, 2005, or Wilson & Gilbert, 2003, for reviews). In particular, healthy people are poor predictors of how sick people view their condition (e.g., Sackett & Torrance, 1978; Ubel, Loewenstein, & Jepson,

2003), even when individuals are asked to predict their own reactions to future illness (Jansen et al., 2000). This research is consistent with numerous studies showing that preferences for life-sustaining medical treatments exhibit substantial instability over time (Danis, Garrett, Harris, & Patrick, 1994; Ditto, Smucker et al., 2003; Fried et al., 2006) and can be affected by changes in the respondent's physical and emotional condition (Ditto, Jacobson, Smucker, Danks, & Fagerlin, 2006; Fried et al., 2006; see Spannhake, chapter 3, this volume) or even the way the questions are asked (Forrow, Taylor, & Arnold, 1992). Thus, even if healthy people could be encouraged to document highly detailed treatment preferences in advance of incapacitating illness, it is not at all clear that these preferences should then be taken as a meaningful representation of the preferences these same individuals would have after they became sick.

Second, even if people were capable of generating highly specific preferences about their hopes for end-of-life medical treatment, research suggests that the majority of people have little desire to exert the kind of tight control over end-of-life decisions that is implied by highly specific advance directives. There is little doubt that most people express positive sentiments toward advance directives in general and laws supporting the general right of individuals to refuse life-prolonging medical treatment if they so desire (Blendon et al., 2005; Pew Research Center, 2006). When asked about their personal wishes, however, many individuals express ambivalence about the need to complete specific instructional directives and instead seem more positively inclined toward informal discussion of wishes and directives that focus on general values and goals rather than specific treatment preferences (Hawkins et al., 2005). Patients often state that they are quite satisfied leaving end-of-life medical decisions to their families (Holley et al., 1997), and this preference for family-centered over individual-centered decision making is particularly true of certain culture groups, such as Asians and Hispanics (Kwak & Haley, 2005). Because individuals are aware that they cannot have all the facts about their future illness when they are completing their living will, many actually state that in the event of a disagreement between their own documented preferences and the opinions of their surrogate, the surrogate's rather than their own directions should be followed (Terry et al., 1999). Similarly, Hawkins et al. (2005) found that over half of the older adults they interviewed wanted their surrogates to have either "compete" or "a lot" of leeway to override their treatment preferences based on their surrogate's assessment of what was in their (the patient's) best interest (see also Sehgal et al., 1992). Only 9% of participants in the Hawkins et al. study believed that surrogates should have no freedom to override the participant's previous stated wishes.

What this suggests is that rather than striving to provide people with tighter and tighter control over their end-of-life care by encouraging the completion of more and more specific living wills, a more psychologically feasible goal, and one more consistent with the degree of control most individuals actually desire over end-of-life medical decisions, would be to encourage general advance directives and thus a more general form of self-determination. A commitment to self-determination does not require that people be forced to make decisions they feel ill-equipped to make, but only that people be provided the level of control they desire. The majority of people seem to have little interest in "micromanaging" their end-of-life treatment (Hawkins et al., 2005) and instead want only to gain some general sense of control over the dying process and to reduce the level of burden on their loved ones.

Toward this end, a number of advance directive forms have been developed that focus on general values and goals underlying end-of-life medical wishes rather than on the documentation of specific treatment preferences (e.g., Doukas & McCollough, 1991), and several others combine an emphasis on specific preferences and general goals (Emanuel, 1991). These general directives can be important because surrogates often have inaccurate beliefs about the values and goals their loved one's wish to guide their end-of-life care. Hawkins et al. (2005), for example, found that in less than one fourth of the patient-surrogate pairs they interviewed could the surrogate correctly guess the one value their patient (typically a spouse or parent who they had known for over 45 years on average) had selected as the most important value guiding their end-of-life medical care. Similarly, fewer than half of surrogates knew the extent of leeway their loved one wanted them to have in end-of-life decision making, with the majority of surrogates believing that patients wanted to maintain tighter control than they actually did.

In addition to refocusing attention on general goals rather than specific treatment preferences, another important step in this regard would be to encourage the completion of proxy advance directives (e.g., durable powers of attorney for health care) or, better yet, directives that combine instructions with the naming of a proxy. What people seem to want most is to have someone they trust make medical decisions for them, in most cases with some general guidance about the values and goals that they want to steer these decisions. Emphasizing the importance of proxy directives thus helps to reconceptualize instructional directives in a more useful way. That is, rather than the traditional (and problematic) way of framing instructional directives as a direct expression of the patient's wishes that can be followed without interpretation, it is more helpful to conceive of them as input into an informed surrogate decision-making process. Viewing living wills as a way to communicate general wishes rather than as an end in themselves captures the way most individuals want their living wills to be used (Hawkins et al., 2005). Moreover, it suggests the importance of embedding the completion of advance directives in a more extensive process of advance care planning. Clearly, the most useful role for instructional advance directives, including specific ones, is as a stimulus for ongoing discussion among one's family members and healthcare providers. Viewing living wills as the beginning of a communication process rather than its end product, and surrogate decision making as guided by patients' desire to inform rather than dictate medical decisions, will lead to an end-of-life decision-making process that is most likely to satisfy the needs and goals of both patients and the loved ones struggling to make decisions on their behalf.

Imagine what might have happened if, prior to her collapse, Terri Schiavo had discussed her wishes about end-of-life care with her husband, parents, and siblings and informed everyone of the person she wished to entrust with the authority to make medical decisions on her behalf. Would this have made the decisions her family faced easy or resolved all of the deeply felt disagreements her family had about her medical care? Almost certainly not. It is not hard to imagine, however, that if everyone in her family knew whose judgment Terri ultimately trusted, and that this individual's decisions were generally consistent with her vision about how she wanted her life to end, her final days would have been much more peaceful, and her story, although still tragic, would no longer be a parable about one way that none of us wants to die.

□ Conclusion

Terri Schiavo became a household name in spring 2005, 15 years after she last took a step, spoke a word, or interacted in any meaningful way with the world around her. Indeed, unlike the brand of celebrity we so often see in today's culture—one based almost solely on self-promotion—it was precisely the fact that Terri Schiavo could tell us nothing about herself that led her to become so famous.

In this chapter, my goal was to use the case of Terri Schiavo to illustrate general problems of surrogate decision making that are most often faced by the loved ones of individuals with chronic and unglamorous diseases like cancer and Alzheimer's disease. It is not surprising that the cases of end-of-life decision making that have generated the most media and legal attention have involved young adults struck down suddenly in the prime of their life and left to languish in persistent vegetative states. Cases like those of Terri Schiavo, Nancy Cruzan, and Karen Ann Quinlan make up only a tiny percentage of all instances when decisions about the use of life-sustaining medical treatment must be made but attract disproportionate attention precisely because they bring into sharp relief the profound and difficult moral and practical questions that often accompany decisions made near the end of life. Such difficult cases will always exist.

No approach to improving end-of-life decisions will ever make it easy, will ever make all families see eye to eye, or will ever allow us to know with certainty the true wishes of individuals too sick to speak for themselves. We can, however, with a concerted and collaborative effort on the part of politicians, health professionals, and researchers, work to develop policy and law that can help many families more effectively negotiate the difficult and inevitable challenges of making decisions for loved ones. We can never know for sure, but I suspect that this would be an outcome that Terri Schiavo would have wanted.

Acknowledgment

This chapter is a revised and expanded version of an article that appeared in *Death Studies*.

Notes

1. It must be noted that decisions about the use of life-sustaining medical technology are really only a relevant concern in the developed world. In the majority of countries around the globe, concerns about stopping medical treatment for individuals who no longer believe their life is worth living are overwhelmed by concerns about providing medical treatment for individuals whose lives are still clearly worth living.
2. Statements offered by the Schindler family suggesting that Terri would not have wanted to be removed from life support were deemed less credible by the court because they occurred when Terri was a child and referred only to Terri's feelings about Karen Ann Quinlan rather than specifically to Terri's wishes for her own medical treatment.

References

Baergen, R. (1995). Revising the substituted judgment standard. *Journal of Clinical Ethics, 6,* 30–38.

Baron, J., & Ritov, I. (2004). Omission bias, individual differences, and normality. *Organizational Behavior and Human Decision Processes, 94,* 74–85.

Blackhall, L. J., Murphy, S. T., Frank, G., Michel, V., & Azen, S. (1995). Ethnicity and attitudes toward patient autonomy. *Journal of the American Medical Association, 274,* 820–825.

Blendon, R. J., Benson, J. M., & Herrmann, M. J. (2005). The American public and the Terri Schiavo case. *Archives of Internal Medicine, 165,* 2580–2584.

Bradley E., Walker, L., Blecher, B. B., & Wettle, T. (1997). Assessing capacity to participate in discussions of advance directives in nursing homes: Findings from a study of the Patient Self Determination Act. *Journal of the American Geriatrics Society, 45,* 79–83.

Brett, A. S. (1991). Limitations of listing specific medical interventions in advance directives. *Journal of the American Medical Association, 266,* 825–828.

Buchanan, A. E., & Brock, D. W. (1990). *Deciding for others: The ethics of surrogate decision-making.* Cambridge, England: Cambridge University Press.

Caralis, P. V., Davis, B., Wright, K., & Marcial, E. (1993). The influence of ethnicity and race on attitudes toward advance directives, life-prolonging treatments, and euthanasia. *Journal of Clinical Ethics, 4,* 155–165.

Coppola, K. M., Bookwala, J., Ditto, P. H., Lockhart, L. K., Danks, J. H., & Smucker, W. D. (1999). Elderly adults' preferences for life-sustaining treatments: The role of impairment, prognosis, and pain. *Death Studies, 23,* 617–623.

Cruzan v. Director, Missouri Department of Health, 497 U.S. 261 (1990).

Danis, M., Garrett, J., Harris, R., & Patrick, D. L. (1994). Stability of choices about life-sustaining treatments. *Annals of Internal Medicine, 120,* 567–573.

Ditto, P. H., Danks, J. H., Smucker, W. D., Bookwala, J., Coppola, K. M., Dresser, R., et al. (2001). Advance directives as acts of communication: A randomized controlled trial. *Archives of Internal Medicine, 161,* 421–430.

Ditto, P. H., Hawkins, N. A., & Pizarro, D. A. (2005). Imagining the end of life: On the psychology of advance medical decision-making. *Motivation and Emotion, 29,* 475–496.

Ditto, P. H., Jacobson, J. A., Smucker, W. D., Danks, J. H., & Fagerlin, A. (2006). Context changes choices: A prospective study of the effects of hospitalization on life-sustaining treatment preferences. *Medical Decision-Making, 26,* 313–322.

Ditto, P. H., Munro, G. D., Apanovitch, A. M., Scepansky, J. A., & Lockhart, L. K. (2003). Spontaneous skepticism: The interplay of motivation and expectation in responses to favorable and unfavorable medical diagnoses. *Personality and Social Psychology Bulletin, 29,* 1120–1132.

Ditto, P. H., Smucker, W. D., Danks, J. H., Jacobson, J. A., Houts, R. M., Fagerlin, A., et al. (2003). Stability of older adults' preferences for life-sustaining medical treatment. *Health Psychology, 22,* 605–615.

Doukas, D. J., & McCollough, L. B. (1991). The values history: The evaluation of the patient's values and advance directives. *Journal of Family Practice, 32,* 145–152.

Dresser, R. (2003). Precommitment: A misguided strategy for securing death with dignity. *Texas Law Review, 81,* 1823–1847.

Eiser, A. R., & Weiss, M. D. (2001). The underachieving advance directive: Recommendations for increasing advance directive completion. *American Journal of Bioethics, 1,* W10.

Emanuel, L. L. (1991). The health care directive: Learning how to draft advance care documents. *Journal of the American Geriatrics Society, 39,* 1221–1228.

Fagerlin, A., Ditto, P. H., Danks, J. H., Houts, R. M., & Smucker, W. D. (2001). Projection in surrogate decision about life-sustaining medical treatments. *Health Psychology, 20,* 166–175.

Forrow, L., Taylor, W. C., & Arnold, R. M. (1992). Absolutely relative: How research results are summarized can affect treatment decisions. *American Journal of Medicine, 92,* 121–124.

Fried, T. R., & Bradley, E. H. (2003). What matters to seriously ill older persons making end-of-life treatment decisions? A qualitative study. *Journal of Palliative Medicine, 6,* 237–244.

Fried, T. R., Bradley, E. H., Towle, V. R., & Allore, H. (2002). Understanding the treatment preferences of seriously ill patients. *New England Journal of Medicine, 346,* 1061–1066.

Fried, T. R., Byers, A. L., Gallo, W. T., Van Ness, P. H., Towle, V. R., O'Leary, J. R., et al. (2006). Prospective study of health status preferences and changes in preferences over time in older adults. *Archives of Internal Medicine, 166,* 890–895.

Haidt, J. (2001). The emotional dog and its rational tail: A social intuitionist approach to moral judgment. *Psychological Review, 108,* 814–834.

Hawkins, N. A., Ditto, P. H., Danks, J. H., & Smucker, W. D. (2005). Micromanaging death: Process preferences, values, and goals in end-of-life medical decision-making. *The Gerontologist, 45,* 107–117.

Holley, J. L., Stackiewicz, L., Dacko, C., & Rault, R. (1997). Factors influencing dialysis patients' completion of advance directives. *American Journal of Kidney Diseases, 30,* 356–360.

Jansen S. J. T, Stiggelbout, A. M., Wakker, P. P., Nooji, M. A., Noordijk, E. M., & Kievit, J. (2000). Unstable preferences: A shift in valuation or an effect of the elicitation procedure? *Medical Decision-Making, 20,* 62–71.

Kish, S. K., Martin, C. G., & Price, K. J. (2000). Advance directives in critically ill cancer patients. *Critical Care Nursing Clinics of North America, 12,* 373–383.

Kwak, J., & Haley, W. E. (2005). Current research findings on end-of-life decision-making among racially or ethnically diverse groups. *The Gerontologist, 45,* 634–641.

Morrison, R. S., Zayas, L. H., Mulvihill, M., Baskin, S. A., & Meier, D. E. (1998). Barriers to completion of health care proxies: An examination of ethnic differences. *Archives of Internal Medicine, 158,* 2493–2497.

Murphy, S. T., Palmer, J. M., Azen, S., Frank, G., Michel, V., & Blackhall, L. J. (1996). Ethnicity and advance care directives. *Journal of Law, Medicine & Ethics, 24,* 108–117.

Pew Research Center for People and the Press. (2006). *Strong public support for right to die.* Retrieved September 16, 2006, from http://people-press.org/reports/display.php3?ReportID=266.

President's Commission for the Study of Ethical Problems in Medicine and Biomedical and Behavioral Research. (1983). *Deciding to forgo life-sustaining treatment: A report on the ethical, medical, and legal issues in treatment decisions.* Washington, DC: Government Printing Office.

Pruchno, R. A., Lemay, E. P., Jr., Feild, L., & Levinksy, N. G. (2005). Spouse as health care proxy for dialysis patients: Whose preferences matter? *The Gerontologist, 45,* 812–819.

Sackett D. L., & Torrance, G. W. (1978). The utility of different health states as perceived by the general public. *Journal of Chronic Disease, 31,* 697–704.

Schneiderman, L. J., Kaplan, R. M., Pearlman, R. A., & Teetzel, H. (1993). Do physicians' own preferences for life-sustaining treatment influence their perceptions of patients' preferences? *Journal of Clinical Ethics, 4,* 28–33.

Sehgal, A., Galbraith, A., Chesney, M., Schoenfeld, P., Charles, G., & Lo, B. (1992). How strictly do dialysis patients want their advance directives followed? *Journal of the American Medical Association, 267,* 59–63.
Spranca, M., Minsk, E., & Baron, J. (1991). Omission and commission in judgment and choice. *Journal of Experimental Social Psychology, 27,* 76–105.
Teno, J. M., Licks, S., Lynn, J., Wenger, N., Connors, A. F., Phillips, R. S., et al. (1997). Do advance directives provide instructions that direct care? *Journal of the American Geriatrics Society, 45,* 508–512.
Terry, P. B., Vettese, M., Song, J., Forman, J., Haller, K. B., Miller, D. J., et al. (1999). End-of-life decision-making: When patients and surrogates disagree. *Journal of Clinical Ethics, 10,* 286–293.
Ubel, P. A., Loewenstein, G., & Jepson, C. (2003). Whose quality of life? A commentary exploring discrepancies between health state evaluations of patients and the general public. *Quality of Life Research, 12,* 599–607.
Weinstein, N. (1980). Unrealistic optimism about future life events. *Journal of Personality and Social Psychology, 39,* 806–820.
Wilson, T. D., & Gilbert, D. T. (2003). Affective forecasting. In M. Zanna (Ed.), *Advances in experimental social psychology* (Vol. 35, pp. 345–411). New York: Elsevier.
Wolfson, J. (2003). *A report to Governor Jeb Bush in the Matter of Theresa Marie Schiavo.* Retrieved September 9, 2005 from http://www.miami.edu/ethics/schiavo/wolfson%27s%20report,pdf

IV

SECTION

Psychosocial Considerations

14

CHAPTER

The Possible Impact of Mental Health Issues on End-of-Life Decision Making

James L. Werth, Jr.

☐ Introduction

End-of-life decisions can be difficult for a variety of reasons, including the obvious association with dying and death, the uncertainty involved (perhaps regarding both the dying process and any sort of afterlife), the frequent need to make profound decisions in a short period of time, the potential for conflict among participants, and the likelihood that the dying person may not be able to speak up for herself or himself. Mental health issues come into play in all of these situations, and more, near the end of life. The impact of physical pain and suffering on medical decisions is fairly obvious, but the various ways that mental health issues can affect decision making are often overlooked or downplayed.

The purpose of this chapter, therefore, is to provide some information regarding the possible impact of mental health issues on end-of-life decision making. Because of space limitations, the full range of mental health issues that have been identified as areas to consider evaluating when people are making end-of-life decisions is not detailed here (for a list, see Table 14.1). However, some of those that appear to be most likely to influence decision making are reviewed, including clinical depression (and the associated condition of hopelessness), types of clinical anxiety disorders (and

TABLE 14.1 Summary of Issues to Consider When Exploring End-of-Life Decisions

1. Assess for presence of capacity to give informed consent to participate in the review and the capacity to make informed healthcare decisions.
2. Decision-making process, including
   a. Physical pain and suffering
   b. Comorbid psychological conditions
   c. Other psychological issues
   d. Fear of loss of control/loss of autonomy/loss of dignity
   e. Financial concerns
   f. Cultural factors
   g. Review possible underlying issues
   h. Overall quality of life
   i. Other issues to explore
3. The person's social support system:
   a. Consideration of significant others
   b. Involvement of significant others
   c. Interviews with significant others
4. Systemic and environmental issues:
   a. Indirect external coercion
   b. Direct external coercion

Source: Report to the Board of Directors, by Working Group on Assisted Suicide and End-of-Life Decisions, 2000, Washington, DC: American Psychological Association, Appendix F.

the associated issue of death anxiety), and other psychological issues (e.g., beliefs about dignity) (Gibson, Breitbart, Tomarken, Kosinski, & Nelson, 2006; Pessin, Rosenfeld, & Breitbart, 2002; Rosenfeld, Abbey, & Pessin, 2006). Although spiritual and religious considerations as well as family dynamics are often discussed in discussions of psychosocial issues near the end of life (e.g., Werth, Gordon, & Johnson, 2002), because there are full chapters on these other topics they are not discussed in depth in this chapter.

☐ Clinical Depression

Although there are actually many different types of mood disorders that could have an impact on end-of-life decision making (e.g., bipolar disorder I and II, dysthymia; see American Psychiatric Association, 2000, for lists and criteria), the research and commentary have focused on clinical depression (Werth et al., 2002). For the purposes of this chapter, and in most professional discussions of depression, the focus is on what mental health professionals call "major depressive disorder," "major depression," or "clinical depression." According to the current edition of the manual used to diagnose mental illnesses (the *Diagnostic and Statistical Manual of Mental Disorders, Fourth Edition, Text Revision*, American Psychiatric Association, 2000, p. 356), there are nine criteria for major depression, and a person needs to have at least one of the first two (i.e., depressed mood or loss of interest or pleasure) and four of the others (e.g., eating problems, sleeping problems, recurrent thoughts of death) for at least 2 weeks before the clinical form of depression can be diagnosed. Some people talk about "minor depression," but this is a vague term that can be a catchall, as can the diagnosis of adjustment disorder with depressed mood, and the layperson's use of the term *depression* (Pessin et al., 2002; Rosenfeld et al., 2006). Basically, what the nonprofessional refers to as depression probably meets just one or two of the official criteria for the diagnosis of major depression.

Prevalence and Treatment of Major Depression Among Dying Persons

The assumption of many people, including some medical and mental health professionals, is that it is normal to be "depressed" if one is dying. However, this assumption mistakes being sad or grieving with being clinically depressed. In other words, although it may be normal to be sad about dying or to be grieving the real and anticipated losses one (and one's significant others) may be experiencing, it is *not* normal for a dying person to be clinically depressed; in fact, most research indicates that only a third or fewer of very ill individuals may meet the stringent criteria for major depression (Block, 2006; Gibson et al., 2006; Rosenfeld et al., 2006). It is important for medical and mental health professionals to accurately diagnose the presence of normal sadness, normal grief, pathological grief, and clinical depression because the treatments, if any, can be radically different. Whereas normal sadness and normal grief may not demand any intervention other than normalization by a professional, pathological (or "complicated") grief may require intervention (Neimeyer, Prigerson, & Davies, 2002; Shear, Frank, Houck, & Reynolds, 2005), and clinical depression almost certainly needs to be addressed immediately (Block, 2006).

If clinical depression is present (once physical conditions, such as pain, are ruled out), treatment should begin as soon as possible, preferably with a combination of medication and psychotherapy and perhaps family counseling (Gibson et al., 2006; Pessin et al., 2002; Rosenfeld et al., 2006).

Depending on the condition of the dying person, psychostimulants or antidepressants may be used (Block, 2006; Rosenfeld et al., 2006), with the psychostimulants having a quicker effect but also being somewhat harder to tolerate by someone who is very ill. If a person has only a few days or weeks left to live, then antidepressants may not have time to take effect, but given the uncertainty about prognosis (Christakis, 1999), some may choose to err on the side of prescribing/taking them as long as they do not have a negative interaction with other medications.

In addition to medication, various types of psychotherapy can be effective with dying individuals (Rosenfeld et al., 2006). There is much research that supports the utility of having a trained, compassionate individual truly listen to a person in distress and utilize what are called the "common factors" (e.g., empathy, drawing on the person's strengths and resources) among nondying individuals (Hubble, Duncan, & Miller, 1999), and there is little reason to believe this style would not work with people near the end of life. One particular humanistic approach, existential therapy, has been used with ill cancer patients in a group format and appears to be effective for many people (Gibson et al., 2006; Greenstein & Breitbart, 2000). Cognitive-behavioral interventions (i.e., examining thinking styles and how those thoughts can affect behavior and then intervening to change both thoughts and behaviors) have been found to be effective with well and ill individuals (Wilson, Chochinov, de Faye, & Breitbart, 2000), although their utility with dying persons has not been directly tested. However, unless the person is cognitively impaired, there is no obvious reason to believe that cognitive-behavioral therapy would not help some people who are dying. Yet, just as not all medications will work with everyone, not all therapies (or therapists) will work with all people; therefore, there needs to be a good match among the dying person, the therapist, and the therapeutic approaches. This is especially true when there are cultural differences between the ill person and the mental health professional.

Ways Major Depression Can Have an Impact on End-of-Life Decision Making

Depression can affect decisions in a variety of ways. Most people are familiar, either given their own personal history or based on interactions with others, with the ways in which depression can alter perceptions and mindset such that no options seem acceptable or even possible or there is only one possibility and it is associated with a negative or bad outcome. It is this tunnel vision that has been associated with suicidality, such that some people who are depressed believe the only way out of the depression is by killing themselves (Bongar, 2002). This may be true among people who are dying as well as those who are not medically ill. However, just as with non-ill individuals, effective treatment of the depression can allow for consideration of more options and therefore reduce or eliminate the suicidality among people near the end of life.

To be more specific, research has clearly indicated that clinical depression is associated with desire for assisted suicide as well as with other end-of-life decisions that may hasten death, such as withholding or withdrawing treatment (Block, 2006; Ganzini, Lee, Heintz, Bloom, & Fenn, 1994). Thus, although much of the focus has been on the link between major depression and assisted death, professionals and loved ones cannot ignore the possibility that clinical depression is influencing an ill person's decision to, for example, discontinue dialysis or use of a ventilator or to stop eating and drinking. In all of these situations a thorough assessment is necessary to determine to what extent, if any, clinical depression or another mental illness, some form of physical suffering, or an interpersonal conflict might be leading to the desire to hasten death (Werth & Rogers, 2005).

Just as the official mental disorder called major depression can affect consideration of options and therefore have an impact on decisions, the associated condition of hopelessness (which is not classified as a mental disorder) can have a significant impact on decision making (Rosenfeld et al., 2006). In fact, among individuals not physically ill, the presence of elevated levels of hopelessness was a better predictor of suicidal ideation (Beck, Steer, Beck, & Newman, 1993) and eventual suicide than was the presence of major depression (Beck, Steer, Kovacs, & Garrison, 1985). As is the case with depression, many people believe that it is natural for a dying person to be hopeless; however, as abundant research has indicated, an individual can be near the end of life and still maintain hope (e.g., Buckley & Herth, 2004; Rosenfeld et al.). The form the hope takes may be different, such that instead of hope for a cure or living an additional 20 years it may take the form of hoping to get a phone call from a loved one or to see the sun rise and set again, but it is still hope; whereas if someone has a fatalistic, pessimistic outlook regarding everything and expresses no hope for anything positive, then this is the type of hopelessness that may indicate a need for intervention. For many people, having a sense of meaning or purpose, even near the end of life, can give them reason to hope (Breitbart & Heller, 2003; Rosenfeld et al.).

There are other ways that major depression and hopelessness can affect end-of-life decision making beyond reducing the consideration of options. A clinically depressed or hopeless person is not enjoyable to be around, not only because they are always down but also because their bad feelings can lead to those around them feeling bad. This can lead to negative interactions among the dying person, loved ones, and health care team; a sense of hopelessness and even clinical depression among all the other participants, which can then have an impact on their decision making;

and avoidance of the dying person, which can lead to more depression and hopelessness by everyone involved. It would make sense that these types of interactions can also lead to more problematic and difficult grief by the loved ones who continue to live.

Further, major depression can interact with other conditions such that it exacerbates them, and they exacerbate it. For example, physical pain can make clinical depression worse, and clinical depression can make physical pain worse (Block, 2000; Gibson et al., 2006; Werth et al., 2002). Thus, treating one condition, such as pain, without also effectively treating major depression can lead to poor quality of life and frustration by all involved because the treatments are not working the way they are "supposed" to work.

Relationship Between Clinical Depression and the Cases in This Book

The possible impact of major depression on end-of-life decision making can be seen in several of the personal stories in this book. The discussion of the power of pain by Spannhake (chapter 3) illustrates not only how important it is to get physical symptoms, perhaps especially pain, under control but also how these symptoms can lead to or interact with major depression in such a way that the ill person, contrary to his or her typical personality, wants to give up. The story also demonstrates, perhaps indirectly, how major depression can affect an individual's perception of other people. Similarly, the story on assisted death by Raye (chapter 5) shows how the presence of what could be clinical depression can have an impact on the dying person as well as how caregiving can lead to major depression among loved ones (there is a substantial body of literature on this point; see, e.g., Zivin & Christakis, 2007). The impact of decision making on depression and vice versa can be seen in both this story and the one involving decision making for others as told by Crow (chapter 4). The author very clearly reveals the toll that the situation took on her mental health.

□ Clinical Anxiety Disorders

Major depression and different clinical anxiety disorders often occur together in nonmedically ill people, and the same may be true of those who are dying (Block, 2006). There are a variety of anxiety disorders (American Psychiatric Association, 2000), including generalized anxiety disorder (a pervasive and overarching sense of dread about many aspects of daily living); panic disorder (episodes of intense fear in the absence of an actual threat, often associated with a fear that one is dying because of physical symptoms that are being experienced); obsessive-compulsive disorder (unwanted thoughts that lead to anxiety and may lead to ritualistic behaviors in an attempt to control the thoughts); acute stress disorder (an intense reaction, which lasts less than 1 month, following a traumatic event); post-traumatic stress disorder (PTSD; an intense reaction to trauma that lasts more than 1 month); and phobias (fear and avoidance of specific things or situations, such as needles). Each of these may affect end-of-life decision making, but little research has been done to determine to what extent and how the various types of clinical anxiety can affect dying people (Pessin et al., 2002).

Prevalence and Treatment of Clinical Anxiety Disorders Among Dying Persons

People who had anxiety problems prior to receiving a life-limiting diagnosis will likely continue to have to deal with the anxiety issues, but the prevalence of the various anxiety disorders among dying people and the extent to which the anxiety issues may be the result of the diagnosis are essentially unknown at this point. Some research has been done on PTSD (Block, 2006), but the variations in rates are significant, although the highest rates still occur in only around one third of people, indicating that a majority of people may not have a clinical anxiety syndrome.

Just as there is less research on the prevalence of anxiety disorders in dying people, there have also been few studies on treatment. However, similar to clinical depression, the combination of medication and psychotherapy may be the best treatment for severe cases (Gibson et al., 2006). With anxiety, either an antidepressant or a benzodiazepine may be indicated (Block, 2006), and as indicated, if anxiety is the result of existential concerns, then a certain type of therapy based on Frankl's work may be useful (Greenstein & Breitbart, 2000), while for others cognitive-behavioral interventions may be in order.

Ways Clinical Anxiety Disorders Can Have an Impact on End-of-Life Decision Making

Fears, and the more intense conditions associated with clinical anxiety, can powerfully affect decision making, whether the intense fear of needles leads to refusing certain treatments or obsessive-compulsive disorder leads to behaviors designed to reduce thoughts that may actually lead to harm, or trauma resulting from witnessing a bad death leads to decisions not to die the same way as that other person. Anxiety that results from or is associated with the treatments a person has received in the past can affect future decisions, such as when the experience of extreme nausea that may be the result of chemotherapy leads a person to decline future chemotherapeutic interventions (Kwilosz, 2005). This type of situation obviously has an impact on treatment decisions. In my experience, many persons with AIDS have been caregivers for others with AIDS who died, and if the person had a "bad" death, the former caregiver who is now dying may choose to hasten death if he or she fears that his or her dying process may also be problematic (see also Sikkema, Hansen, Meade, Kochman, & Lee, 2005).

Another type of anxiety in the end-of-life literature that is not an official diagnosis but that has received significant attention is death anxiety (Neimeyer, Wittkowski, & Moser, 2004). Many authors have hypothesized that people, perhaps especially European American citizens of the United States, have a significant fear of death that can be so extreme that they may actually deny that they will eventually die (Becker, 1973). This may not be a problem in most situations and with most people, but in an end-of-life setting or with a person who is dying, severe death anxiety can lead to treatment choices that may result in significant suffering and cost (emotional and financial) for the dying person and those around that person. Relatively low hospice use rate and the late referrals to hospice may be examples of how death anxiety may affect end-of-life decision making.

Relationships Among Clinical Anxiety Disorders and the Cases in This Book

The four personal stories in this book all have some elements that could be indicative of clinical anxiety disorders in the ill or dying person or the caregivers. The case of the adolescent, Richard (chapter 2), clearly demonstrates how anxiety can lead to not wanting to address certain end-of-life issues that, although perhaps not obvious at the time, may have significant repercussions if decisions have to be made at a later date by someone other than the ill person (see Ditto, chapter 13, this volume). In the case of Spannhake (chapter 3), the trauma associated with the pain and treatments for his condition led him to consider stopping treatment and dying, while the trauma associated with his failing health may have contributed to Raye's father's decision (chapter 5). Both Raye and Crow (chapter 4) seem to have experienced some anxiety both before the decision was made and after their loved one died, illustrating that end-of-life decision making can lead to clinically significant anxiety conditions in caregivers and loved ones as well.

Other Psychosocial Issues

There are a host of other psychological, interpersonal, spiritual, and societal issues that may affect end-of-life decision making (see Werth et al., 2002, for a review), but many have been covered elsewhere in this book. There are, however, two that are regularly mentioned in the end-of-life literature that have only been touched by other chapter authors—autonomy and dignity—so they are discussed next.

Autonomy

Concern about maintaining autonomy or self-determination is significant in the United States, especially among European American men, who hold most of the power in this country and therefore make most of the decisions and have written most of the rules in this country and in the medical system. As a result, the predominant culture in the United States is individualistic and built around making one's own decisions. As Hayslip and his colleagues discuss elsewhere in this book (chapter 17), this style is not universal within the United States and certainly is not the norm around the globe. The law and the rules and regulations related to medical care are built on this foundation of a person making his or her own decisions in as many situations as possible for as long as possible. In fact, a person who is of legal age is considered able (i.e., competent) to make decisions unless legally determined otherwise in a court of law, and even teenagers are being given a say in their treatment decisions (Freyer, 2004).

This emphasis on autonomy means that many people go through life expecting to have control over themselves and their choices. This way of living does not automatically change as death approaches (Shneidman, 1978), so that people who have had control over most aspects of their life will continue to expect to have such power near the end of life. Rules and laws are designed to help people maintain control by protecting confidentiality of records and preparing advance directives.

For some people, dying can be a severe threat to their autonomy because suddenly it is the medical team or the institution or ultimately the disease or condition that is in charge of the process. As a result, to maintain autonomy and control, the person may make end-of-life decisions that may seem ill-advised to others but make complete sense to the dying person who is trying to maintain control (see, e.g., Kastenbaum, 1978; Williams & Koocher, 1998). This is often discussed in terms of assisted suicide, but the same type of thinking and decision making can influence decisions to withhold or withdraw treatment or to continue aggressively treating a condition.

Whether this style of thinking and decision making should be questioned or interfered with is a matter of debate, depending on the perspective one takes (and the experiences one may have had). Some have asserted that a compromise can be reached between the extreme civil libertarian who would grant any person the power to end his or her life and the extreme interventionist who believes that one should always take actions to lengthen life through the use of a thorough assessment of the decision-making process used by the dying person (Werth & Rogers, 2005). These authors believe that although the dying person would need to give up some autonomy in the process by going through the assessment, the possibility of being able to carry out one's wishes without interference once the evaluation is done may ameliorate the resistance to some degree.

Regardless of one's beliefs about autonomy, the fact is that this idea is a part of the end-of-life decision-making process and must be considered when working with people who are dying and their loved ones.

Dignity

Perhaps associated with autonomy for some, dignity is a nebulous concept that necessarily must be defined for each person. Although originally used by proponents of assisted death, the issue of dignity near the end of life has been discussed more broadly recently (Chochinov, 2002), and a whole approach to helping people who are dying maintain dignity as they define it has been developed ("dignity-conserving care"; Chochinov). Broadly speaking, *dignity* can be defined as one's perception of being "worthy, honored, or esteemed" (*Webster*, 1946, p. 730, as cited in Chochinov, 2002, p. 2254). Thus, what is dignified for one person may be undignified for another for a variety of personal, interpersonal, cultural, spiritual/religious, or other reasons. Thus, it is important to get a sense of what the dying person considers to be a dignified death to try to understand better the decisions that the person is making. This can also help with troubleshooting regarding interventions and mediating interpersonal conflict between the dying person and other participants in the end-of-life arena.

How Autonomy and Dignity Relate to the Cases in This Book

Both autonomy and dignity are clearly present in Raye's account (chapter 5). Her description of her father and his decision-making process indicates that these were preeminent concerns for him and for his family, even if they did not necessarily agree with his decisions or definitions. Crow (chapter 4) also takes into account what she thinks her brother's beliefs would be about his position and the lack of autonomy in it and whether he would see it as a dignified way to continue to live. Richard (chapter 2), as an adolescent, is still trying to develop his sense of place in the world; therefore, what autonomy and dignity mean to him and his lack of deep thought about these issues are evident in his commentary. Finally, Spannhake (chapter 3) alluded to autonomy and dignity when he described the treatments he was receiving and how he did or did not want to be a part of the decision making regarding them.

□ Conclusion

If we want to try to truly understand the end-of-life decisions that people are making, we must consider the mental health issues that may be affecting what they are considering and why when making these choices. If we do not understand the decision or the process to arrive at the decision, it may be our own values getting in the way, or it may be that the person is experiencing a mental disorder that is affecting his or her judgment. In such cases, intervention may be in order to allow the person to make choices that are consistent with who he or she really is as opposed to the decisions being ruled by clinical depression or anxiety.

Similarly, a dying person's beliefs about autonomy and dignity may be influencing personal decision making, and these beliefs, almost by definition, defy gross assumptions or determinations. Each person must be considered unique in his or her belief systems on these issues and asked how they may be affecting decision making. Then, we may be better able to understand what is influencing the choices made.

Merely considering the physical pain and suffering of a dying person is incomplete, just as only looking at mental health issues would be incomplete without including the physical, interpersonal, spiritual, and societal influences on the individual. We must consider each person holistically; for many, this means considering how mental health issues may be having an impact on their end-of-life decision making.

□ References

American Psychiatric Association. (2000). *Diagnostic and statistical manual of mental disorders* (4th ed., text revision). Washington, DC: Author.

Beck, A. T., Steer, R. A., Beck, J. S., & Newman, C. F. (1993). Hopelessness, depression, suicidal ideation, and clinical diagnosis of depression. *Suicide and Life-Threatening Behavior, 23,* 139–145.

Beck, A. T., Steer, R. A., Kovacs, M., & Garrison, B. (1985). Hopelessness and eventual suicide: A 10-year prospective study of patients hospitalized with suicidal ideation. *American Journal of Psychiatry, 142,* 559–563.

Becker, E. (1973). *The denial of death.* New York: Free Press.

Block, S. D. (2000). Assessing and managing depression in the terminally ill patient. *Annals of Internal Medicine, 132,* 209–218.

Block, S. D. (2006). Psychological issues in end-of-life care. *Journal of Palliative Medicine, 9,* 751–772.

Bongar, B. (2002). *The suicidal patient: Clinical and legal standards of care* (2nd ed.). Washington, DC: American Psychological Association.

Breitbart, W., & Heller, K. S. (2003). Refraining hope: Meaning-centered care for patients near the end of life. *Journal of Palliative Medicine, 6,* 979–988.

Buckley, J., & Herth, K. (2004). Fostering hope in terminally ill patients. *Nursing Standard, 19*(10), 33–41.

Chochinov, H. M. (2002). Dignity-conserving care—a new model for palliative care. *Journal of the American Medical Association, 287,* 2253–2260.

Christakis, N. A. (1999). *Death foretold: Prophecy and prognosis in medical care.* Chicago: University of Chicago Press.

Freyer, D. R. (2004). Care of the dying adolescent: Special considerations. *Pediatrics, 113,* 381–388.

Ganzini, L., Lee, M. A., Heintz, R. T., Bloom, J. D., & Fenn, D. S. (1994). The effect of depression treatment on elderly patients' preferences for life-sustaining medical therapy. *American Journal of Psychiatry, 151,* 1613–1616.

Gibson, C. A., Breitbart, W., Tomarken, A., Kosinski, A., & Nelson, C. J. (2006). Mental health issues near the end of life. In J. L. Werth Jr. & D. Blevins (Eds.), *Psychosocial issues near the end of life: A resource for professional care providers* (pp. 137–162). Washington, DC: American Psychological Association.

Greenstein, M., & Breitbart, W. (2000). Cancer and the experience of meaning: A group psychotherapy program for people with cancer. *American Journal of Psychotherapy, 54,* 486–500.

Hubble, M. A., Duncan, B. L., & Miller, S. D. (1999). *The heart and soul of change: What works in therapy.* Washington, DC: American Psychological Association.

Kastenbaum, R. (1978). In control. In C. A. Garfield (Ed.), *Psychosocial care of the dying patient* (pp. 227–240). New York: McGraw-Hill.

Kwilosz, D. M. (2005). Patient as teacher. *Death Studies, 29,* 737–744.

Neimeyer, R. A., Prigerson, H. G., & Davies, B. (2002). Mourning and meaning. *American Behavioral Scientist, 46,* 235–251.

Neimeyer, R. A., Wittkowski, J., & Moser, R. P. (2004). Psychological research on death attitudes: An overview and evaluation. *Death Studies, 28,* 309–340.

Pessin, H., Rosenfeld, B., & Breitbart, W. (2002). Assessing psychological distress near the end of life. *American Behavioral Scientist, 46,* 357–372.

Rosenfeld, B., Abbey, J., & Pessin, H. (2006). Depression and hopelessness near the end of life: Assessment and treatment. In J. L. Werth Jr. & D. Blevins (Eds.), *Psychosocial issues near the end of life: A resource for professional care providers* (pp. 163–182). Washington, DC: American Psychological Association.

Shear, K., Frank, E., Houck, P. R., & Reynolds, C. F., III. (2005). Treatment of complicated grief: A randomized controlled trial. *Journal of the American Medical Association, 293,* 2601–2608.

Shneidman, E. S. (1978). Some aspects of psychotherapy with dying persons. In C. A. Garfield (Ed.), *Psychosocial care of the dying patient* (pp. 202–218). New York: McGraw-Hill.

Sikkema, K. J., Hansen, N. B., Meade, C. S., Kochman, A., & Lee, R. S. (2005). Improvements in health-related quality of life following a group intervention for coping with AIDS-bereavement among HIV-infected men and women. *Quality of Life Research, 14,* 991–1005.

Werth, J. L., Jr., Gordon, J. R., & Johnson, R. R., Jr. (2002). Psychosocial issues near the end of life. *Aging and Mental Health, 6,* 402–412.

Werth, J. L., Jr., & Rogers, J. R. (2005). Assessing for impaired judgment as a means of meeting the "duty to protect" when a client is a potential harm-to-self: Implications for clients making end-of-life decisions. *Mortality, 10,* 7–21.

Williams, J., & Koocher, G. P. (1998). Addressing loss of control in chronic illness: Theory and practice. *Psychotherapy, 35,* 325–335.

Wilson, K. G., Chochinov, H. M., de Faye, B. J., & Breitbart, W. (2000). Diagnosis and management of depression in palliative care. In H. M. Chochinov & W. Breitbart (Eds.), *Handbook of psychiatry in palliative medicine* (pp. 25–49). New York: Oxford University Press.

Working Group on Assisted Suicide and End of Life Decisions. (2000). *Report to the board of directors.* Washington, DC: American Psychological Association. Retrieved January 25, 2004, from http://www.apa.org/pi/aseolf.html

Zivin, K., & Christakis, N. A. (2007). The emotional toll of spousal morbidity and mortality. *American Journal of Geriatric Psychiatry, 15,* 772–779.

15

CHAPTER

Family End-of-Life Decision Making

Sharla Wells-Di Gregorio

Introduction

Health care in the United States continues to be dominated by an individualistic, patient-centered perspective despite the fact that most medical decisions from symptom recognition to withdrawal of life support are made in the context of the family.[1] Discussion of family end-of-life (EOL) decision making tends to focus rather narrowly on patient completion of advance directives (e.g., living will, healthcare power of attorney) and family understanding of these documents. However, the fact that advance directives are founded on the ethical principle of autonomy, or self-determination, can be problematic given that one person's dying process typically involves many other people (Breslin, 2005).

As a result of this emphasis on patient autonomy in decision making, families are frequently unaware of patient EOL values and preferences. Family members are often excluded from patient–healthcare provider communication, limiting the information they have available to make informed decisions as a family (see Crow, chapter 4, this volume). Foster and McLellan (2002) described the immense moral uncertainty that family members experience in making the "right" decisions and fears of "killing" another human being with their decisions. Families must simultaneously evaluate past, present, and future, including what has happened medically, the present choices to be made, the future implications of these choices, and the meaning of the patients' life, amidst anguish "envisioning a future as they contemplate their loss" (p. 48). Consequently many families live with persistent doubts and regrets regarding EOL decisions made for loved ones in the absence of shared advance care plans (Teno, Stevens, Spernak, & Lynn, 1998). Several quotations from bereaved family members convey this sense of overwhelming responsibility and doubt: "The reality of making those decisions is something that you have to live with, always." "You are making all the decisions and in such an emotional state and you are hoping and praying you are making the right decisions." "All of her medical care, all those decisions had to be made by me, and if I made the wrong decision, then I was going to be the one that had to suffer as well" (Teno, Casey, Welch, & Edgman-Levitan, 2001, p. 743).

Family EOL decision making involves much more than patient completion of advance directives and family adherence to these documents. In addition to making decisions regarding the use of life-sustaining technologies at the EOL, families are faced with choices about home care, hospice care, nursing home placement, nutritional status, clinical trials, second opinions, the possibility of additional surgery, medication continuation or discontinuation, and hospital transfers. Simultaneously, families are faced with additional financial decisions, family event planning around illness, work arrangements, transportation, child care, and family coordination of care/visits. These decisions often must be made rapidly, with limited time for information seeking and processing (Hiltunen, Medich, Chase, Peterson, & Forrow, 1999) and limited awareness of patients' values, goals of care, or specific preferences (Emanuel & Emanuel, 1992).

Family member decision making does not end here. After the patient dies, family members are faced with many additional decisions that are most often tragically not anticipated or planned in advance. Postdeath, families must decide on the date and type of service, if any, to mark the person's death and perhaps to celebrate the individual's life, cremation versus burial, where to place the remains, how to pay for such services, how to manage family finances in the absence of the deceased (made especially difficult in the absence of a will or trust), how to maintain family communication without the deceased, understanding the nature of grieving, how to support one another in grief, and how to maintain connection with the deceased in memory while moving forward with life. All of these decisions are influenced by the specific cultural context of the person who died and those who continue to live, with cultural differences within a family system making such decisions even more complex.

Decision making at the EOL can be incredibly complex, particularly in the absence of advance care planning. Advance care planning is an ongoing dialogue with patients, family members, and healthcare providers regarding choices for care near the EOL. Advance care planning is designed to clarify the patient's questions, fears, and values and thus improve the patient's well being by reducing the frequency and magnitude of overtreatment and undertreatment as defined by the patient and family. Advance care planning that focuses only on specific treatment decisions or does not include family members in the discussion is unlikely to be satisfactory to patients and their families (Hines et al., 1999; Tulsky, Chesney, & Lo, 1995). Many patients feel comfortable leaving EOL decisions to family members rather than structured advance care planning (Hawkins, Ditto, Danks, & Smucker, 2005; Holley, Stackiewicz, Dacko, & Rault, 1997; Sehgal et al., 1992), particularly as illness progresses or if the patient is unable to speak for himself or herself (Nolan et al., 2005; Rosenfeld, Wenger, & Kagawa-Singer, 2000). Some do not complete advance directives because they believe family members understand their wishes (Hamel, Guse, Hawranik, & Bond, 2002). Despite only moderate agreement between patients and surrogates in the SUPPORT (Study to Understand Prognoses and Preferences for Outcomes and Risks of Treatment) trial (SUPPORT principal investigators, 1995), 78% of patients indicated willingness for their surrogate to make treatment decisions for them if they were unable to speak for themselves. Congruence between patient and family wishes may be less important than patient trust of family to make decisions based on family needs. Patients may be more interested in the process of exploring or explaining preferences, such as who will make decisions and how much latitude decision makers should have, versus specific treatment preferences (Ditto & Hawkins, 2005; Hawkins et al., 2005; Ott, 1999).

Patients may in fact only complete advance directives to protect family welfare versus the standard notion of patients utilizing advance directives to protect patient autonomy (Nolan & Bruder, 1997). Patients may view advance care planning as a means of protecting their families from burden in the future. A study by Nolan and Bruder (1997) found that 74% of patients thought having an advance directive would prevent family disagreements over patient treatment at the EOL. Seventy-eight percent thought an advance directive would help reduce guilt over treatment decisions for family members at the EOL. Over 70% also thought having an advance directive would prevent costly medical expenses for their family at the EOL. This chapter provides evidence that a family-based approach to advance care planning could circumvent many of the problems resulting from an exclusive focus on patient autonomy as the central goal in advance care planning. Family-based advance care planning would better match the preferences of most Americans for family-centered EOL decision making. Both Volicer (chapter 18, this volume) and Lyon (Richard & Lyon, chapter 2, this volume) describe processes for families to be involved in advance care planning. In fact, Richard explicitly engaged in the process both to express his preferences for care and to ensure that his family would not make decisions that would increase their burden.

☐ Role of Families in Health Care Decision Making

Families play an integral role in the health of their members from birth until death. Family membership often determines the type and extent of healthcare resources available, such as nutritious foods, insurance coverage, or a safe neighborhood for exercise or play. Family ties can exert a strong influence on health behaviors (Umberson, 1992). Marriage and the presence of children in the home serve as a deterrent to negative health behaviors, with divorce associated with an increase in these behaviors (Umberson, 1987, 1992). Families frequently play a role in disease detection, treatment decisions, and adherence (or lack of adherence) to physician recommendations (Denberg, Beaty, Kim, & Steiner, 2005; Stanton, 1987). Families provide the majority of care to a loved one when the loved one becomes ill (Emanuel et al., 1999), and contrary to what might be expected from an individualist nation, families continue to provide care until they are no longer able to physically or emotionally manage the care of their loved one at home (Gaugler, Kane, Kane, Clay, & Newcomer, 2003). Fewer than 10% of older adults are placed in the permanent care of a nursing home; most of these individuals are over the age of 85 and have no living relatives (Spillman, Liu, & McGilliard, 2002).

The National Survey of Families and Households indicated that there are approximately 54 million caregivers in the United States. The majority of these caregivers are female (75%) with an average age of 46 years old. Many (41%) have children under age 18 in the home, and more than half (52%) work full time outside the home (Arno, Levine, & Memmott, 1999). Some report caregiving a few hours per week, but 20% of caregivers report full-time or constant care with no reimbursement for their services (Donelan et al., 2002; Hayman et al., 2001).

Family caregivers often assume numerous roles, including transportation assistance, shopping, homemaking, emotional support, nutritional care, nursing care, personal care, and financial management. They must manage numerous medications, appointments, and field phone calls from concerned family members (Emanuel, Fairclough, Slutsman, & Emanuel, 2000). Family caregivers are members of the medical team who are often required to administer medications and make complex medical decisions with little training and no compensation (Donelan et al., 2002; Rabow, Hauser, & Adams, 2004). Having just provided care at home to my mother at the end of her life after her long battle with metastatic breast cancer, I can say from experience that the statistics do not do justice to the emotional and physical exhaustion of this endeavor. Coordination of care can be exasperating, ranging from multiple phone calls to obtain prior authorization for release of much-needed medication to difficulty coordinating appointment times for a loved one living with tremendous fatigue and increasing disability, limiting physical tolerance for travel and waiting.

Near the EOL, approximately half of all Americans may be decisionally incapacitated, requiring others, typically family members, to make medical decisions with or without advance specifications (Lynn et al., 1997). In the intensive care unit (ICU) setting, 95% of patients may lack decisional capacity (Cohen et al., 2005). In situations of incapacity, the patient-designated healthcare power of attorney is asked to make decisions for the individual. In most but not all states, in the absence of such a designee, the order of surrogacy is spouse, adult children, parents, or adult siblings, with the last three categories requiring unanimous decision.

☐ Factors Influencing Family End-of-Life Decision Making

For families to make the most effective EOL decisions, patients and families must have current information on the patient's diagnosis, prognosis, and disease course; must understand the certainties and uncertainties associated with each recommended course of action; and must have sufficient time as well as the mental and emotional capacity to process their options. In addition, patients and families must have an active and influential voice in healthcare decision making. The following factors can limit or have an impact on family decision making near the EOL and are important for families and healthcare providers to understand:

Patient Optimistic Bias

Many patients demonstrate an *optimistic bias*, rating their own chances of survival as better than the statistics they have been given (Brundage et al., 2001). In one study of patients with metastatic colon and lung cancer, patients who overestimated their survival time were more likely to favor life-extending treatments over comfort care (Weeks et al., 1998). A closer exploration of this false optimism indicates that patient optimism may represent a collusion in doctor-patient communication by which the "doctor does not want to pronounce a 'death sentence' and the patient does not want to hear it" (The, Hak, Koeter, & van der Wal, 2001, p. 247). Such overestimates of life expectancy or treatment effectiveness can limit advance care planning and EOL preparation of the family (Emanuel & Emanuel, 1998). Stewart (1994) provided a moving example of the impact of collusion, overoptimism, and lack of communication on one family member postbereavement:

> Because we didn't talk about his dying. I keep thinking to myself, I just wish I had him back so that we could hug and kiss and say goodbye. We never said goodbye. We faked the whole thing. We fooled each other. We fooled no one. I think I would have rather been able to say goodbye with a hug and our crying together. I don't know, maybe that would have been more devastating for me to live with. I just feel there was no ending, no finish. We played a game and lost. Yet, he never took the lead. I waited for him to say something. And he never said, "Ma, I'm dying." (p. 343)

Absence or Ambiguity of Family Communication with Healthcare Providers

Fewer than 25% of Americans have completed advance directives (Eiser & Weiss, 2001). The most essential factor enabling such communication is patient, family, and staff availability for such discussions. Family members are often unable to attend patient care meetings that conflict with work or child care responsibilities. Families may be expected to attend meetings at an institution that is geographically distant, on short notice, and with limited time to gather and review information that might help them to further understand the choices at hand. Surrogates may find it difficult to obtain leave time from work, particularly if they have been providing long-term care and have utilized available sick and vacation time.

The following excerpt demonstrates this barrier and the consequent advocacy burden of one husband in a busy hospital setting:

> I think it's a very complicated situation to be an advocate in a world where you are not an equal. … Sometimes it used to annoy me if I went to the nurse's station and they were busy, and they wouldn't even look up, but I would say, "Excuse me, excuse me, I have a question" or "I need some help with something." And you are there when she is calling the nurse and the nurse doesn't respond. And you are thinking if they are not doing it while I'm here, being the advocate, what are they doing when I'm not here? (Teno et al., 2001, p. 743)

Another barrier to advance care planning is the healthcare providers use of medical jargon. For example, in response to a physician's statement, "The bilirubin is going up. The bilirubin is going up," one daughter/caregiver comments, "We had no context for that. We knew it was bad, but we didn't know if that meant that in 6 months he was going to be in trouble, or in a week he might be in trouble" (Rabow et al., 2004, p. 484). When discussing do not resuscitate (DNR) orders with patients, residents may frequently use jargon, provide minimal information regarding patient survival, and may fail to discuss patients' values and emotional concerns (Tulsky et al., 1995). At other times, assumptions of care providers regarding family medical expertise may severely limit dialogue with family members. Laura Crow's narrative in this book (chapter 4) portrays this situation, "My own loss of faith in the medical system began when we asked Josh's neurosurgeon to detail the areas of injury, and he replied, 'You wouldn't possibly understand. That's a seminar-level medical school discussion.' End of conversation." To achieve a level of information that will be most useful for family decision making, an initial question such as, "How much do you understand about your family member's condition and prognosis?" and "What would you like to know?" would allow providers to better gauge family member understanding and areas in need of clarification.

Lack of Prognostication and Physician Optimistic Bias

Prognostic information in situations of imminent death is rarely provided in practice. Physicians may think they are poorly prepared for prognostication, find it stressful to make predictions, and believe that patients and families expect more certainty than they are able to provide (Christakis & Iwashyna, 1998). They may fear destroying hope (Baile, Lenzi, Parker, Buckman, & Cohen, 2002; Gordon & Daugherty, 2003). Physicians may also be susceptible to the same optimistic bias demonstrated by patients. In their analysis of survival estimates provided by 343 physicians at the time of hospice referral, Christakis and Lamont (2000) found that doctors overestimated survival in 63% of cases by a factor of 5.3.

Overestimation of response and survival can have dire outcomes for patients and their family members, as demonstrated in the following description:

> Well, none of us would have made the decisions we did (to continue treatment) if we had known the truth about her illness. ... You have got to wonder why they put her through all that—I mean the chemo and especially the radiology and all those burns. She was in pain and had burns everywhere from the radiation. It was awful. She wouldn't have gone through it if she had known what they knew, but they told us it was curable; so what are you going to do? How can you know? I mean, we are not the experts in medical things. Should we be? We didn't really have any decisions to make because we didn't know anything. And they told us that her disease was

> curable. They even said the cancer was gone. That still has me wondering even now. What did they know? (Cherlin et al., 2005, p. 1182)

Crow (chapter 4, this volume) asked similar questions reflecting back on the early medical decisions she and her father made for Josh.

The problem likely lies among patient, family, and healthcare providers. Lack of communication may in fact represent collusion between the physician and family by which the physician's discomfort with such discussions and the family's difficulty hearing bad news inhibit these discussions. One study of 218 family caregivers of patients enrolled in hospice found great variability regarding what information families wanted and when they wanted it (Cherlin et al., 2005). Some families thought physicians withheld information; others were glad not to discuss EOL concerns, and some families were ambivalent about further discussion. Careful assessment and documentation of family informational needs and wishes are essential.

Lack of Direct End-of-Life Communication Between Patient and Family

Despite the perceived benefits of EOL discussions and advanced care planning reported by patients and family members (i.e., increased comfort, reduced burden and stress, and increased sense of control) (Butow, Maclean, Dunn, Tattersall, & Boyer, 1997; Ditto et al., 2001; Sutherland, Llewellyn-Thomas, Lockwood, Tritchler, & Till, 1989; Tilden, Tolle, Nelson, & Fields, 2001), family members frequently lack the information necessary from patients to make effective EOL decisions for them (Diamond, Jernigan, Moseley, Messina, & McKeown, 1989; Emanuel & Emanuel, 1992). Without advance directives, surrogates demonstrate limited accuracy in predicting patient treatment preferences (Uhlmann, Pearlman, & Cain, 1988). Without prior discussion or exposure to a patient's living will, surrogates are often left to struggle with understanding the patient's condition and prognosis while trying to interpret isolated, out-of-context patient statements made earlier in life (Lang & Quill, 2004; see Ditto, chapter 13, this volume). Lack of EOL discussions can increase family burden and fear of making decisions incompatible with patient wishes at the EOL. This anguish is very clearly demonstrated in Crow's story (chapter 4, this volume), "Decision Making in the Absence of Advance Directives." She relied heavily on information from her brother's friends regarding his wishes but experienced considerable ambivalence throughout the decision-making process because of the absence of direct discussion of his wishes prior to his injury and decisional incapacity.

Patients' and family members' conversations regarding EOL preferences are often infrequent and too general to aid family members in making very specific decisions at the EOL (Hines et al., 1999). In their study of 242 pairs of dialysis patients and their designated surrogates, Hines and colleagues (2001) found that surrogates were more likely than patients to want patient preferences expressed verbally and in writing (62% vs. 39%). Surrogates, more than patients, thought it was important to discuss preferences for the location of death, worst-case scenarios, and the option of stopping treatment. Both patients and surrogates tended to overestimate surrogates' knowledge of patients' wishes.

Many factors conspire to limit patients and family members from participating together in advance care planning. First, the patients' overoptimism regarding their prognosis may inhibit discussions prior to decisional incapacity or death (Brundage et al., 2001). Second, family members may be excluded from decision making based on models of shared decision making that focus heavily on the patient and physician dyad (Whitney, 2003). Even policies and systems designed to protect patients' privacy can prevent information sharing with family members. For instance, with the recent implementation of the Health Information Portability and Accountability Act's (HIPPA) Privacy Rule, many family members have reported to me that they have found it difficult to obtain information via telephone in emergency situations about loved ones due to HIPAA regulations, escalating their uncertainty and anxiety.

Although family members may regard communication about cancer or terminal disease to be one of their most urgent needs (Kilpatrick, Kristjanson, Tataryn, & Fraser, 1998), many families report emotional, interpersonal, and attitudinal barriers to such discussions with their loved ones. In their study of advanced-stage lung cancer patients and caregivers, Zhang and Siminoff (2003) found that 65% of families reported communication difficulties. The most frequent reasons for avoiding discussion included the inability to manage intense affect or psychological distress, mutual protection, and beliefs about positive thinking.

Caregivers who observed that the patient was already upset or distressed were reluctant to raise the topic of illness (Zhang & Siminoff, 2003). Both patients and caregivers demonstrated "mutual protection" in which each tried to protect the other from being exposed to "harmful" discussions. The authors reported that "family members endured a great deal of worry, anger, and fear about their loved one's dying, but they fought hard to conceal their emotions to avoid upsetting patients" (p. 423).

Another reason for families' avoidance of communication at the EOL is the "tyranny of positive thinking" (Holland & Lewis, 2000) in which thoughts about the disease, about treatment termination, or about death are considered to be negative and self-destructive. Patients and families may believe that positive thinking is an antidote to cancer, and that frank discussions of EOL will promote disease progression. Cultural beliefs and expectations regarding family communication at the EOL may also have an impact on conversations, particularly which family members should be included in such discussions.

Fears of Burdening Caregivers

Numerous studies described the difficulties patients experience at the EOL related to their physical limitations and fears of burdening others with their care. One study of 60 patient/caregiver dyads facing advanced cancer revealed that patient depression and more hours of required caregiving were independent predictors of patients' increased desires for hastened death (Ransom, Sacco, Weitzner, Azzarello, & McMillan, 2006). This represents one of the few studies that considered both patient and caregiver perspectives at the EOL, but it suggests the unique role that patient fears of burdening caregivers play in their own EOL decision making.

Imprecision of Advance Directives

An additional impediment to implementation of advance directives is the need for surrogates to understand patients' wishes once expressed. Several studies have now demonstrated only low-to-moderate accuracy between patient preferences and surrogate prediction of those preferences (Hare, Pratt, & Nelson, 1992; Seckler, Meier, Mulvihill, & Paris, 1991; Suhl, Simons, Reedy, & Garrick, 1994; Uhlmann et al., 1988; Zweibel & Cassel, 1989). Even with patient and surrogate discussion of advance directives, the accuracy of predicting patient preferences may not be improved (Ditto et al., 2001; see Ditto, chapter 13, this volume).

Decisions regarding artificial nutrition and hydration are particularly challenging for family members (Daly, 2000). The primitive role of the family to feed and shelter its members may outweigh a rational analysis of the costs and benefits of EOL feeding and hydration. For example, in one study in which patients were decisionally incapacitated at the time of feeding tube placement, only 47.9% of surrogates felt confident that the patient would have wanted this procedure. The surrogates understood the benefits (83%) but not the risks of tube feeding (48.9%) (Mitchell, Berkowitz, Lawson, & Lipsitz, 2000).

A major difficulty for families utilizing living wills in EOL decision making is the vagueness and lack of congruence of the living will with the clinical situation at hand (Teno et al., 1997). Current advance directives focus heavily on what not to do (I *do not* want CPR [cardiopulmonary resuscitation], I *do not* want artificial nutrition and hydration) and "reflect a poverty of vision about what *can* and ought to be done to *support* patients who have ultimately fatal conditions" (Zuckerman & Wollner, 1999, p. 95, emphasis original). Patients often believe that living wills provide more information than the living will actually does to surrogates faced with EOL decisions (Keysar & Barr, 2002). A narrative recorded by one of the SUPPORT trial nurses clarifies this point:

> At that time, the patient's wife expressed concern that the patient not be kept alive if there was no hope of recovery, that those were his wishes, and she wanted to honor them. ... Her question was, how would she know when to stop? (Teno et al., 1998, p. 441)

Although impossible to list all specific treatment and outcome possibilities (Brett, 1991), families would benefit from a better understanding of patient preferences in the face of illness/symptom progression, functional capacity changes, mental status impairment, and other psychosocial considerations confronting families at the EOL (Zuckerman & Wollner, 1999).

In situations of limited or ambiguous communication about patient EOL wishes, projection bias is likely to ensue. Projection bias is well known in the social psychology literature; it is also known as the false consensus effect (Marks & Miller, 1987). Projection bias results when a person "projects" their own characteristics or beliefs onto others, assuming that others are likely to behave and believe as they themselves do. For example, a series of studies involving 361 elderly outpatients and their chosen surrogates demonstrated that surrogates' predictions more closely resembled their own life-sustaining treatment wishes than the wishes of the individual they were trying to predict (Fagerlin, Ditto, Danks, Houts, & Smucker, 2001). Families could benefit from education regarding the projection bias and overoptimistic bias that occur at the EOL as these have a significant impact on the lack of urgency for family discussions of EOL issues.

Family Member Perceptual Biases and Psychological Distress

Family member perceptual biases and mood may also influence their interpretation of advance directives. Family surrogates overestimate patients' desire for life-sustaining treatment (Ditto et al., 2001; Fagerlin et al., 2001; Uhlmann et al., 1988). Surrogate decision makers also show systematic bias in underestimating patient quality of life (Scales, Tansey, Matte, & Herridge, 2006). This may be particularly true for surrogates experiencing depression. In a study of 40 caregivers of patients with mild-to-moderate dementia, caregiver depression and burden negatively affected their assessment of the patients' quality of life. This bias could ultimately affect their ability to make EOL decisions consistent with patient preferences (Karlawish, Casarett, Klocinski, & Clark, 2001).

This is a concern as the risk of psychological disorders is greatly elevated among caregivers. In the year before the patient's death, the prevalence of anxiety is 46%, and the prevalence of depression is 39% among cancer caregivers (Ramirez, Addington-Hall, & Richards, 1998). This contrasts with rates of anxiety and depression in the general population of 3% to 5% and 2% to 9%, respectively (American Psychiatric Association, 2000). However, African American caregivers report less depression and burden (Haley, Han, & Henderson, 1998; Haley et al., 1995) and are less likely to institutionalize elderly family members (Friedman, Steinwachs, Rathouz, Burton, & Mukamel, 2005; Stevens et al., 2004).

A further limiting factor in the implementation of advance directives is the surrogates' ability to make decisions corresponding to patient preferences in a highly distressing context. EOL decision making can be a tremendously difficult process for surrogates as they are simultaneously faced with the task of both advocating for the patient and accepting that a loved one is dying (Teno et al., 1998). Frequently surrogates will require several conversations with treatment providers to fully process and move toward a decision. They may also need to hear information from multiple sources. For surrogates, the life of their loved one rests in their hands. It is unreasonable to expect that they might be able to disengage from a lifetime of memories following a brief family conference.

Family Sense of Burden

The National Longitudinal Caregiver Study (Buhr, Kuchibhatla, & Clipp, 2006) has identified several factors predictive of institutionalization of a loved one with dementia. These include the need for more skilled care (65%), particularly related to lower-extremity weakness, the caregiver's health (49%), and patient dementia-related behaviors such as psychosis and behavioral dysregulation (46%). Greater task burden and lower life satisfaction of caregivers were also associated with institutionalization.

These factors are consistent with previous research indicating that the number of caregiving hours is not associated with institutionalization (Gaugler, Kane, Kane, Clay, & Newcomer, 2005), but rather role captivity or feelings of being trapped in the caregiving role (Gaugler et al., 2000), bowel incontinence (Friedman et al., 2005), and economic strain predict nursing home placement (Aneshensel, Pearlin, & Schuler, 1993). In fact, the Caregiver Health Effects Study has also demonstrated that caregiver strain is associated with increased mortality among caregivers. Caregivers experiencing strain related to caregiving had mortality risks 63% higher than noncaregiving control participants (Schulz & Beach, 1999). Notably, hospice care may reduce the risk of death of the patient's bereaved spouse, even if services are utilized for only 3 to 4 weeks (Christakis & Iwashyna, 2003).

Family Support

Social support is an important predictor of caregiver burden. Zarit, Reever, and Bach-Peterson (1980) found that the frequency of visits from other family members was significantly related to lower caregiver burden, more so than patient cognitive impairments, memory and behavior problems, patient functional abilities, and duration of illness. Caregivers receiving more visits from children, grandchildren, and siblings reported less burden. The most beneficial type of support may be engaging in social interaction for fun and recreation. This type of support demonstrates the strongest relationship with lowered caregiver burden compared to other types of support, such as practical or emotional support (Thompson, Futterman, Gallagher-Thompson, Rose, & Lovett, 1993). This may be particularly important for spouse caregivers providing care for an individual with aphasia or memory impairment that limits the caregivers' communication or relationship with the care recipient. Unfortunately, some caregivers report a social death long before the death of their loved one. In fact, for daughters and daughters-in-law, quitting work may be a precursor to social isolation and negative reactions to caregiving (Pohl, Given, Collins, & Given, 1994).

Patient Mental Status

In their study of hypothetical treatment preferences, Allen-Burge and Haley (1997) found that surrogates were less likely to desire life-sustaining treatments such as CPR, CPR and ventilation, and CPR and tube feeding if the hypothetical relative were described as moderately demented versus cognitively intact.

Financial Difficulties

One third of families experience significant loss of income and savings related to the patient's illness (Covinsky et al., 1994). Families may need to sell assets, take out loans, or obtain second jobs to pay for healthcare costs (Emanuel et al., 2000). Twenty percent quit work or make other major life changes, with African American and Hispanic families more at risk of financial burden than White families (Covinsky et al., 1994, 2001). Although the Family Medical Leave Act (1993) has made it possible for many family members to obtain time to care for an ill family member, this leave often involves the use of unpaid sick time. Family economic hardship can have a great impact on family decision making for EOL care. Financial hardship of family caregivers has been associated with a preference for "comfort care only" over life-prolonging care (Covinsky et al., 1996).

Family Member/Surrogate Race

Several studies have also confirmed the important role of race in EOL decision making. African and Latino Americans report being less knowledgeable regarding advance directives, rely more on family-centered approaches to EOL decision making, and use formal documentation for expressing healthcare preferences less frequently than European Americans (Caralis, Davis, Wright, & Marcial, 1993). Across many studies, Caucasians are less likely to desire life-sustaining treatments than African Americans (Allen-Burge & Haley, 1997; Blackhall, Murphy, Frank, Michel, & Azen, 1995; Eleazer et al., 1996). In one focus group study of African American perspectives on EOL planning and decision making, Waters (2001) described many historical, spiritual, and cultural factors contributing to such preferences. These include reliance on God above contracts and lack of trust of healthcare providers and insurers related to past and current experiences of racism in medical care.

□ Patient and Family Values at the End of Life

The following studies describe what is most valued at the EOL from the family perspective. Several common themes emerge through these studies. The first study conducted by Steinhauser and colleagues (2000) involved patients, recently bereaved family members, physicians, and other healthcare providers. Six areas of care emerged as most important at the EOL across all groups: (a) attention to symptoms and personal care (freedom from pain, anxiety, and shortness of breath; being kept clean; and having physical touch); (b) preparation for EOL (financial affairs in order, feeling prepared to die, believing that the family is prepared for the death, and knowing what to expect about the patients' physical condition); (c) achieving a sense of completion (saying good-bye to important people, remembering personal accomplishments, and resolving unfinished business); (d) decisions about treatment preferences (having treatment preferences in writing and naming someone to make decisions in the event that one cannot); (e) being treated as a whole person (maintaining one's dignity, maintaining a sense of humor, having a physician who knows one as a whole person, presence of close friends, not dying alone, and having someone who will listen); and (f) relationships with healthcare professionals (receiving care from one's personal physician, trusting one's physician, having a nurse with whom one feels comfortable, knowing that one's physician is comfortable talking about death and dying, and having a physician with whom one can discuss personal fears).

A second study conducted by Teno and colleagues (2001) analyzed the dialogue from six focus groups with 42 family members 3–12 months postbereavement. Bereaved family members defined high-quality medical care at the EOL as (a) physical comfort, (b) increasing patient control, (c) relieving family members of the burden of being present at all times to advocate for their loved one, (d) educating family members so they felt confident to care for their loved ones at home, and (e) providing family members with emotional support both before and after the patient's death. Many felt unprepared for tasks at home, such as giving medications. One family member stated:

> All of a sudden now she is on all this morphine and all this whatever it is. And that kind of bothered me too. It really did. Because it was like, my God, I'm giving her this stuff. Am I giving her too much? I'm not a trained medical person. (Teno et al., 2001, p. 743)

Family members wanted information regarding what to expect as the patient is dying, but also information regarding what to expect during the process of bereavement. Patient control was highly valued by family members—not simply control over medical decisions, but control over daily activities. Patients with advanced disease often experience weakness, fatigue, and limited control of their environment such that even simple choices can make a difference.

The third study, reported by Vohra and colleagues (Vohra, Brazil, Hanna, & Abelson, 2004) utilized the Family Perception of Care Scale with 203 family members (mostly daughters) who had lost a loved one while the loved one lived in a long-term care facility. The most important priorities of family members for staff were (a) easing of patient pain, (b) treating the patient with dignity, (c) being sensitive to the needs of the patient, (d) informing family members when they thought death was at hand, and (e) providing comfort to the patient. In rating the level of care they received, family members were most dissatisfied with staffing levels, family support, updating the family on the status of the loved one, and involvement of the family in care planning and decision making.

According to these studies, families have several goals for EOL care. Families are seeking adequate pain and symptom management for the patient, including relief of emotional distress. Patient dignity and control are essential, ranging from focusing on the whole person rather than the disease process to ensuring that personal care needs are met in a gentle and sensitive manner. Both patients and families emphasize needs for assistance that will relieve family members of the physical and emotional burdens of caregiving and letting go. Families, in general, report needs for more information on providing personal and medical care, symptom management, and preparation for what to expect during dying and bereavement. Ideally, advance care planning would facilitate these goals, enabling families to focus on strengthening relationships and achieving a sense of completion during the patient's final days. As Byock (1997) has emphasized, dying is an important developmental phase, with opportunities to experience "the love of self and others, the completion of relationships, the acceptance of the finality of one's life, and the achievement of a new sense of self despite one's impending demise" (p. 33).

□ Family End-of-Life Decision-Making Process

Families are making multiple decisions from the point of diagnosis to the eventual death of the patient. Stewart (1994) described three phases of family movement from diagnosis with terminal disease to loss. Stage I involves impact or movement from despair to hope, role disruption, search for meaning, informing others and managing others' emotional reactions, and remaining emotionally engaged. During this time, families are incorporating the life-threatening illness into their lives. Families begin to experience the additional physical and emotional fatigue encountered as a result of adding multiple caregiving roles to their lives. During stage II (the living-dying interval), families experience reorganization, framing memories including EOL conversations, last travels, and separation. This stage is often foreshortened because of the patient/family/physician communication difficulties described. A primary difficulty experienced by family members during this stage is the desire to set boundaries on visitors to protect quality time with the dying member while also experiencing increasing needs for assistance. Stewart presented very harrowing and moving tales of what many families experience at the EOL prior to the death of their loved one. The final stage, bereavement, involves individuals' approaches to mourning, alignment of the social network while living in a "shadow of grief that never leaves them" (p. 349).

Another excellent review of the process of family decision making at the EOL includes critical incident descriptions of 13 of the 18 nurses participating in the SUPPORT study (Hiltunen et al., 1999). They reported that families were required to make the majority of decisions because of the severity of the patients' illnesses and limited capacity. These families faced significant *decisional conflict* or "simultaneous opposing tendencies within the individual to accept and reject a given course of action" (Janis & Mann, 1977, p. 46). Symptoms of such decisional conflict include hesitation, wavering back and forth, feelings of uncertainty, and acute emotional distress when the decision becomes the focus of attention. The process involves four phases: (a) recognition of a dilemma and consequent burden, (b) a period of vacillation, (c) moving to a turning point, and (d) letting go.

The following nurse's narrative represents each of the phases in this process. The patient in this story was intubated, ventilated, sedated, and unable to communicate. Her husband made short visits as a result of his own poor health.

> The physicians felt that the patient would surely not recover ... withdrawal of the ventilator was also discussed. During this discussion the family members listened intently, all except the husband. He was very teary, and kept turning from one person to the next asking, "What do you think? What should I do?" The team retreated and allowed the husband time to think and process. I spent a great amount of time allowing him to grieve and talk. He expressed that he knew his wife would not want the type of treatment she was receiving, but it was very difficult for him to be the one to make the decision to stop. This process went on for several hours on and off. After this time had passed, the husband summoned me and said, "I'm ready, it'll be okay now. We should stop the machine," he said. I helped him walk to his wife's bedside, and lowered the side rail. She was unresponsive and still on the ventilator. ... The husband gently leaned forward and kissed his wife on the cheek. There were tears streaming down his face. He somehow found the strength to stop his tears, and then said to his wife, "I love you." ... She was extubated that evening, and passed away shortly after. Clearly more than a patient's autonomy was involved in this case. (Hiltunen et al, 1999, p. 128)

Family members may waver between ongoing aggressive treatment and palliative measures because of known patient fears of dying and desires to prevent further suffering. They may have limited information about patients' wishes, including the quality of life for which the decision to pursue curative treatment would be unwarranted. Family vacillation may be more pronounced if they are presented with discrepant perceptions of the patients' condition and chances for survival. Forbes, Bern-Klug, and Gessert (2000) reported that many family members were unaware of the dying trajectory expected for dementia patients, which seriously impeded effective decision making. Family vacillation may also be more prominent if members have not been present to observe the patients' decline or degree of injury and if they are anticipating future family events (e.g., births, marriages) near a time close to the patients' demise.

Moving to a turning point requires a great deal of emotional energy and strength of family members. It requires time to talk to other family members and friends who might have discrepant views or wish to visit with the patient prior to final decisions. This period of turning also involves framing the dying individual's life and experiences. Family members may find it helpful to communicate with others about the trajectory of the dying persons' life and personal habits, personality, and values and meaning of their life. Crow's description in chapter 4 of this book demonstrates such framing:

> As I attempted to reconcile this information and my own observations of his declining condition, I journeyed through a lifetime of memories. Josh and I grew up in the same household and had never strayed very far from each other. … It was the most alone I had ever felt for the one person I needed to talk to could not hear me. (pp. 38–39)

Family members may find it helpful during this phase if medical personnel are able to make a recommendation based on their opinion or expertise as this can help lift the total burden of decision making from family members and alleviate some of the postbereavement feelings of guilt for "giving up" or letting go.

Letting go involves giving permission to medical personnel and to the dying individual to stop prolonging the dying experience. As Saunders (in Saunders & Baines, 1989), the founder of the modern hospice movement stated, "Those who visit the bereaved will be only too aware how the last hours become imprinted on the memory" (p. 41). Memories of the last days of a patient's life follow families into bereavement, sometimes complicating their grief and leaving them with feelings of regret. Crow's story (chapter 4, this volume) exemplifies the intense pain and doubt associated with letting go. She states:

> Our concern had shifted from prolonging Josh's life to alleviating his suffering, from how to handle our own loss to honoring what we believed would be his wishes. The pain of our decision to withdraw care was devastating, not only because we would miss our family member, but also from an ethical perspective. Josh's life was in our hands, and we were choosing to end it. What if we were wrong? … I had to accept that allowing him to die did not mean that I loved him less or that I killed him. (pp. 40, 44)

Families experience both the anticipation of grief in which they try to imagine living in a world without the valued family member and "executioner's guilt," in which they may feel responsible for deciding for that family member's fate in the absence of guidance from the deceased. Many families feel abandoned in letting go—left with the total burden of decision making rather than a shared process with physicians, nurses, and others.

Although most individuals will come to terms with bereavement over time without professional intervention (Schut & Stroebe, 2005), most individuals experience distressing emotional and physical symptoms during the grieving process. Some of the more common changes during bereavement include depression, sleep disorders, and cognitive changes, especially concentration difficulties (Galloway, 1990; Stroebe, Hansson, Stroebe, & Schut, 2002). A recent study (Maciejewski, Zhang, Block, & Prigerson, 2007) evaluating Kübler-Ross's stage theory of grief among 233 bereaved individuals found that yearning was the predominant distressing emotional response during the first 2 years postbereavement. Although less frequent, the bereaved reported the highest levels of each emotional response in the sequence proposed by Kübler-Ross's theory (i.e., disbelief, yearning, anger, depression, and acceptance), with depression peaking at approximately 6 months postloss. However, other important emotional responses such as confusion and anxiety were not assessed in this study (Rando, 2000).

Some (5% to 22%) experience a more difficult adjustment to bereavement and may require professional intervention. Two systems have been proposed for defining "complicated grief." Criteria proposed by Prigerson et al. (1999) include persistent separation distress (e.g., preoccupation with thoughts of the deceased, longing and searching for the deceased, loneliness) and traumatic distress (e.g., feeling disbelief about the death, mistrust, anger, feeling shocked by the death, and the experience of somatic symptoms that the deceased experienced). The distress must be sufficient to cause clinically significant functional impairment. Horowitz and colleagues (1997) described three sets of symptoms associated with complicated grief including: (a) intrusion (e.g., unbidden memories, emotional spells, strong yearning); (b) avoidance (e.g., avoiding places that are reminders of the deceased, emotional numbness toward others); and (c) failure to adapt symptoms (e.g., feeling lonely or empty, having trouble sleeping).

Complicated grief predicts greater health problems, such as cancer, cardiac events, increased alcohol consumption, and suicidal ideation, among survivors. Complicated grief symptoms are also less responsive to standard treatments for depression (Lichtenthal, Cruess, & Prigerson, 2004). Eight factors may predispose families to complicated mourning: (a) sudden, unanticipated deaths (especially if traumatic, violent, or random); (b) death from a lengthy illness; (c) death of a child; (d) deaths associated with perceived preventability; (e) relationships with the deceased that were characterized as markedly angry, ambivalent, or dependent; (f) prior or concurrent unaccommodated losses; (g) prior or concurrent mental health problems; or (h) the mourner's perception of lack of support (Rando, 2000).

□ Improving Family End-of-Life Communication

Communication remains one of the most frequently cited areas in need of improvement at the EOL (Hanson, Danis, & Garrett, 1997; Institute of Medicine, 1997; Lynn, 1997; Mangan, Taylor, Yabroff, Fleming, & Ingham, 2003; Russ & Kaufman, 2005; see Csikai, chapter 11, this volume). Such difficulties are not surprising given the often highly charged situation during EOL decision making. Families are reentering the healthcare system often when they are most distressed and depleted and at a time when healthcare professionals are challenged in caring for a patient for whom current knowledge and skills have not brought cure or recovery. Being informed about EOL prospects gives back a sense of control, reduces anxiety, improves compliance, and creates realistic expectations for families (Jacobson, 1997). Earlier discussion allows families to make more informed choices, to achieve better symptom palliation, and to work toward life closure (Quill, 2000). Depending on their cultural beliefs, some families may want to have the opportunity to prepare for impending death; to be present at death; to give their loved ones permission to die; and to have consistent, thorough, and honest communications with healthcare providers (Berns & Colvin, 1998; Steinhauser et al., 2001).

Family members' communication needs parallel their views about what constitutes quality EOL care. Family members need information on adequate pain and symptom management and where to seek assistance in the face of uncontrollable symptoms. Patients and family members can both benefit from family education on symptom management (Keefe et al., 2005; McMillan, 2005; Northouse, Kershaw, Mood, & Schafenacker, 2005; Warner, 1992).

Many patients, family, and staff members are not aware of the distinction between palliative and hospice care and believe erroneously that palliative and hospice care mean "giving up" hope and inviting death. Patients, family, and staff members need to understand that palliative care means symptom management and is available throughout the disease process.

Family members also have a limited understanding of hospice services. In one study of families referred to hospice, only 31% of family members could describe the goals of care at their initial hospice visit. Only 11% were aware of the focus on comfort care and symptom management as a goal, and only 15% were aware of the availability of multidisciplinary staff (Casarett, Crowley, & Hirschman, 2004). Far fewer are likely aware of more recent evidence that suggests that among certain terminally ill patient groups, those referred to hospice survive an average of 29 days longer than those not receiving hospice care (Connor, Pyenson, Fitch, Spence, & Iwasaki, 2007).

Family members most often desire basic information about hospice services, including information on visit frequency (60%), payment for hospice (59%), and practical assistance provided at home (52%) (Casarett, Crowley, Stevenson, Xie, & Teno, 2005). The timing of hospice discussions is very important. One study (Cherlin et al., 2005) found that 41% of providers discussed hospice just 1 month before the patient's death, many less than 2 weeks before. This leaves limited time for families to complete personal, relational, and financial business. Sixty-eight percent of families did not understand that the patients' disease was incurable until the physician told him or her. Only 24% already suspected, so reliance on family members to raise questions about hospice is unlikely to meet the needs of most families.

In addition to information on symptom management and hospice services, family members also want assurances that the patient will not be abandoned by the primary care team. Families would prefer open discussions with the patients' primary attending physician. Family members do not want discussion with physicians with limited previous contact with the patient and the presence of unknown medical personnel, and they hope to avoid collusion between the physician and patient to discuss only positive aspects of patient's condition or treatment (Pentz, Lenzi, Holmes, Khan, & Verschraegen, 2002). Although family members may feel overwhelmed with decision making, they are rarely overwhelmed by medical information. Most families prefer as much information as possible about the patient's condition, potential care options, and what to expect in the future (Fallowfield, Ford, & Lewis, 1995; Jacobson, 1997). However, there are cultural exceptions. For example, some Asian cultures may perceive it as inhumane to discuss a terminal diagnosis with the patient and prefer that all communication takes place between the healthcare team and select family members (Searight & Gafford, 2005).

Although in 2000 the American Medical Association (AMA) recommended involvement of the patient and family member or proxy "early and often" in advance care planning, a rather large number of studies on family-healthcare provider advance care communication occur in the context of the ICU. This is unfortunately where many family EOL discussions begin. Curtis and colleagues have published widely on the content and style of communication with family members during ICU family conferences. One of the most notable findings of this group (McDonagh et al., 2004) is the association they have found between family satisfaction with physician communication and increased proportion of family member speech during family ICU conferences. The average time allotted for these conferences was 32 minutes, during which family members spoke 29% of the time, and clinicians spoke 71% of the time.

Focus groups with palliative care patients, caregivers, and professionals indicated the need for earlier discussions of potential treatment decisions, possible future symptoms or problems, preferences for the place of death, the process of dying, what needs to be done after the death, and existential issues. Dying patients recommend discussion of fears of dying and dispelling myths, description of likely final days and the likely unconscious period, and the reduced need for food and fluids (Clayton, Butow, Arnold, & Tattersall, 2005). The primary focus of discussions about the use of life-sustaining technologies should be on the realistic and achievable goals of care (Singer, Martin, & Kelner, 1999). For example, family members may agonize over DNR decisions without having information that very few patients with multiple, severe, chronic illness who receive CPR survive to discharge (Quill, 2000). Families also need to understand that their role is not to "pull the plug" but to answer the question, "What would my loved one decide?" (Teno et al., 1998).

Curtis and colleagues (2005) have explored missed opportunities for communication with families during family conferences, such as opportunities to listen and respond to the family, acknowledge and address family emotions, and provide affirmations of nonabandonment. They have suggested several strategies for supporting families, including showing caring in the words used, acknowledging the physical and emotional care provided by the family, the emotional difficulty of the situation, and reassurance of patient comfort. Such conferences provide an opportunity to learn more about the values and hobbies of the patient and to humanize the care provided in an otherwise potentially dehumanizing environment. Other simple but powerful actions include ensuring privacy of discussions and starting with introductions of all staff and family members. It is important to acknowledge that withholding or withdrawing treatment is not withdrawing care. Providers can also anticipate and accept periods of silence, acknowledge strong emotions, and try to ease family guilt or burden by making recommendations based on medical EOL expertise.

It is also important to offer a waiting period to give the family time to adjust to the news, a private space for continued discussions, a follow-up meeting, and easy accessibility to staff for discussion (Ruark & Raffin, 1988). Introduction to professional staff trained to provide emotional or spiritual support, such as chaplains, psychologists, or social workers, is also helpful, particularly if followed up by a caring phone call to assess family questions, conflicts, or concerns. Duggleby and Wright (2004) outlined several hope-fostering communication strategies for families faced with quantity- and quality-of-life decisions.

Care for the family should not end with the withdrawal of life support or the EOL-prolonging treatments. Bereaved family members highly value a physician condolence telephone call, letter, or visit as well as attendance at the patient's funeral (Bedell, Cadenhead, & Graboys, 2001; Main, 2000). Family members may also benefit from education to anticipate the resurgence of grief during holidays, birthdays, and anniversaries of the patient's death. For most bereaved family members, depression and other negative affect may not peak for 4–6 months (Maciejewski et al., 2007) or, for some, even years later. It is helpful for families to know that there is no acceptable time limit to grieving—that for most it is a lifelong process and to have someone to contact if needed well beyond the patient's death. One bereaved spouse, in writing about his hospice experience, stated:

> When my wife died, it was in hospice. They were so sympathetic, probably for two or three months after my wife passed away they would be calling me wanting to know if I was okay and if my children were okay. Would I like to come in to talk to somebody? (Teno et al., 2001, p. 744)

In the months of loneliness following the death of a loved one, such contact can be very meaningful and supportive.

☐ Family-Based End-of-Life Policy

Healthcare decisions occur primarily in the context of the family. Families assume multiple roles in providing care for patients at the EOL, often resulting in financial, psychosocial, and additional health burdens. Any system of advance care planning that does not include family members from the outset is likely to be poorly received by patients and family members and unlikely to meet the needs of the family as a decision-making unit. The current "top-down" model of advance care planning with its emphasis on patient autonomy does not meet the needs of families. Advance care planning founded on a "bottom-up" or family-based model would base legal, ethical, and policy decisions on the values, needs, and goals of patients and family members. Lyon's model (Richard & Lyon, chapter 2, this volume) is an example of one such approach. Such decisions must be firmly rooted in empirical data from the healthcare consumer/family perspective. EOL policies should reflect the fact that all healthcare decisions ultimately affect all members of a family system—from the time required to provide care at home, the crucial impact on employment, and the financial and emotional devastation experienced by many families at the EOL. Family-based advance care planning would define the unit of planning as between the patient and his or her family, with communication of values, preferences, and goals to healthcare providers at regular intervals.

Future EOL research must shift from healthcare system needs to more adequately address patient and family needs at the EOL. Future research must demonstrate a greater awareness of healthcare system biases in the approach to EOL studies. For example, is dying at home a family-based or healthcare system-based value? Dying at home may not always be the best option or preference for families (Phipps & Braitman, 2004). Sixty percent of patients will die in the hospital—many times based on the preference of families. Hospitals must no longer be judged based on the rate of mortality but the quality of mortality.

Research and institutional policy needs to reflect the phases through which families transition at the EOL—from recognition of terminal illness, to letting go, to bereavement. Recommendations for communication at the EOL must be based on empirical data regarding what is most and least helpful to families during the movement from treatments focused on cure to palliation. Grief-focused interventions must also be supported by empirical observations regarding what is effective and for whom. Healthcare systems should be concerned about EOL and postbereavement care from an ethical and financial perspective as bereaved family members are the future and often imminent consumers of institutional health care. Families' consequent avoidance of health care because of complicated bereavement or a poor experience with patient EOL care in a medical setting means greater late-stage diagnosis for family members in the future and ultimately higher incidence of health problems in the population.

The future of health care will be family based from diagnosis to the EOL. The assumption of patient desires for autonomy at the EOL complicates the dying process. It is contrary to the preferences of the majority of Americans, especially among the increasing population of Latinos and African Americans in the United States, but also among non-Latino Caucasians. Family-based advance care planning would likely increase the rate of advance directive completion and increase family understanding of the benefits and risks of life-sustaining treatments before a crisis occurs and emotion overwhelms reason in decision making. And, most important, family-based advance care planning could decrease family anxiety and burden that occur in the absence of prior EOL family conversations and planning.

Note

1. For the purposes of this chapter, *family* is defined as "enduring relationships in which people's interests are complexly entwined and in which people care deeply about each other" (Nelson, 1992) or families of choice (Stewart, 1994), regardless of whether they are blood relatives.

References

Allen-Burge, R., & Haley, W. E. (1997). Individual differences and surrogate medical decisions: Differing preferences for life-sustaining treatments. *Aging and Mental Health, 1,* 121–131.

American Medical Association. (2000). *End of life care ethics: What is advance care planning?* Retrieved June 30, 2008 from http://virtualmentor.ama-assn.org/2000/11/elce1-0011.html

American Psychiatric Association. (2000). *Diagnostic and statistical manual of mental disorders* (4th ed., text revision). Washington, DC: Author.

Aneshensel, C. S., Pearlin, L. I., & Schuler, R. H. (1993). Stress, role captivity, and the cessation of caregiving. *Journal of Health and Social Behavior, 34,* 54–70.

Arno, P. S., Levine, C., & Memmott, M. M. (1999). The economic value of informal caregiving. *Health Affairs, 18,* 182–188.

Baile, W. F., Lenzi, R., Parker, P. A., Buckman, R., & Cohen, L. (2002). Oncologists' attitudes toward and practices in giving bad news: An exploratory study. *Journal of Clinical Oncology, 20,* 2189–2196.

Bedell, S. E., Cadenhead, K., & Graboys, T. B. (2001). The doctor's letter of condolence. *The New England Journal of Medicine, 344,* 1162–1164.

Berns, R., & Colvin, E. R. (1998). The final story: Events at the bedside of dying patients as told by survivors. *American Nephrology Nurses' Association Journal, 25,* 583–587.

Blackhall, L. J., Murphy, S. T., Frank, G., Michel, V., & Azen, S. (1995). Ethnicity and attitudes toward patient autonomy. *Journal of the American Medical Association, 274,* 820–825.

Breslin, J. M. (2005). Autonomy and the role of the family in making decisions at the EOL. *Journal of Clinical Ethics, 16,* 11–19.

Brett, A. S. (1991). Limitations of listing specific medical interventions in advance directives. *Journal of the American Medical Association, 266,* 825–828.

Brundage, M. D., Feldman-Stewart, D., Cosby, R., Gregg, R., Dixon, P., Youssef, Y., et al. (2001). Phase I study of a decision aid for patients with locally advanced non-small-cell lung cancer. *Journal of Clinical Oncology, 19,* 1326–1335.

Buhr, G. T., Kuchibhatla, M., & Clipp, E. C. (2006). Caregivers' reasons for nursing home placement: Clues for improving discussions with families prior to the transition. *Gerontologist, 46,* 52–61.

Butow, P. N., Maclean, M., Dunn, S. M., Tattersall, M. H., & Boyer, M. J. (1997). The dynamics of change: Cancer patients' preferences for information, involvement and support. *Annals of Oncology, 8,* 857–863.

Byock, I. (1997). *Dying well: Peace and possibilities at the end of life.* New York: Riverhead.

Caralis, P. V., Davis, B., Wright, K., & Marcial, E. (1993). The influence of ethnicity and race on attitudes toward advance directives, life-prolonging treatments, and euthanasia. *Journal of Clinical Ethics, 4,* 155–165.

Casarett, D., Crowley, R., Stevenson, C., Xie, S., & Teno, J. (2005). Making difficult decisions about hospice enrollment: What do patients and families want to know? *Journal of the American Geriatrics Society, 53,* 249–254.

Casarett, D. J., Crowley, R. L., & Hirschman, K. B. (2004). How should clinicians describe hospice to patients and families? *Journal of the American Geriatrics Society, 52,* 1923–1928.

Cherlin, E., Fried, T., Prigerson, H. G., Schulman-Green, D., Johnson-Hurzeler, R., & Bradley, E. H. (2005). Communication between physicians and family caregivers about care at the end of life: When do discussions occur and what is said? *Journal of Palliative Medicine, 8,* 1176–1185.

Christakis, N. A., & Iwashyna, T. J. (1998). Attitude and self-reported practice regarding prognostication in a national sample of internists. *Archives of Internal Medicine, 158,* 2389–2395.

Christakis, N. A., & Iwashyna, T. J. (2003). The health impact of health care on families: A matched cohort study of hospice use by decedents and mortality outcomes in surviving, widowed spouses. *Social Science and Medicine, 57,* 465–475.

Christakis, N. A., & Lamont, E. B. (2000). Extent and determinants of error in doctors' prognoses in terminally ill patients: Prospective cohort study. *British Medical Journal, 320,* 469–472.

Clayton, J. M., Butow, P. N., Arnold, R. M., & Tattersall, M. H. N. (2005). Discussing end of life issues with terminally ill cancer patients and their carers: A qualitative study. *Supportive Care in Cancer, 13,* 589–599.

Cohen, S., Sprung, C., Sjokvist, P., Lippert, A., Ricou, B., Baras, M., et al. (2005). Communication of end-of-life decisions in European intensive care units. *Intensive Care Medicine, 31,* 1215–1221.

Connor, S. R., Pyenson, B., Fitch, K., Spence, C., & Iwasaki, K. (2007). Comparing hospice and nonhospice patient survival among patients who die within a three-year window. *Journal of Pain and Symptom Management, 33,* 238–246.

Covinsky, K. E., Eng, C., Lui, L. Y., Sands, L. P., Sehgal, A. R., Walter, L. C., et al. (2001). Reduced employment in caregivers of frail elders: Impact of ethnicity, patient clinical characteristics, and caregiver characteristics. *Journals of Gerontology, 56,* M707–M713.

Covinsky, K. E., Goldman, L., Cook, E. F., Oye, R., Desbiens, N., Reding, D., et al. (1994). The impact of serious illness on patients' families. *Journal of the American Medical Association, 272,* 1839–1844.

Covinsky, K. E., Landefeld, C. S., Teno, J., Connors, A. F., Jr., Dawson, N., Youngner, S., et al. (1996). Is economic hardship on the families of the seriously ill associated with patient and surrogate care preferences? SUPPORT investigators. *Archives of Internal Medicine, 156,* 1737–1741.

Curtis, J. R., Engelberg, R. A., Wenrich, M. D., Shannon, S. E., Treece, P. D., & Rubenfeld, G. D. (2005). Missed opportunities during family conferences about end-of-life care in the intensive care unit. *American Journal of Respiratory and Critical Care Medicine, 171,* 844–849.

Daly, B. J. (2000). Special challenges of withholding artificial nutrition and hydration. *Journal of Gerontological Nursing, 26*(9), 25–31.

Denberg, T. D., Beaty, B. L., Kim, F. J., & Steiner, J. F. (2005). Marriage and ethnicity predict treatment in localized prostate carcinoma. *Cancer, 103,* 1819–1825.

Diamond, E. L., Jernigan, J. A., Moseley, R. A., Messina, V., & McKeown, R. A. (1989). Decision-making ability and advance directive preferences in nursing home patients and proxies. *Gerontologist, 29,* 622–626.

Ditto, P. H., Danks, J. H., Smucker, W. D., Bookwala, J., Coppola, K. M., Dresser, R., et al. (2001). Advance directives as acts of communication: A randomized controlled trial. *Archives of Internal Medicine, 161,* 421–430.

Ditto, P. H., & Hawkins, N. A. (2005). Advance directives and cancer decision-making near the end of life. *Health Psychology, 24*(4 Suppl.), S63–S70.

Donelan, K., Hill, C. A., Hoffman, C., Scoles, K., Feldman, P. H., Levine, C., et al. (2002). Challenged to care: Informal caregivers in a changing health system. *Health Affairs, 21,* 222–231.

Duggleby, W., & Wright, K. (2004). Elderly palliative care cancer patients' descriptions of hope-fostering strategies. *International Journal of Palliative Nursing, 10,* 352–359.

Eiser, A. R., & Weiss, M. D. (2001). The underachieving advance directive: Recommendations for increasing advance directive completion. *American Journal of Bioethics, 1*(4), W10.

Eleazer, G. P., Hornung, C. A., Egbert, C. B., Egbert, J. R., Eng, C., Hedgepeth, J., et al. (1996). The relationship between ethnicity and advance directives in a frail older population. *Journal of the American Geriatrics Society, 44,* 938–943.

Emanuel, E. J., & Emanuel, L. L. (1992). Proxy decision-making for incompetent patients. An ethical and empirical analysis. *Journal of the American Medical Association, 267,* 2067–2071.

Emanuel, E. J., & Emanuel, L. L. (1998). The promise of a good death. *Lancet, 351,* 21–29.

Emanuel, E. J., Fairclough, D. L., Slutsman, J., Alpert, H., Baldwin, D., & Emanuel, L. L. (1999). Assistance from family members, friends, paid care givers, and volunteers in the care of terminally ill patients. *New England Journal of Medicine, 341,* 956–963.

Emanuel, E. J., Fairclough, D. L., Slutsman, J., & Emanuel, L. L. (2000). Understanding economic and other burdens of terminal illness: The experience of patients and their caregivers. *Annals of Internal Medicine, 132,* 451–459.

Fagerlin, A., Ditto, P. H., Danks, J. H., Houts, R. M., & Smucker, W. D. (2001). Projection in surrogate decisions about life-sustaining medical treatments. *Health Psychology, 20,* 166–175.

Fallowfield, L., Ford, S., & Lewis, S. (1995). No news is not good news: Information preferences of patients with cancer. *Psycho-oncology, 4,* 197–202.

Family Medical Leave Act of 1993, Pub. L. No. 103-3, U.S. Department of Labor.

Forbes, S., Bern-Klug, M., & Gessert, C. (2000). End-of-life decision-making for nursing home residents with dementia. *Journal of Nursing Scholarship, 32,* 251–258.

Foster, L. W., & McLellan, L. J. (2002). Translating psychosocial insight into ethical discussions supportive of families in end-of-life decision-making. *Social Work in Health Care, 35*(3), 37–51.

Friedman, S. M., Steinwachs, D. M., Rathouz, P. J., Burton, L. C., & Mukamel, D. B. (2005). Characteristics predicting nursing home admission in the program of all-inclusive care for elderly people. *The Gerontologist, 45,* 157–166.

Galloway, S. C. (1990). Young adults' reactions to the death of a parent. *Oncology Nursing Forum, 17,* 899–904.

Gaugler, J. E., Edwards, A. B., Femia, E. E., Zarit, S. H., Stephens, M. A., Townsend, A., et al. (2000). Predictors of institutionalization of cognitively impaired elders: Family help and the timing of placement. *Journals of Gerontology, 55,* P247–P255.

Gaugler, J. E., Kane, R. L., Kane, R. A., Clay, T., & Newcomer, R. (2003). Caregiving and institutionalization of cognitively impaired older people: Utilizing dynamic predictors of change. *The Gerontologist, 43,* 219–229.

Gaugler, J. E., Kane, R. L., Kane, R. A., Clay, T., & Newcomer, R. C. (2005). The effects of duration of caregiving on institutionalization. *The Gerontologist, 45,* 78–89.

Gordon, E. J., & Daugherty, C. K. (2003). "Hitting you over the head": Oncologists' disclosure of prognosis to advanced cancer patients. *Bioethics, 17,* 142–168.

Haley, W. E., Han, B., & Henderson, J. N. (1998). Aging and ethnicity: Issues for clinical practice. *Journal of Clinical Psychology in Medical Settings, 5,* 393–409.

Haley, W. E., West, C. A. C., Wadley, V. G., Ford, G. R., White, F. A., Barrett, J. J., et al. (1995). Psychological, social, and health impact of caregiving: A comparison of black and white dementia family caregivers and noncaregivers. *Psychology and Aging, 10,* 540–552.

Hamel, C. F., Guse, L. W., Hawranik, P. G., & Bond, J. B., Jr. (2002). Advance directives and community-dwelling older adults. *Western Journal of Nursing Research, 24,* 143–158.

Hanson, L. C., Danis, M., & Garrett, J. (1997). What is wrong with end-of-life care? Opinions of bereaved family members. *Journal of the American Geriatrics Society, 45,* 1339–1344.

Hare, J., Pratt, C., & Nelson, C. (1992). Agreement between patients and their self-selected surrogates on difficult medical decisions. *Archives of Internal Medicine, 152,* 1049–1054.

Hawkins, N. A., Ditto, P. H., Danks, J. H., & Smucker, W. D. (2005). Micromanaging death: Process preferences, values, and goals in end-of-life medical decision-making. *The Gerontologist, 45,* 107–117.

Hayman, J. A., Langa, K. M., Kabeto, M. U., Katz, S. J., DeMonner, S. M., Chernew, M. E., et al. (2001). Estimating the cost of informal caregiving for elderly patients with cancer. *Journal of Clinical Oncology, 19,* 3219–3225.

Hiltunen, E. F., Medich, C., Chase, S., Peterson, L., & Forrow, L. (1999). Family decision-making for end-of-life treatment: The SUPPORT nurse narratives. *Journal of Clinical Ethics, 10,* 126–134.

Hines, S. C., Glover, J. J., Babrow, A. S., Holley, J. L., Badzek, L. A., & Moss, A. H. (2001). Improving advance care planning by accommodating family preferences. *Journal of Palliative Medicine, 4,* 481–489.

Hines, S. C., Glover, J. J., Holley, J. L., Babrow, A. S., Badzek, L. A., & Moss, A. H. (1999). Dialysis patients' preferences for family-based advance care planning. *Annals of Internal Medicine, 130,* 825–828.

Holland, J. C. & Lewis, S. (2000). *The human side of cancer: Living with hope, coping with uncertainty.* New York: HarperCollins.

Holley, J. L., Stackiewicz, L., Dacko, C., & Rault, R. (1997). Factors influencing dialysis patients' completion of advance directives. *American Journal of Kidney Diseases, 30,* 356–360.

Horowitz, M. J., Siegel, B., Holen, A., Bonanno, G. A., Milbrath, C., & Stinson, C. H. (1997). Diagnostic criteria for complicated grief disorder. *American Journal of Psychiatry, 154,* 904–910.

Institute of Medicine. (1997). *Approaching death: Improving care at the end of life.* Washington, DC: National Academy Press.

Jacobson, J. A. (1997). Preaching to the choir: New voices in the end of life discussion. *Journal of Clinical Oncology, 15,* 413–415.

Janis, I. L., & Mann, L. (1977). *Decision-making: A psychological analysis of conflict, choice, and commitment.* New York: Free Press.

Karlawish, J. H., Casarett, D., Klocinski, J., & Clark, C. M. (2001). The relationship between caregivers' global ratings of Alzheimer's disease patients' quality of life, disease severity, and the caregiving experience. *Journal of the American Geriatrics Society, 49,* 1066–1070.

Keefe, F. J., Ahles, T. A., Sutton, L., Dalton, J., Baucom, D., Pope, M. S., et al. (2005). Partner-guided cancer pain management at the end of life: A preliminary study. *Journal of Pain and Symptom Management, 29,* 263–272.

Keysar, B., & Barr, D. J. (2002). Self-anchoring in conversation: Why language users do not do what they "should." In T. Gilovich, D. Griffin, & D. Kahneman (Eds.), *Heuristics and biases: The psychology of intuitive judgment* (pp. 150–166). New York: Cambridge University Press.

Kilpatrick, M. G., Kristjanson, L. J., Tataryn, D. J., & Fraser, V. H. (1998). Information needs of husbands of women with breast cancer. *Oncology Nursing Forum, 25,* 1595–1601.

Lang, F., & Quill, T. (2004). Making decisions with families at the end of life. *American Family Physician, 70,* 719–723.

Lichtenthal, W. G., Cruess, D. G., & Prigerson, H. G. (2004). A case for establishing complicated grief as a distinct mental disorder in *DSM-V. Clinical Psychology Review, 24,* 637–662.

Lynn, J. (1997). Measuring quality of care at the end of life: A statement of principles. *Journal of the American Geriatrics Society, 45,* 526–527.

Lynn, J., Teno, J. M., Phillips, R. S., Wu, A. W., Desbiens, N., Harrold, J., et al. (1997). Perceptions by family members of the dying experience of older and seriously ill patients. *Annals of Internal Medicine, 126,* 97–106.

Maciejewski, P. K., Zhang, B., Block, S. D., & Prigerson, H. G. (2007). An empirical examination of the stage theory of grief. *Journal of the American Medical Association, 297,* 716–723.

Main, J. (2000). Improving management of bereavement in general practice based on a survey of recently bereaved subjects in a single general practice. *British Journal of General Practice, 50,* 863–866.

Mangan, P. A., Taylor, K. L., Yabroff, K. R., Fleming, D. A., & Ingham, J. M. (2003). Caregiving near the end of life: Unmet needs and potential solutions. *Palliative & Supportive Care, 1,* 247–259.

Marks, G., & Miller, N. (1987). Ten years of research on the false-consensus effect: An empirical and theoretical overview. *Psychological Bulletin, 102,* 72–90.

McDonagh, J. R., Elliott, T. B., Engelberg, R. A., Treece, P. D., Shannon, S. E., Rubenfeld, G. D., et al. (2004). Family satisfaction with family conferences about end-of-life care in the intensive care unit: Increased proportion of family speech is associated with increased satisfaction. *Critical Care Medicine, 32,* 1484–1488.

McMillan, S. C. (2005). Interventions to facilitate family caregiving at the end of life. *Journal of Palliative Medicine, 8* (Suppl. 1), S132–S139.

Mitchell, S. L., Berkowitz, R. E., Lawson, F. M., & Lipsitz, L. A. (2000). A cross-national survey of tube-feeding decisions in cognitively impaired older persons. *Journal of the American Geriatrics Society, 48,* 391–397.

Nelson, J. L. (1992). Taking families seriously. *The Hastings Center Report, 22*(4), 6–12.

Nolan, M. T., & Bruder, M. (1997). Patients' attitudes toward advance directives and end-of-life treatment decisions. *Nursing Outlook, 45,* 204–208.

Nolan, M. T., Hughes, M., Narendra, D. P., Sood, J. R., Terry, P. B., Astrow, A. B., et al. (2005). When patients lack capacity: The roles that patients with terminal diagnoses would choose for their physicians and loved ones in making medical decisions. *Journal of Pain and Symptom Management, 30,* 342–353.

Northouse, L., Kershaw, T., Mood, D., & Schafenacker, A. (2005). Effects of a family intervention on the quality of life of women with recurrent breast cancer and their family caregivers. *Psycho-oncology, 14,* 478–491.

Ott, B. B. (1999). Advance directives: The emerging body of research. *American Journal of Critical Care, 8,* 514–519.

Pentz, R. D., Lenzi, R., Holmes, F., Khan, M. M., & Verschraegen, C. (2002). Discussion of the do-not-resuscitate order: A pilot study of perceptions of patients with refractory cancer. *Supportive Care in Cancer, 10,* 573–578.

Phipps, E. J., & Braitman, L. E. (2004). Family caregiver satisfaction with care at end of life: Report from the Cultural Variations Study (CVAS). *American Journal of Hospice and Palliative Care, 21,* 340–342.

Pohl, J. M., Given, C. W., Collins, C. E., & Given, B. A. (1994). Social vulnerability and reactions to caregiving in daughters and daughters-in-law caring for disabled aging parents. *Health Care for Women International, 15,* 385–395.

Prigerson, H. G., Shear, M. K., Jacobs, S. C., Reynolds, C. F., 3rd, Maciejewski, P. K., Davidson, J. R., et al. (1999). Consensus criteria for traumatic grief. A preliminary empirical test. *British Journal of Psychiatry, 174,* 67–73.

Quill, T. E. (2000). Initiating end-of-life discussions with seriously ill patients: Addressing the "elephant in the room." *Journal of the American Medical Association, 284,* 2502–2507.

Rabow, M. W., Hauser, J. M., & Adams, J. (2004). Supporting family caregivers at the end of life: "They don't know what they don't know." *Journal of the American Medical Association, 291,* 483–491.

Ramirez, A., Addington-Hall, J., & Richards, M. (1998). ABC of palliative care. The carers. *British Medical Journal, 316,* 208–211.

Rando, T. A. (2000). *Clinical dimensions of anticipatory mourning: Theory and practice in working with the dying, their loved ones, and their caregivers.* Champaign, IL: Research Press.

Ransom, S., Sacco, W. P., Weitzner, M. A., Azzarello, L. M., & McMillan, S. C. (2006). Interpersonal factors predict increased desire for hastened death in late-stage cancer patients. *Annals of Behavioral Medicine, 31,* 63–69.

Rosenfeld, K. E., Wenger, N. S., & Kagawa-Singer, M. (2000). End-of-life decision-making: A qualitative study of elderly individuals. *Journal of General Internal Medicine, 15,* 620–625.

Ruark, J. E., & Raffin, T. A. (1988). Initiating and withdrawing life support. Principles and practice in adult medicine. *New England Journal of Medicine, 318,* 25–30.

Russ, A. J., & Kaufman, S. R. (2005). Family perceptions of prognosis, silence, and the "suddenness" of death. *Culture, Medicine and Psychiatry, 29,* 103–123.

Saunders, C., & Baines, M. (1989). *Living with dying: The management of terminal disease.* Oxford, England: Oxford University Press.

Scales, D. C., Tansey, C. M., Matte, A., & Herridge, M. S. (2006). Difference in reported pre-morbid health-related quality of life between ARDS survivors and their substitute decision makers. *Intensive Care Medicine, 32,* 1826–1831.

Schulz, R., & Beach, S. R. (1999). Caregiving as a risk factor for mortality: The caregiver health effects study. *Journal of the American Medical Association, 282,* 2215–2219.

Schut, H., & Stroebe, M. S. (2005). Interventions to enhance adaptation to bereavement. *Journal of Palliative Medicine, 8* (Suppl. 1), S140–S147.

Searight, H. R., & Gafford, J. (2005). Cultural diversity at the end of life: Issues and guidelines for family physicians. *American Family Physician, 71,* 515–522.

Seckler, A. B., Meier, D. E., Mulvihill, M., & Paris, B. E. (1991). Substituted judgment: How accurate are proxy predictions? *Annals of Internal Medicine, 115,* 92–98.

Sehgal, A., Galbraith, A., Chesney, M., Schoenfeld, P., Charles, G., & Lo, B. (1992). How strictly do dialysis patients want their advance directives followed? *Journal of the American Medical Association, 267,* 59–63.

Singer, P. A., Martin, D. K., & Kelner, M. (1999). Quality end-of-life care: Patients' perspectives. *Journal of the American Medical Association, 281,* 163–168.

Spillman, B. C., Liu, K., & McGilliard, C. (2002, Nov.). *Trends in residential long-term care: Use of nursing homes and assisted living and characteristics of facilities and residents.* Washington, DC: U.S. Department of Health and Human Services.

Stanton, A. L. (1987). Determinants of adherence to medical regimens by hypertensive patients. *Journal of Behavioral Medicine, 10,* 377–394.

Steinhauser, K. E., Christakis, N. A., Clipp, E. C., McNeilly, M., Grambow, S., Parker, J., et al. (2001). Preparing for the end of life: Preferences of patients, families, physicians, and other care providers. *Journal of Pain and Symptom Management, 22,* 727–737.

Steinhauser, K. E., Christakis, N. A., Clipp, E. C., McNeilly, M., McIntyre, L., & Tulsky, J. A. (2000). Factors considered important at the end of life by patients, family, physicians, and other care providers. *Journal of the American Medical Association, 284,* 2476–2482.

Stevens, A., Own, J., Roth, D., Clay, O., Bartolucci, A., & Haley, W. (2004). Predictors of time to nursing home placement in White and African American individuals with dementia. *Journal of Aging and Health, 16,* 375–397.

Stewart, B. M. (1994). End-of-life family decision-making from disclosure of HIV through bereavement. *Scholarly Inquiry for Nursing Practice, 8,* 321–352.

Stroebe, M. S., Hansson, R. O., Stroebe, W. & Schut, H. (2002). *Handbook of bereavement research: Consequences, coping, and care.* Washington, DC: American Psychological Association.

Suhl, J., Simons, P., Reedy, T., & Garrick, T. (1994). Myth of substituted judgment. Surrogate decision-making regarding life support is unreliable. *Archives of Internal Medicine, 154,* 90–96.

SUPPORT principal investigators. (1995). A controlled trial to improve care for seriously ill hospitalized patients: The study to understand prognoses and preferences for outcomes and risks of treatments. *Journal of the American Medical Association, 274,* 1591–1598.

Sutherland, H. J., Llewellyn-Thomas, H. A., Lockwood, G. A., Tritchler, D. L., & Till, J. E. (1989). Cancer patients: Their desire for information and participation in treatment decisions. *Journal of the Royal Society of Medicine, 82,* 260–263.

Teno, J. M., Casey, V. A., Welch, L. C., & Edgman-Levitan, S. (2001). Patient-focused, family-centered end-of-life medical care: Views of the guidelines and bereaved family members. *Journal of Pain and Symptom Management, 22,* 738–751.

Teno, J. M., Licks, S., Lynn, J., Wenger, N., Connors, A. F., Jr., Phillips, R. S., et al. (1997). Do advance directives provide instructions that direct care? *Journal of the American Geriatrics Society, 45,* 508–512.

Teno, J. M., Stevens, M., Spernak, S., & Lynn, J. (1998). Role of written advance directives in decision-making: Insights from qualitative and quantitative data. *Journal of General Internal Medicine, 13,* 439–446.

The, A. M., Hak, T., Koeter, G., & van der Wal, G. (2001). Collusion in doctor-patient communication about imminent death: An ethnographic study. *Western Journal of Medicine, 174,* 247–253.

Thompson, E. J., Futterman, A., Gallagher-Thompson, D., Rose, J., & Lovett, S. (1993). Social support and caregiving burden in family caregivers of frail elders. *Journals of Gerontology, 48,* S245–S254.

Tilden, V. P., Tolle, S. W., Nelson, C. A., & Fields, J. (2001). Family decision-making to withdraw life-sustaining treatments from hospitalized patients. *Nursing Research, 50,* 105–115.

Tulsky, J. A., Chesney, M. A., & Lo, B. (1995). How do medical residents discuss resuscitation with patients? *Journal of General Internal Medicine, 10,* 436–442.

Uhlmann, R. F., Pearlman, R. A., & Cain, K. C. (1988). Physicians' and spouses' predictions of elderly patients' resuscitation preferences. *Journal of Gerontology, 43,* M115–M121.

Umberson, D. (1987). Family status and health behaviors: Social control as a dimension of social integration. *Journal of Health and Social Behavior, 28,* 306–319.

Umberson, D. (1992). Gender, marital status and the social control of health behavior. *Social Science and Medicine, 34,* 907–917.

Vohra, J. U., Brazil, K., Hanna, S., & Abelson, J. (2004). Family perceptions of end-of-life care in long-term care facilities. *Journal of Palliative Care, 20,* 297–302.

Warner, J. E. (1992). Involvement of families in pain control of terminally ill patients. *Hospice Journal, 8*(1–2), 155–170.

Waters, C. M. (2001). Understanding and supporting African Americans' perspectives of end-of-life care planning and decision-making. *Qualitative Health Research, 11,* 385–398.

Weeks, J. C., Cook, E. F., O'Day, S. J., Peterson, L. M., Wenger, N., Reding, D., et al. (1998). Relationship between cancer patients' predictions of prognosis and their treatment preferences. *Journal of the American Medical Association, 279,* 1709–1714.

Whitney, S. N. (2003). A new model of medical decisions: Exploring the limits of shared decision-making. *Medical Decision-making, 23,* 275–280.

Zarit, S. H., Reever, K. E., & Bach-Peterson, J. (1980). Relatives of the impaired elderly: Correlates of feelings of burden. *The Gerontologist, 20,* 649–655.
Zhang, A. Y., & Siminoff, L. A. (2003). Silence and cancer: Why do families and patients fail to communicate? *Health Communication, 15,* 415–429.
Zuckerman, C., & Wollner, D. (1999). End of life care and decision-making: How far we have come, how far we have to go. *Hospice Journal, 14*(3–4), 85–107.
Zweibel, N. R., & Cassel, C. K. (1989). Treatment choices at the end of life: A comparison of decisions by older patients and their physician-selected proxies. *The Gerontologist, 29,* 615–621.

16
CHAPTER

Religious and Spiritual Perspectives on Life-Threatening Illness, Dying, and Death

Kenneth J. Doka

Once, a king of small independent kingdom in the Indian Subcontinent experienced the birth of a son and heir. A seer prophesized to the king that his child was destined for greatness. However, the nature of the greatness was unclear. The child might become a great monarch or a truly enlightened religious sage. The king had no desire to raise a monk so he immersed the child in every conceivable pleasure. The child grew into manhood surrounded by comfort and beauty. He married and had a son of his own.

Yet, one day as the prince rode outside the palace, he viewed an aged person, an ill person, and a corpse. Overwhelmed by the suffering he had witnessed, Prince Siddhartha abandoned his kingdom and family to search for answers to the distress he had seen. So began Buddha's quest.

Introduction

In many ways, Buddha's struggle represents the existential quest that many face as they encounter life-threatening illness and possible death.

Inevitably, these experiences raise deeply spiritual questions: What is the nature of life? Why does one need to suffer and die? Where is fairness?

One cannot understand life-threatening illness as only a medical crisis. It is a psychological, social, and family crisis as well. Yet, even more than that, it is a spiritual crisis—fraught with existential questions.

This chapter attempts to address, at least in part, those questions. The chapter begins by defining both spirituality and religion and exploring the ways that spirituality and religious faith influence the experience of life-threatening illness and death. It seeks to offer tools for assessing and utilizing the spiritual strengths of those who face illness and the prospect of death—recognizing that in this final encounter an individual needs to marshal all resources.

□ Religion, Spirituality, and Life-Threatening Illness

Religion and spirituality are often elusive concepts that are difficult to define and differentiate. The International Work Group on Death, Dying, and Bereavement defined *spirituality* as "concerned with the transcendental, inspirational, and existential way to live one's life" (1990, p. 75). Miller's (1994) definition is more poetic:

> *Spirituality* relates to our souls. It involves the deep inner essence of who we are. It is an openness to the possibility that the soul within each of us is somehow related to the Soul of all that is. Spirituality is what happens to us that is so memorable that we cannot forget it, and yet we find it hard to talk about because words fail to describe it. Spirituality is the act of looking for meaning in the very deepest sense; and looking for it in a way that is most authentically ours. (handout, p. 2)

To Miller (1994), spirituality is inherently individual, personal, and eclectic. Religion, however, is more collective. *Religion* is a belief shared within a group of people. Miller again offers a lyrical perspective:

> Now *religion* works in a very different way. While spirituality is very personal, religion is more communal. In fact, if you take the words back to its origins, religion means "that which binds together," "that which ties things into a package." Religion has to do with collecting and consolidating and unifying. Religion says, "Here are special words that are meant to be passed on. Take them to heart." Religion says, "Here is a set of beliefs that form a coherent whole. Take them

> as your own." Religion says, "Here are people for you to revere and historical events for you to recall. Remember them." Religion says, "Here is a way for you to act when you come together as a group, and here's a way to behave when you're apart." (handout, pp. 2–3)

Thus, although spirituality is very personal, a person's spirituality may very well be shaped by an individual's religious beliefs. Yet, because of the individual nature of spirituality, religious affiliation is not likely to be the sole determinant of spiritual beliefs. Often, developmental outlooks, personal experiences, and cultural perspectives will join with religious beliefs in shaping an individual's spirituality.

However, whatever these beliefs are, they are likely to be challenged by life-threatening illness. As stated, a life-threatening illness can be an existential crisis. The encounter with the possibility or even the probability of death raises a series of questions. Why do I have this diagnosis, and why now? Is life worth this suffering, treatment, and uncertainty? Is it consistent with my belief system, my spirituality to cease treatment or forgo certain types of treatment? If I recover, what did I learn, what will I take, and what will I do with this experience? If I die, did my life have meaning, how do I wish to die, and what will happen after?

A life-threatening illness then is a teachable moment—a time when one's spirituality can be extremely important. Spirituality may offer answers and reassurance, breeding resilience. Or, spirituality may seem empty, leading to an existential despair or a new quest for a deeper spiritual sense that can sustain one in this crisis.

☐ Religion and Spirituality: Complicating and Facilitating Factors

Research has indicated that religion and spirituality can both facilitate and complicate responses to life-threatening illness. In reviewing this research, it is well to link both terms as the operational definitions of spirituality and religion vary considerably among the researchers. Nonetheless, this research has indicated that spirituality and religion can have positive roles in assisting individuals who struggle with life-threatening illness.

For example, research has supported the fact that religion and spirituality can assist persons in finding a sense of meaning in the illness (Siegel & Schrimshaw, 2002). Often, the diagnosis of a life-threatening illness challenges an individual's assumptive world as the person struggles with attempting to make sense of the illness. Later in the illness, individuals may seek to make sense of their suffering, their death, or their life. Throughout this existential endeavor, religious and spiritual perspectives can offer meanings. Religious and spiritual perspectives may reassure persons with life-threatening illness that their illness is part of a larger plan or that the illness experience may offer lessons to self or others. Even with death, there is some evidence that religious and spiritual beliefs may minimize fear and uncertainty (Siegel & Schrimshaw). In short, spiritual and religious perspectives can assist individuals in making sense of the illness.

It may also allow a sense of a larger connection. Even in the inherent existential isolation of an illness, there may be a sense that a god or some higher power will sustain and protect. This connection may be more tangible as well. Many individuals may benefit from the social support available through the ministries of a chaplain, clergy, spiritual advisor, ministry team, or even within the larger faith community. The sense that one is not alone—that others are caring, visiting, and praying—seems to provide benefit (Siegel & Schrimshaw, 2002; Townsend, Kladder, & Mulligan, 2002). Spannhake (chapter 3, this volume) talked about the importance of the social support he received while hospitalized, although at times it was also a source of stress.

Religious and spiritual practices and beliefs may even enhance health. Most spiritual belief systems suggest either abstinence or moderation in certain behaviors, such as alcohol or tobacco use. Such practices and beliefs may discourage inappropriate coping techniques throughout the course of the illness. Spiritual and religious beliefs also may enhance coping by encouraging self-esteem. Most religious and spiritual systems stress the inherent worth of the individual. Such beliefs may be especially important in a life-threatening illness, during which self-blame may loom large and self-acceptance is threatened. There is also some speculation that spiritual and religious beliefs may have physiological benefits, such as lowering blood pressure or enhancing immune function, though here the research has shown some inconsistency (Dane, 2000; Lin & Bauer-Wu, 2003; Miller & Thoresen, 2003; Olive, 2004; Sephton, Koopman, Shaal, Thoresen, & Spiegel, 2001; Stefanek, McDonald, & Hess, 2005).

Religious and spiritual beliefs also may influence an individual's sense of control. In a time of life-threatening illness, individuals may feel that they have little or no control. Religious and spiritual beliefs may reaffirm a sense of personal control. This can be expressed in a number of ways. Individuals may have a sense of interpretive control—the ability to find meaning or benefit from the experience. They may have a sense of vicarious control, leaving the illness in the hands of a higher power. In some cases, the control may be of a predictive nature, perhaps believing that God will cure them or be with them throughout this experience.

Yet, this discussion also demonstrates the ways that religious and spiritual beliefs may complicate the response to a life-threatening illness. For example, a person with life-threatening illness may be convinced that he or she may be cured by a divine intervention. If death ensues, such an individual or other family members may become immobilized, unrealistic in decisions, or even despondent.

Certain religious or spiritual beliefs may serve to increase rather than decrease death anxiety. For example, fears over divine judgment or uncertainty in an afterlife may not offer comfort to a dying person. The certainty with which religious and spiritual beliefs are held as well as the nature of such beliefs is a factor in the reasons that the relationship of religiosity and spirituality to death anxiety is inconsistent (Neimeyer, 1994). Moreover, religious and spiritual perspectives can sometimes conflict with medical practices and advice. For example, some spiritual systems, such as Christian Science, may eschew any medical treatment, while others such as the Jehovah Witnesses may prohibit certain medical practices, such as blood transfusions or blood-based therapies. In other cases, a fatalistic spirituality may inhibit health-seeking behaviors or adherence to a medical regimen. It is little wonder that Pargament, Koenig, Tarakeshwar, and Hahn (2004) found in a longitudinal study that certain types of religious coping, such as seeking spiritual support or believing in a benevolent God, were related with better health, while other spiritual coping behaviors and beliefs, such as a perspective of a punishing God or religious discontent, were predictive of declines in health.

Religious and spiritual beliefs also may be evident in reactions to illness. For example, anger could be directed toward God. There may be anger that one has the disease or that the disease has come at an inopportune or unfair time. One's reaction may be clouded by a moral guilt—a belief that this illness is a punishment for some transgression. Fear and anxiety, as mentioned, can also have a religious or spiritual root, as one may fear the wrath of God in this world or the next. There may even be an existential sense of abandonment—a sense that one is facing the crisis alone, alienated from God. Such responses can emerge at any time in the illness. For example, after a relapse there may be an emerging sense of anger or despair as an individual perceives that his or her spiritual practices or beliefs are no longer viable. In all of these cases, religious and spiritual beliefs may intertwine with psychological and affective reactions to the illness.

Throughout the illness, an individual may have to cope with distinctly spiritual tasks. In an earlier work (Doka, 1993b), I proposed, building on the work of both Pattison (1978) and Weisman (1980), that life-threatening illness can best be viewed as a series of phases: prediagnostic, diagnostic, chronic, terminal, and recovery. In any particular disease, individuals may jump from one phase to another. For example, in some cases, a successful removal of a tumor may place an individual right into a recovery phase with virtually no chronic phase. In another disease, diagnosis may be immediately followed by a steep and inexorable decline toward death.

In each phase, there are distinct medical, psychological, social, and spiritual tasks.

For example, in the first two phases, the prediagnostic and diagnostic, individuals have to deal with the diagnosis of a life-threatening illness. Weisman (1980) noted that even when the diagnosis is expected or feared, it still comes as a shock, creating a sense of "existential plight" in which one's very existence is threatened. Often, it is a life divide. Even if the person survives the encounter, he or she will often talk about this as a turning point, wrought with implications that follow for the rest of life.

Here, the spiritual issue is incorporating the present reality of illness into one's sense of past and future. Questions such as, Why did I get this disease, now? arise here. An individual now struggles to make sense of the disease and of the new reality of his or her life. Spiritual and religious beliefs may offer an answer to these questions or at least provide direction for further quest. And, spiritual strengths and practices such as prayer and meditation may be mobilized as the individual prepares for the battle, literally, of his or her life.

The chronic phase centers around the time of treatment. Here, the individual must not only cope with the disease but also with the burdens and side effects of treatment. Often, as persons continue such treatment, they may resume some of their prior roles—returning to work or functioning within their families. Frequently, this is a lonely time. The crisis of the diagnosis is now past, so family, friends, and other social support may not be as available. This phase can also be a time of great uncertainty as individuals cope with the ambiguities of both the disease and treatment. The disease may or may not progress. Treatment may or may not be successful.

In the chronic phase, suffering may become a major spiritual issue. Why am I suffering through this disease and treatment? Is it all worth it? Persons will often look to their religious or spiritual beliefs to make sense of this suffering. Their beliefs may vary. Again, some may see the suffering as retribution for sins in this or another life. Some may even find comfort in that, believing that suffering now may offer recompense or even purification that will mollify God or better prepare them for an afterlife. Others may see suffering as random. Another group may see their suffering as a learning experience, allowing greater empathy. Some may see it as sacrifice, offering it as a way to gain a greater connection to God or other people.

Not everyone dies from life-threatening illness. Many individuals may fully recover, resuming their lives, and others may face long, even permanent, periods of remission. Yet, the encounter with disease leaves all types of residues. Individuals may have an enhanced sense of their fragility, feeling that they are living under a sword that can strike at any time (Koocher & O'Malley, 1981). The experience with illness may affect everything from relationships with other people to career mobility. The sense of one's own mortality was clearly illustrated in Spannhake's (chapter 3, this volume) account of his experience with untreatable pain and the physiological reactions to the medications he was taking.

There also are spiritual residues. Individuals may struggle with a sense of "the bargain." It is not unusual for persons to make spiritual commitments and promises in a cosmic deal to surmount the illness. Now that they have recovered from this threat, they may believe they have to fulfill their promises. For example, Martin Luther, a promising law student, felt compelled, despite the entreaties from family and friends, to enter a monastery as he had promised when he was frightened for his life during a ferocious storm. A failure to fulfill such commitments may loom large should a person experience a relapse or even encounter another disease.

There may be other spiritual changes as well. Some individuals may move closer to their religion or become more spiritually aware and active. Others may feel alienated either from their God or their spiritual community. Another group may actively seek a new spirituality, perceiving that their past beliefs did not serve them well in this crisis.

In the terminal phase, the goals of treatment move from extending life or curing the individual to being strictly palliative. In this phase, people often struggle with three spiritual needs (Doka, 1993a, 1993b). The first is to have lived a meaningful life. Individuals may assess their life to find a sense of meaning and purpose. Here, people may struggle, seeking forgiveness for tasks unaccomplished or for hurtful acts that they may have committed. Individuals may struggle with a second goal—to die an appropriate death, however that is individually defined. As discussed in the next section, religious and spiritual beliefs may be a significant factor in how an individual chooses to die and in what end-of-life decisions are made. A final spiritual need is to find hope beyond the grave. This means that the individual needs a sense that life will continue—in whatever appropriate way is supported by the person's spiritual sense. This can include living on the memories of others, in the genes of family members, within one's community, in the creations and legacies left, in a sense of "eternal nature" (that is, that one returns to the cycle of life), in some transcendental mode, or in an afterlife (Doka, 1993b; Lifton & Olsen, 1974).

In summary, then, throughout the course of an illness individuals may struggle with a variety of spiritual issues or tasks. Their success in dealing with these spiritual concerns may very well affect how well they cope with the disease.

Families also may experience similar spiritual issues. Even after the individual dies, the family may still struggle spiritually, trying to reconstruct their own faith or spiritual system that may have been challenged by that loss (Doka, 1993a).

☐ Religion, Spirituality, End-of-Life Decisions, and Ethics

Throughout the course of a life-threatening illness, patients and their families will have to make critical decisions about care. What strategies should be used to manage pain? Is it appropriate to use palliative sedation? Should a patient be placed on a ventilator? How long should active medical treatment persist even if it is perceived as futile? When should treatment cease, and who should be empowered to make such determinations? Should the patient receive artificial hydration and nutrition? Can treatments be withheld or, if administered, withdrawn? Is assisted suicide ever a valid ethical choice in life-threatening illness? All of these questions arose across the personal stories in the beginning of this volume.

Health professionals have long realized that religious and spiritual systems play a significant role in the ways that patients and their families make end-of-life decisions and resolve ethical dilemmas (Koenig, 2004). As patients and their families struggle with these decisions, they often turn to their religious and spiritual values, and even to their clergy or spiritual mentors, for guidance. The investigation, then, of religious and spiritual perspectives of these end-of-life dilemmas is clearly warranted. It is in fact a mandate that frames this chapter.

Yet, it is a daunting challenge. Such a section could only trace in broad lines major religious and spiritual themes that frame such decision making. It is important to discuss the significant limitations of this undertaking.

First, within each religion or faith system (e.g., Christianity, Buddhism, Judaism, Hinduism, Islam), there are numerous divisions and denominations. Some perspectives are more fundamentalist and conservative, holding fast to historical traditions and placing great weight on a very literal interpretation of holy texts. Others are more liberal—attempting to apply the basic tenets of faith to contemporary circumstances.

Beyond this literalist/modernist divide, each faith system may have a variety of sects and denominations that have different histories. For example, the Shiite/Sunni division in Islam dates back to 661 A.D. in a dispute regarding the succession of caliphs. Within each branch are numerous sects and schools. Similarly, the Orthodox and Catholic branches of Christianity divided in schism in 1054, while the Protestant branch separated from the now Roman Catholic Church beginning in 1517.

Moreover, each of these denominations may emphasize different themes or facets of their faith. For example, charismatic and Pentecostal Christians will emphasize the shared and present gifts of the Holy Spirit to an extent not found in other denominations. In fact, sometimes it is even difficult to decide where to place a denomination in the spectrum of religious systems. The Church of Jesus Christ of Latter-day Saints, popularly known as the Mormons, considers itself part of the Christian tradition. Some other Christians, though, might dispute such an affiliation, asserting that Mormon beliefs and additional books of revelation effectively remove it from that tradition.

Complicating the issues even more, with few exceptions, such as the Roman Catholic papacy, most denominations and religious systems are highly decentralized. Hence, it can be very difficult to determine their stance on ethical issues at the end of life. Of course, such opinions may vary as new circumstances and conditions arise. For example, in the recent Terri Schiavo case, statements of the Pope seemed to suggest a greater support for artificial nutrition and hydration than had previously been the case. In short, it is critical to remember that any attempts to discuss the historic responses of faith systems to end of life necessarily have to be painted in very broad strokes.

Moreover, it is important to recognize that the religious and spiritual perspectives are but one, albeit important, factor in such ethical decisions. People make ethical decisions based on many factors. Culture and history, for example, play a significant role. For example, many African Americans, although predominantly Christian, tend to be reluctant to withhold or withdraw medical treatment (Mouton, 2000). Although this certainly reflects spiritual emphases such as suffering and survival, it also reflects an historical and cultural mistrust in the medical system (Mouton).

Although there is value in reviewing the ways that major faith systems approach ethical decisions at the end of life, it is also important to remember the limitations of such an approach. In the end, spirituality is inherently personal. It matters less what religious systems or denominations say about these issues than what the individual believes that his or her faith commends him or her to do in this situation.

□ Overview of Major Religious Perspectives on End-of-Life Issues

Judaism

Judaism is the most ancient of the Western faiths, dating back nearly 3,500 years. In the United States, Jews were among the earliest immigrants, but significant migrations did not begin until the 1880s. Judaism is divided into Orthodox, Conservative, Reform, and Reconstructionist movements. In addition, many individuals may identify with Judaism as a cultural identity. Although the Torah and other biblical books popularly identified as the Old Testament constitute the Jewish Canon, other books such as the Talmud and various commentaries and encyclopedic codes are also considered authoritative.

Jewish thought tends to place a high emphasis on the sanctity of life. Life is a gift from God that must be nurtured and preserved. The story in which God stills the patriarch Abraham's hand before he can sacrifice his son Isaac (i.e., Genesis 22:1–18) is often seen as a defining moment in the evolution of Judaism—a rejection of the common practice in that area of child sacrifice—that set aside the Hebrew people with a distinct set of values in the preservation of life.

Such a position generally abhors any form of active euthanasia. Although life is generally to be preserved, there are debates within the Jewish community regarding how far this concept should be applied. For example, much Jewish thought affirms the principle of double effect—adequate pain medication can be given even at the risk of shortening life as long as the intent is to relieve pain rather than hasten death. This also is applied to withholding or withdrawing treatment. Such a response, many Jewish scholars hold, can be undertaken near the end of life to minimize pain and suffering (Kavesh, 2000). However, this consensus is not so apparent in cases of artificial hydration and nutrition, for which more orthodox scholars tend to emphasize the importance of maintaining food and liquids, while other scholars tend to see artificial nutrition and hydration as a medical treatment that can be halted (Kavesh, 2000; Tiano & Beyer, 2005). Adherence to the value of life generally makes organ transplants acceptable, and the emphasis on compassionate care and pain relief sees no conflict with hospice.

Christianity

Christianity began nearly 2,000 or so years ago as an offshoot of Judaism. The Christian church began as Jewish disciples of Jesus proclaimed him as the long-promised Messiah. In the first decades of the church's life, it ceased to view itself solely as an expression of Judaism, actively proselytizing Gentiles. By the fourth century, Christianity had become the dominant religion within the Roman Empire. Soon, it dominated all of Europe and was spread by missionaries and settlers throughout the rest of the world. However, the unity of the church was not preserved. The Great Schism in 1054 between Rome and Constantinople divided the church into Roman Catholic and Orthodox Churches. The Protestant Reformation later divided Catholic Europe. Despite these divisions, most Christian churches accept the Bible's Old and New Testaments as authoritative even though they may vary on the precise formulation of the canon, the validity of certain translations, and the role of tradition and writings of Church fathers.

Christians are the prevailing religious group in North America, including Canada and the United States. In the United States, somewhere around 76–90% of the U.S. population identify as Christian (depending how the term is defined or the question is asked) (www.adherents.com). It is important to note that Christianity is extremely diverse in the United States, with hundreds of discrete denominations reflecting different faiths, distinct cultures, and divergent histories. There is little unanimity on end-of-life ethics.

Nonetheless, it is important to remember the Jewish roots of Christianity. As with Judaism, Christians have tended to place a significant value on the sanctity of life. Like Jews, there is a general, but incomplete, consensus that assisted suicide is morally wrong (Cohen, 2005). Beyond that, consensus tends to be elusive. Many Christians would tend to make a distinction between actively killing and letting an individual naturally die. However, the application of this principle in denominational statements and specific ethical cases shows considerable divergence. Generally, the divide places more evangelical and conservative Protestant churches, along with the Roman Catholic and Orthodox Churches, on one end of a spectrum and the more liberal Protestant churches on the other end of this continuum. Again, culture plays a significant role. For example, although black churches have historically been in the forefront of progressive social issues, a number of prominent African American clergy, such as the Reverend Jesse Jackson, actively opposed the withdrawal of artificial nutrition in the Schiavo case.

The more conservative churches, as a whole, would favor artificial hydration and nutrition and would be skeptical (but not fully or uniformly opposed) to the withdrawal or withholding of other medical treatments. The more liberal churches would as a whole be more accepting of withdrawing or withholding treatments, including artificial hydration and nutrition. There might be a similar division on palliative sedation, although both would probably accept a notion that intent is critical. Both groups would generally adhere to a similar principle—that extraordinary treatment to prolong life is not necessary. The question between them would be where to draw these lines.

There are other elements of a shared consensus. Christians in general would support both hospice care and organ transplantation. Recently, many Christian ethicists on both sides of this conservative/liberal divide have begun to question the primacy that many contemporary ethicists give to autonomy—affirming that individuals are not fully autonomous but in their decisions need to be responsive to their connections to family, community, and God (Cohen, 2005).

Islam

As of the 2000 census, Islam is now one of the largest non-Christian religions in the United States. From its beginnings in Arabia by the Prophet Mohammad in the early seventh century, Muslims accept the Koran to be authoritative, and the Old and New Testaments are considered Holy Books. Muslims in the United States are divided into a number of sects, of which the Sunni and Shiite are the largest; within these divisions there are various schools of interpretation.

The very name *Islam* literally means submission to God. Muslims believe that at death the soul separates from the body and will rejoin the body on the day of judgment. With other Western religions, Islam emphasizes the sanctity of life. Generally then, Muslims oppose suicide, physician-assisted suicide, and active euthanasia. Muslims also believe that individuals should seek treatment for disease, affirming that Allah can always provide a cure if He wishes. However, advance directives and do not resuscitate orders are acceptable for persons with a terminal condition when further treatment is futile. The prolongation of life with artificial means is not morally necessary and in fact may thwart God's will. However, food and water may not be withdrawn, so many Islamic ethicists, such as the Islamic Medical Association of North America, oppose withholding or withdrawing nutrition or hydration (Cohen, 2005).

Muslims have traditionally viewed donating blood as an act of piety. Many Islamic ethicists would hold organ donation in a similar light.

Islamic tradition emphasizes that a person should die in a peaceful, quiet setting surrounded by family and friends and where the spiritual practices surrounding the dead body can be observed. Hospice then can be a desirable option. However, it is preferable that the person remains conscious until death, so there may be a concern with the use of pain medication.

Buddhism

Buddhism derives from the teachings of Siddhartha, a prince who renounced his throne in the Indian Subcontinent some 2500 years ago. In the United States, Buddhism has grown in a number of ways—the migration of Buddhists from Asia into Hawaii and the U.S. mainland over the past two centuries, but especially in the past 40 years since the Immigration Act of 1965, as well as conversion and intermarriage. Although the Buddhist community remains relatively small in North America, many traditional Buddhist beliefs such as reincarnation and practices such as meditation have strongly influenced New Age and nontraditional spiritualities.

In understanding the ways that Buddhists approach end-of-life decisions, a few concepts are central. A fundamental thesis of Buddhism is that life is transient and impermanent. Although life is a gift, it also has an illusionary quality—death is inevitable. Buddha also emphasizes balance—seeking a middle way between renunciation and asceticism and immersion in the pleasures of life.

These principles guide the Buddhist perspective on end-of-life decisions. Because life is essentially transient, little is gained from artificial extension of life. Buddhists would generally support withholding and withdrawing medical treatment, including artificial hydration and nutrition, if such procedures would artificially lengthen life and prolong suffering. There also would be little objection for pain medication even if that should hasten death. Under some circumstances, even suicide, physician-assisted suicide, or forms of active euthanasia could be morally appropriate if done with a selfless concern for others and if there is suffering and no hope of recovery.

Palliative care such as hospice fits well within Buddhist tradition. Such care, especially centered on the family, is preferred at the final stages of life to active medical treatment that simply seeks to delay the inevitable.

Buddhists emphasize that it is difficult to create general guidelines—each case has to be evaluated on its own merits. For example, in Buddha's teachings there are two incidences when monks ask his advice on suicide. In one case, Buddha reproves the monk for seeking death, but in the other he commends the monk for a selfless act as this monk was motivated by a realistic understanding of his condition and a concern for others (Nakasone, 2000).

For Buddhists, process is important. Balance and consensus join as both spiritual and cultural values. Family consensus is to be sought as one attempts to balance individual wishes with the family's needs and larger societal values.

Concepts of brain death and organ transplantation remain controversial to most Buddhists. Buddhists traditionally define death as the absence of a heartbeat. For organ transplantation, generally the person is declared brain dead even as the heart still (albeit artificially) beats. Organ transplantation may cause cultural conflicts as well. Filial piety, strongly supported throughout many Asian countries where Buddhism predominates, emphasizes that all parts of the body are gifts from parents and thus are to be preserved. Beyond this discomfort, many Buddhists would hold that with life being transient, little good can come from artificially extending life through transplantation. Yet, other Buddhists would argue that because a body is merely a vessel, it is a great gift to donate organs—giving life to another (Nakasone, 2000). In any case, the individual should not make such decisions alone. Family consensus ensures that balance is achieved.

Hinduism

Hinduism, the majority religion in India and one of the oldest faith systems, has gained a small foothold in the United States and North America as Indians and other adherents have migrated to North America. Hinduism has no single founder, universal creed, or hierarchy. It is polytheistic and quite diverse in its beliefs and practices.

Like other faiths, Hinduism holds life sacred and thus is wary of acts that destroy life. Nonviolence is a treasured belief. Moreover, actively seeking or causing one's death through suicide may interfere with one's karma, thus affecting rebirth.

However, there are also traditions within the faith in which suicide and "self-willed" deaths are culturally and spiritually acceptable. A good death is defined when one is fully aware of one's fate and in control of one's mental faculties. So, it may be permissible under circumstances of great suffering to take action to hasten death. In fact, there are traditions that hold that when one senses death is imminent, an individual may refuse nourishment and participate in rituals that ready one to die. It would seem, then, that Hindus would be free to refuse artificial hydration and nutrition.

Hinduism is generally practiced within India, where, for most, medical resources may be more limited. Hence, Hindu ethicists have yet to grapple with the dilemmas posed by modern medical technology. As more Hindus migrate and establish themselves in North America and as India itself develops, it is likely that there will be more commentary on such issues.

Individualistic, Eclectic, and Diverse Spiritualities

Naturally, in concluding this section it is important to emphasize a number of points. The faith traditions discussed may present general themes or emphases that may guide adherents in the decisions they make at the end of life. However, these traditions themselves are still grappling with the dilemmas posed by technological advances. As seen, many of these faiths offer divergent perspectives. Moreover, although the faiths discussed here represent the religious affiliations of most North Americans, there are many individuals who would affiliate with other beliefs. The Baha'i faith, which attempts to honor and combine all major faiths as a move toward global peace and unity, is small but growing in the United States, both from migration and conversion. New Age spiritualities have revived, for example, a range of spiritual beliefs, some of which (e.g., Wicca or Druidism) claim an old history. Other New Age beliefs try to fuse Western and Eastern religious insights, practices, and beliefs. In addition, other groups such as the Ethical Cultural Society have sought to create a moral and spiritual system devoid of theistic assumptions. Others may have no explicit belief system identifying as agnostic or atheistic.

The preceding discussion should not obscure the fact that although each major faith system or religion has developed principles to assist persons in dealing with ethical dilemmas and decisions faced at the end of life, spirituality is ultimately individual. A person's spirituality is ultimately what he or she says it is. These individual spiritualities are eclectic, often drawing from that person's perception of the teachings of his or her faith, as well as cultural, generational, and other influences. Spirituality, in short, can never be assumed by a religious affiliation. It needs to be assessed.

Finally, it is important to remember the rich diversity of spirituality that exists even within a family or intimate network. Decisions at the end of life often are discussed with others, such as surrogates, family members, and friends (Doka, Jennings, & Corr, 2005). All of these individuals' spiritualities may be involved in consideration and resolution of the ethical dilemmas and choices that emerge as one faces death.

☐ Assisting Individuals and Families at the End of Life: Utilizing Spirituality

Because spirituality is so central as individuals and their families struggle with later life, it is important that holistic care includes spiritual assessment. Although there are a variety of tools to assist assessment (Hodge, 2005; Ledger, 2005), the key really is to engage both the individual and family in an exploration of their individual and collective spiritual histories. The goal is to understand the collective and individual spiritual journeys. Do they identify with a particular faith? Do they actively practice that faith—engaging in public and private rituals and practices? Do they belong to a church, temple, synagogue, or mosque? How important is their faith system in making decisions?

However, such an assessment should go beyond religious affiliation. It might be worthwhile to explore with individuals when and where they feel most spiritually connected; what practices they utilize when they are stressed, anxious, or depressed; and what stories, prayers, or songs offer spiritual comfort. Such approaches may allow a larger exploration of the very distinct ways that individuals find meaning and hope. Even persons who claim no belief system such as atheists or agnostics may respond to questions about what offers them a sense of meaning or home or what practices, perhaps even a walk in the woods or on the beach, assist them when they are troubled. An assessment may yield information on spiritual strengths that an individual possesses, themes within an individual's spirituality (such as grace, karma, fate, or retribution), and experiences that have tended to challenge that person's spirituality. Occasionally, such an assessment may uncover forms of spiritual abuse—spiritual beliefs, practices, or behaviors of spiritual mentors that have resulted in a sense of spiritual alienation.

Once an assessment of spirituality is made, individuals can be encouraged to connect with their spiritual strengths. Often, this involves their clergy, chaplains, spiritual mentors, or faith community. Clergy, chaplains, and other spiritual mentors can play an important supportive (and sometimes an unsupportive) role as an individual responds to a life-threatening illness. Their visits throughout the illness may be valued. Clergy, chaplains, and other spiritual advisors may be sought as an individual or family member responds to the spiritual questions inherent in the illness. They may be consulted as individuals and family members struggle with treatment decisions and ethical dilemmas.

Because clergy, chaplains, and other spiritual members play such an important role for patients and families, healthcare institutions may wish to review the ways that they incorporate and interact with religious and spiritual communities. Despite the importance of ministry to the ill, dying, and bereaved, many clergy report little formal seminary education on dealing with dying patients and their families (Abrams, Albury, Crandall, Doka, & Harris, 2005; Doka & Jendreski, 1985). Clergy and other spiritual care workers gave positive evaluations to a statewide project in Florida sponsored by the Hospice Foundation of America that provided such education. Interestingly, they especially valued medical information on pain management, active dying, and palliative and hospice care that shed light on ethical dilemmas that they regularly face in their ministries (Abrams et al., 2005). Such programs can serve as a model for smaller-scale endeavors that healthcare organizations might wish to sponsor to connect and strengthen relationships with spiritual and religious organizations within their area of service.

Although clergy, chaplains, and other spiritual mentors play an important role, faith communities also can play a critical role. Often, such groups can offer spiritual comfort and connection; visits, calls, cards, and letters that show support and ease isolation; and assistance with tangible tasks such as cooking, home maintenance, transportation, and caregiving.

Spiritual beliefs and practices also may be sources of strength. A person's spiritual beliefs may be critical in making meaning throughout an illness and for family after the death. Often, a simple question such as, "How do your beliefs speak to you in this situation?" can engage the person in spiritual exploration. It may also be useful to investigate the ways that the individual's beliefs assisted and helped the person make sense of the experience in earlier crises. There may be situations when the individual's beliefs seem inadequate or dysfunctional. In such situations, it may help if the individual receives spiritual support from a member of his or her own spiritual community. For example, in one case, a bereaved father whose adult son was an intravenous drug user dying of AIDS feared that his son's decision to forgo further treatment, including artificial nutrition and hydration, would result in eternal damnation. A chaplain from the father's fundamentalist Christian denomination led him in a Biblical study of the story of Sampson, a self-destructive judge of Israel whose salvation is noted in the New Testament, in a successful attempt for the father to address his spiritually based fears.

Spiritual practices such as prayer and meditation also may have a role in the illness. At the very least, intercessory prayer (the prayer of others) is a visible sign that the individual is not facing this crisis alone. It offers family and friends a tangible thing to do—reaffirming a form of vicarious control in an unsettled time. Individuals who are struggling with physical illness often use prayer as a form of coping (Ribbentrop, Altmaier, Chen, Found, & Keffala, 2005). There is some evidence that prayer and meditation do affect physical health in a number of ways, including lowering stress levels and blood pressure (Mayo Clinic Health Letter, 2005). Schroeder-Sheker (1994) has even pioneered the field of musical thanatology, using spiritual music as a way to ease the transition to death.

Rituals also can be a source of comfort to both the ill or dying patient as well as family. Many faith traditions that have rituals for the sick and the dying, such as the Roman Catholic rite for anointing of the sick (popularly known as "last rites") or rituals at the time of death, such as washing or preparing the body. Individuals who do not have distinctive rituals as part of their tradition may still be invited to create one at the time of death, such as lighting a candle, anointing the dead person, joining in prayer or meditation, singing a spiritual hymn or song, or other individual ways of saying a final good-bye to mark the transition from life to death. Rituals work well in these liminal or transitional moments—offering participants a way to acknowledge loss and transition.

□ Conclusion: The Challenge of Spiritual Support

There is challenge and opportunity in offering spiritual support as individuals and their families struggle with life-threatening illness and, perhaps, death. Illness, dying, and death are crises on many levels, including spiritually. The spiritual perspectives of persons will not only influence the ways they find, or fail to find, meaning in the illness; these perspectives will affect their reactions and adaptation to the illness. More than that, spiritual considerations will play a critical role in the choices they make throughout their illness and the ethical decisions they encounter near the end of life.

Yet, spiritual support can be a challenge. Many health professionals have little specialized training in spirituality. Moreover, there may be concern lest one impose one's own spirituality on a patient or family member. Sometimes, out of respect for the diversity and individuality of a person's spiritual beliefs, health professionals may be reluctant to enter into conversations involving religion or spirituality. Thus, there often is temptation to leave these issues to chaplains, clergy, or other spiritual mentors. This is unlikely to suffice. Spiritual concerns arise throughout the entire experience of the illness. Patients and families will choose when, where, and with whom they will share these spiritual concerns. These choices may not always fit into neat organizational charts or job descriptions. These spiritual concerns also cannot be neglected. Holistic care entails that spiritual concerns are both acknowledged and validated. A true respect for spirituality means that such concerns and struggles need to be addressed by every professional. Spirituality therefore cannot be ignored. Death, after all, may be the ultimate spiritual journey.

□ References

Abrams, D., Albury, S., Crandall, L., Doka, K., and Harris, R. (2005). The Florida Clergy End-of-Life Education Enhancement Project: A description and evaluation. *American Journal of Hospice and Palliative Medicine, 22,* 181–187.

Cohen, C. (2005). Religious, spiritual and ideological perspectives of ethics at the end-of-life. In K. Doka, B. Jennings, & C. Corr (Eds.), *Living with grief: Ethical dilemmas at the end-of-life* (pp. 19–40). Washington, DC: The Hospice Foundation of America.

Dane, B. (2000). Thai women: Meditation as a way to cope with AIDS. *Journal of Religion and Health, 38,* 5–21.

Doka, K. (Ed.). (1993a). *Death and spirituality.* Amityville, NY: Baywood Press.

Doka, K. (1993b). *Living with life-threatening illness: A guide for patients, their families, and caregivers.* Lexington, MA: Lexington Books.

Doka, K., & Jendreski, M. (1985). Clergy understandings of grief, bereavement and mourning. *Research Record, 2,* 105–114.

Doka, K, Jennings, J., & Corr, C. (Eds.). (2005) *Living with grief: Ethical dilemmas at the end-of-life.* Washington, DC: The Hospice Foundation of America.

Hodge, D. (2005). Developing a spiritual assessment toolbox: A discussion of the strengths and limitations of five different assessment methods. *Health and Social Work, 30,* 314–323.

International Work Group on Death, Dying, and Bereavement (Spiritual Care Work Group). (1990). Assumptions and principles of spiritual care. *Death Studies, 14,* 75–81.

Kavesh, W. (2000). Jewish perspectives in end-of-life decision-making. In K. Braun, J. Pietsch, & P. Blanchette (Eds.), *Cultural issues in end-of-life decision-making* (pp. 181–197). Thousand Oaks, CA: Sage.

Koenig, H. (2004). Religion, spirituality, and medicine: Research findings and implications for clinical practice. *Southern Medical Journal, 97,* 1194–1200.

Koocher, G. P., & O'Malley, J. E. (1981). *The Damocles syndrome: Psychological consequences of surviving childhood cancer.* New York: McGraw-Hill.

Ledger, S. (2005). The duty of nurses to meet patients' spiritual and/or religious needs. *British Journal of Nursing, 14,* 220–225.

Lifton, R., & Olsen, G. (1974). *Living and dying.* New York: Bantam Books.

Lin, H., & Bauer-Wu, S. (2003). Psycho-spiritual well being in patients with advanced cancer: An integrative review of the literature. *Journal of Advanced Nursing, 44,* 69–90.

Mayo Clinic Health Letter. (2005). *Meditation, 23*(3), 3–4.

Miller, J. (1994, November). *The transforming power of spirituality.* Presentation to a conference on transformative grief, Burnsville, NC.

Miller, W., & Thoresen, C. (2003). Spirituality, religion, and health: An emerging research field. *American Psychologist, 58,* 1–19.

Mouton, C. (2000). Cultural and religious issues for African-Americans. In K. Braun, J. Pietsch, & P. Blanchette (Eds.), *Cultural issues in end-of-life decision-making* (pp. 71–82). Thousand Oaks, CA: Sage.

Nakasone, R. (2000). Buddhist issues in end-of-life decision-making. In K. Braun, J. Pietsch, & P. Blanchette (Eds.), *Cultural issues in end-of-life decision-making* (pp. 213–228). Thousand Oaks, CA: Sage.

Neimeyer, R. (Ed.). (1994). *Death anxiety handbook: Research, instrumentation, and application.* Washington, DC: Taylor & Francis.

Olive, K. (2004). Religion and spirituality: Important psychosocial variables frequently ignored in clinical research. *Southern Medical Journal, 97,* 1152–1153.

Pargament, K., Koenig, H., Tarakeshwar, N., & Hahn, J. (2004). Religious coping methods as predictors of psychological, physical, and spiritual outcomes among medically ill elderly patients: A two-year longitudinal study. *Journal of Health Psychology, 9,* 713–730.

Pattison, E. M. (1978). The living-dying process. In C. Garfield (Ed.), *The psychosocial care of the dying patient* (pp. 133–168). New York: McGraw-Hill.

Ribbentrop, E., Altmaier, E., Chen, J., Found, E., & Keffala, V. (2005). The relationship between religion/spirituality and physical health, mental health, and pain in a chronic pain population. *Pain, 116,* 311–321.

Schroeder-Sheker, T. (1994). Music for the dying: A personal account of the new field of music-thanatology—history, theory and clinical narratives. *Journal of Holistic Nursing, 12,* 83–99.

Siegel, K., & Schrimshaw, E. (2002). The perceived benefits of religious and spiritual coping among older adults living with HIV/AIDS. *Journal for the Scientific Study of Religion, 41,* 91–102.

Sephton, S., Koopman, C., Shaal, M., Thoresen, C., & Spiegel, D. (2001). Spiritual expression and immune status in women with metastatic cancer: An exploratory study. *Breast Journal, 7,* 345–353.

Stefanek, M., McDonald, P., & Hess, S. (2005). Religion, spirituality and cancer: Current status and methodological challenges. *Psycho-oncology, 14,* 450–463.

Tiano, N., & Beyer, E. (2005). Cultural and religious views on non-beneficial treatment. In K. Doka, B. Jennings, & C. Corr (Eds.), *Living with grief: Ethical dilemmas at the end-of-life* (pp. 41–59). Washington, DC: The Hospice Foundation of America.

Townsend, M., Kladder, V., & Mulligan, T. (2002). Systematic review of clinical trials examining the effects of religion on health. *Southern Medical Journal, 95,* 1429–1434.

Weisman, A. (1980). Thanatology. In H. Kaplan & B. Sadock (Eds.), *Comprehensive textbook of psychiatry* (pp. 1277–1286). Baltimore, MD: Williams & Williams.

17

CHAPTER

Culture, Individual Diversity, and End-of-Life Decisions

Bert Hayslip, Jr., Robert O. Hansson,
Jon D. Starkweather, and Diana C. Dolan

☐ Introduction

In this chapter, we discuss cultural, racial, ethnic, and individual differences in end-of-life decision making. Such variation is important to recognize in that it helps us understand (a) why persons from various backgrounds feel and behave the way they do regarding end-of-life choices and (b) which barriers interfere with the making of such choices. At the same time, this very sensitivity should alert us to the fact that many of the assumptions we make about persons whose life experiences and cultural heritages are different from our own often are inaccurate. We end up walking a fine line between appreciating the unique perspective that people may have (e.g., how their race or ethnicity differentiates them from others); relying on overgeneralizations about them to the exclusion of other influences on their views, feelings, and behaviors related to end-of-life issues; and appreciating individual differences among persons, taking into consideration not only race, ethnicity, and culture but also age, gender, sexual orientation, socioeconomic status, religion/spirituality, and health/disability status. Consequently, our discussion will interface with chapters dealing with caregiving, hospice care, the influence of religion and spirituality, legal considerations, and competence.

Central to our discussion is what Kastenbaum (1998) has termed *decontextualization*, reflecting the fact that, in the context of cultural shifts in values about life and death (see Hayslip & Peveto, 2005), parameters influencing end-of-life issues have been redefined independent of the context in which they formerly existed. This imposes on individuals the responsibility and freedom of choice to make decisions that were previously not possible, such as when the criteria for death were well defined through the Harvard Medical Criteria for Death (Harvard Medical School Ad Hoc Committee, 1968; see also Corr, Nabe, & Corr, 2006). This creates anxiety, uncertainty, ambivalence, guilt, and anger—common emotions among those whose must make end-of-life choices, as evidenced by the public's response to the Terri Schiavo case in 2005.

In this light, it is noteworthy that in 1996 a telephone survey of over 1,000 adults by the Gallup Organization on behalf of the National Hospice Foundation found that (a) 6 of 10 persons had given some thought to preparing for the possible death of a family member or loved one, and that (b) 9 of 10 persons believed that it was the family's responsibility to care for a loved one and that they would prefer to die at home. The ambivalence and conflict people felt regarding end-of-life choices were reflected in the fact that although 62% said they would continue to seek curative treatment should they become terminally ill, 35% said they would ask their physician to end their lives under such circumstances. A similarly oriented poll conducted by the Health Communication Research Institute in California suggested that most respondents thought that the family should play a central role in decisions about the quality of the dying person's life, based on the pain and suffering an individual may endure, and that comfort measures rather than aggressive life-sustaining treatments were preferable, although the latter were endorsed if they would benefit the patient (Values Near the End of Lives, 2001).

Interestingly, there was little variation across race/ethnicity, gender, religion, and age in such opinions. A focus group-based study of nearly 400 people across the United States found that participants feared dying in hospital environments, that they were increasingly distrustful of their physicians' investment in their best interests, and that they feared losing control over the end of their lives (American Health Decisions, 1997; Values Near the End of Lives, 2001). In this case, however, ethnicity appears to have played a role in influencing such feelings in that African American, Hispanic, or Native American persons were less likely to trust the healthcare system and terminate life support than were Caucasians or Asian Americans, and that African Americans were more suspicious of language used to describe quality of life than were others (American Health Decisions).

It has been noted that there exists a paradox between the seemingly homogeneous picture painted by public health surveys and focus groups and the importance of acknowledging different value systems across racial and ethnic subgroups regarding end-of-life issues, perhaps because such individuals were underrepresented in such work (Values at the End of Lives, 2001). Such views may also be intensely personal or seem strange to express in a specific cultural setting, and the language people use to symbolize their feelings and attitudes serves, at least on the surface, as an impediment to sharing one's views with others who do not speak one's language (Values at the End of Lives). Indeed, as culture shapes views on the importance of pain and how pain is experienced, the role of the family in making end-of-life decisions, and the meaning attributed to death and suffering (see Values at the End of Lives; Werth, Blevins, Toussaint, & Durham, 2002), differences of opinion can arise between families and physicians regarding whether the patient should be told of a terminal illness, appreciation for what constitutes essential qualities of life, or whether someone is in pain, leading to an imbalance of power in decision making. The increasing salience of being in pain and its relationship to the fine line between life and death is vividly expressed by Spannhake (chapter 3, this volume), who nearly choked to death on his own phlegm fighting Guillian-Barre syndrome. Yet, an overemphasis on culture can obscure the individual patient's rights to, and preferences for, quality end-of-life care (Values at the End of Lives).

□ Culture as Context

The cultural environments into which we are born shape the nature of our experience, and they rest on assumptions and values that become fundamental to how we lead our lives. Because cultures can be viewed to have evolved as their members learned to cope with problems of adaptation (see Schein, 2004), it follows that different cultures would exhibit quite different sets of values, religious meaning systems, norms concerned with social responsibility, interpersonal and family relations, and informal and formal coping resources. From this perspective, then, the meaning of death, cultural scripts for handling the dead, the formation of policy and law on the topic, emotional expectations, as well as our understandings of rites of passage, rituals, grief, and mourning, can be viewed as social constructions (Klass, 2001; Rosenblatt, 2001, in press).

□ Observations on Diversity and Culture

A number of trends have focused our efforts to understand the changing demography of the United States and its implications for health and social policy. As of the 2000 census, 33% of the population identified themselves as other than White, with 13% identifying as African American, 1.5% as American Indian or Alaskan Native, 4.5% as Asian/Pacific Islander, 13% Hispanic, and 7% other (U.S. Census Bureau, 2001). Of particular interest as well are the increases among Hispanic and Asian Americans, leading to assertions that national policy must take this into account (American Psychological Association, 2003). Much of this effort has reflected the concern that in a diverse society, one's minority status could be associated with the experience of stereotyping, cumulative disadvantage, and disenfranchisement (see Doka, 2002), but it may also be true that cultural issues might threaten the validity of our assumptions about diverse populations (Fiske, 2004).

The implications of diversity for end-of-life choices are many if we expect human and cultural diversity to influence end-of-life coping, planning, and decision making. Culture, race, and country of origin have received considerable attention in this area. In addition, other variables such as gender, religious/spiritual beliefs, sexual orientation, and physical and mental health status also play a role in end-of-life decision making (American Psychological Association, 2003).

The Complex Nature of Human Diversity

It is important to understand the complexities inherent in the notion of diversity itself and the manner in which general assumptions regarding categories of people may confound efforts to conduct research, develop social policy and design, and implement intervention programs. A first assumption is that nonmajority populations should always be assumed to be at risk. Although it is important to focus on the implications of relative disadvantage that accrue to minority and stigmatized populations, it is equally important to appreciate areas of relative advantage. Individual and cultural differences can also result in a rich and varied mix of coping resources, important to successful aging and to fostering personal control near the end of life. They may contribute, for example, to collaboration in meaning making and in spiritual and emotional preparation as well as provide a context for the development of cultural and religious belief systems, rituals, support for bereaved survivors, social integration, and care (Klass, 2001).

A second problematic assumption is that diverse populations are homogeneous regarding characteristics that influence their well-being. This would overlook the presence of considerable variation within any ethnic population with respect to age, gender, educational or economic status, degree of acculturation into the majority population, or unique personal history of cumulative disadvantage resulting from group membership. Meyerowitz, Richardson, Hudson, and Leedham (1998), for example, noted that American Hispanics may have come from as many as 30 different countries of origin, reflecting considerable variation with respect to language, cultural and religious tradition, and economic status. Asian/Pacific Islanders residing in the United States speak as many as 100 different languages or dialects. Native Americans may have up to 200 different languages. The ancestors of African Americans likewise came from many regions of Africa, but many have also arrived in the United States via other countries in the Caribbean and at one time may have spoken their first language, but then also some combination of English, Spanish, or French. Furthermore, increasing numbers of Americans are now of multiple races and ethnicities (Meyerowitz et al.).

Such complexity has resulted in a growing awareness among researchers that little can be learned from studies that simply compare health or adjustment outcomes among members of populations categorized on the basis of race, ethnicity, gender, age, and other characteristics. Meyerowitz and colleagues (1998) reviewed the empirical literature on ethnicity and cancer outcomes (a topic at the center of our concern for end-of-life decision making), finding that certain populations (e.g., Asian and Native Americans) were less likely to be included in this research. However, although many of the studies reviewed did find substantial ethnicity-related differences (i.e., in population rates for certain cancers, 5-year survival rates, anatomical site of the cancer, likelihood of screening and early disease detection, follow-up, and adherence to prescribed treatments), across these studies there were few discernible and reliable patterns. This leads to the conclusion that for such work to be useful, one's focus would need to go beyond demographic variables, examining psychological variables (e.g., experienced culture, ethnic identity, and minority status). In this light, Meyerowitz et al. proposed a framework for predicting cancer outcomes (survival and quality of life) in which second-order variables (e.g., socioeconomic status, education and fluency in the primary language of the culture, traditional ethnic beliefs, the influence of family members prior to engaging in certain treatment) mediate the relationship between ethnicity and cancer outcomes.

A third assumption is that ethnic identity is not a complex construct. In a pluralistic society, we interact with many different kinds of people; this can raise important questions: Do we understand one another? Can we respect and tolerate one another? What are the cumulative consequences of being advantaged—or disadvantaged—by membership in our own particular group? Psychological researchers are now also asking more fundamental questions that go beyond those related to discrimination and stereotyping. For example, how (and to what extent) does one's cultural (e.g., religious, gender) identity shape one's self-concept and influence psychological functioning? Do we really understand the components and structure of ethnic identity? How might any of our identities (viewed as psychological constructs) influence end-of-life decision making?

A review by Phinney (1990) provided a number of insights into these issues. There is consensus, for example, that ethnicity becomes more salient when one's group may be underrepresented in, or exploited by, the dominant culture. A heightened ethnic consciousness and involvement can be adaptive, to include an increased focus and attention to the language, values, and history of one's own group. A person of minority status may also have choices regarding acculturation into the dominant culture; acculturation need not simply involve adopting the values and mores of the majority and abandoning those of one's minority group. Instead, there appear at least four possibilities: (a) moving to a strong identification with the majority and weakening ties with the ethnic group; (b) retaining a strong identification with the ethnic group only; (c) adopting a strong identification with both cultures (becoming bicultural/integrated); or (d) moving to a weak identification with both cultures (and becoming marginalized) (Berry, Trimble, & Olmedo, 1986).

To understand the construct of social identity, we must understand its components and their relationship to one another. These include self-identification, sense of belonging, attitude toward one's group, and degree of ethnic involvement. *Self-identification* is the degree to which a person adopts a self-label related to membership in the group, reflecting the individual's personal choice. Its awareness should increase if negative treatment of one's group by society is perceived to increase. It may also reflect an acknowledgment of and resignation to the labels assigned by the dominant cultural group. The *sense of belonging* is the degree felt of belonging to the minority group, a sense of "peoplehood" and shared fate. The *attitude toward one's group* reflects positive or negative evaluations of the group, its members, its values, and other variables, involving pride in membership. Finally, *degree of ethnic involvement* is the extent to which an individual participates in the social life of the group, speaks its language, practices its religion, has formed significant friendship relations within the group, and endorses the group's political goals (Phinney, 1990).

Culture and Problem Solving

There is reason to believe that culture plays a role in the fundamental process of problem solving, and this has implications for end-of-life preparations and decision making. Sternberg (2004) proposed the concept of *successful intelligence*, with the goal of predicting success in life, by which a mix of analytical, creative, and practical abilities learned within one's own culture could be identified that would foster successful performance and adaptation within the confines of that culture. His view, then, is that a number of core components of intellectual functioning are universal to our species. Our discussion of culture and problem solving becomes central as we turn to the kinds of challenges faced near the end of life, for example, the notion of preparing for a "good death." In culturally diverse societies such as the United States, individuals nearing death and their families find themselves interacting with institutional environments (e.g., hospitals, hospice, Medicare, religious institutions, funeral homes).

These entities and the processes they oversee can be instrumental to successfully living out the remainder of one's life, which is assumed to involve maintenance of one's emotional and cognitive health, social competence, sense of personal control, and life satisfaction. They can also influence an individual's efforts to achieve a good death. A good death (at least in Western culture) might be assumed to involve an acceptance of and being at peace, accepting the timeliness of death, embracing one's family, being of little burden to loved ones, minimizing pain to self and trauma to family members, and having opportunities to communicate final goodbyes (Carr, 2003; Hansson & Stroebe, 2007). It is important to heed the advice of Rosenblatt (in press), who stressed that it is our culture that provides us with meanings of death (embedded in our own belief—perhaps religious meaning systems), prescribing the cultures' understood characteristics of a good death, and providing traditional scripts concerned with caring for the dying, the deceased, and continuing relationships between deceased and surviving family members.

□ Cultural Shifts in End-of-Life Decision Making

Just as people do, cultures change over time. Indeed, the literature on sociocultural (cohort) effects in developmental change has highlighted our sensitivity to the relativity of our findings in such arenas as causes of death, grandparenthood, intelligence, family caregiving, and personality (e.g., Connidis, 2001; Lamb, 2003; Mrozeck, Spiro, & Griffin, 2006; Schaie, 2005; Uhlenberg & Kirby, 1998). Thus, it would not be surprising to observe that the United States has changed over time in ways that not only influence attitudes toward end-of-life issues but also create many personal dilemmas for such individuals in making decisions about the quality of their own or others' lives. For example, the decision to abandon further treatment and the availability of hospice care have likely altered the context in which families make decisions about the quality of care provided to terminally ill family members (Hayslip & Hansson, 2006). Similarly, the rise in deaths because of AIDS, the passage of the Patient Self-Determination

Act in 1990, the implementation of advanced directive legislation by many states, and the growth of consumer groups and private foundations (e.g., Project Death in America of the Open Society Institute, Hospice Foundation of America, Nathan Cummings Foundation, Robert Wood Johnson Foundation) advocating for recognition of patients' rights and improvements in end-of-life care have all come together to bring end-of-life issues to the forefront of the public's consciousness.

In the context of Brofenbrenner's (1979) notion of structural lag, it is relevant to discuss the impact of cultural change on end-of-life decision making. *Structural lag* refers to the delay between an event's occurrence and that event's impact on individuals. In the context of the above cultural events driving attitudinal changes, as well as several high-profile cultural events (e.g., the controversy surrounding Dr. Jack Kevorkian, who was ultimately convicted of murder in 1999 for his role in ending the life of Thomas Youk; the passage of the Oregon Death With Dignity Act in 1994; the deaths of Karen Ann Quinlan in 1975, Nancy Cruzan in 1983, and Terri Schiavo in 2005), questions regarding the moral and legal parameters defining end-of-life decisions have been raised (see Cerminara, chapter 8, this volume). They present physicians, healthcare personnel, lawyers, ethicists, and perhaps most poignantly, dying persons and their families with choices that are unprecedented in terms of their impact on the quality of life for such individuals, their families, and those persons for whom such decisions are both possible and inevitable (see Kleespies, Miller, & Preston, chapter 9, this volume). This situation can clearly be seen in Raye's (chapter 5, this volume) accounting of her father's death and the interactions between family members and medical providers.

The gravity of such cultural changes is highlighted by findings from a 30-year time lag study of two heterogeneous groups of approximately 600 adults each. The groups' opinions regarding end-of-life issues were ascertained over time, with the results stratified by race and ethnicity (African American, Hispanic American, Asian American, Caucasian), age, and gender (Hayslip & Peveto, 2005). These data clearly suggest that race and ethnicity are powerful influences on attitudes toward end-of-life issues, and that cultural shifts in their influence have taken place. For example, in the 1970 sample of Kalish and Reynolds (Kalish & Reynolds, 1976), Caucasians and Japanese Americans were more likely to want to be told that they were dying; Caucasians, and to a lesser extent Blacks, Japanese Americans, and Mexican Americans (in that order), were more likely to endorse telling dying persons that they were dying. Each is a prerequisite for informed decision making about matters relating to the preparation of a will, or one's wishes regarding life-sustaining medical interventions and treatments. Mexican Americans were least likely to endorse the possibility that people hasten or slow their death via their own will, while causing grief in others was a principal reason for not wanting to die. On the other hand, persons across ethnicities were equally likely to state that it was the physician's role to inform patients of a terminal illness, that avoiding pain was not key in not wanting to die, and that people who were terminally ill (with cancer) knew about their diagnosis before being told. Generally, African Americans' views on death were most different from those of other ethnic groups in the Kalish and Reynolds (1976) study. Among the Japanese, death attitudes were dominated by themes of reciprocity among family and cohesiveness among family members. Mexican Americans' views were the most homogeneous (see Hayslip & Peveto, 2005).

Similar to Kalish and Reynolds's (1976) findings, Hayslip and Peveto's 2000 sample findings again suggested that Caucasians and Asian American remained most likely to want to be told that they were dying. Moreover, generally Hayslip and Peveto's participants (irrespective of ethnicity) were less likely to say that they would tell someone they were dying (suggesting then, that someone else should assume this responsibility). Critical to understanding people's views about life-sustaining treatments and procedures, these participants were also less likely to say that they would accept death peacefully and that they would change their behavior dramatically if they were told they were dying. However, they were more likely to say that they would show concerns for others if they themselves were dying and were more likely over time to state that reducing uncertainty about death was most important to them. More Asian Americans and African Americans indicated they would accept death peacefully, while Hispanic Americans were most likely to say they would "fight" death; Caucasians were most ambivalent in this respect. Relevant to cultural shifts in the impact of ethnicity on death attitudes, Hayslip and Peveto (2005) found that experience with dying people had changed most (increased) over time for Caucasians and African Americans, and that these groups also evidenced the greatest historical increase in showing concern for others in the event of their dying, versus Hispanic and Japanese Americans, whose responses to this question decreased relative to those in 1970. African Americans' and Hispanic Americans' concerns that their death would cause others to grieve increased the most over time. Although gender did not emerge as a salient influence in a comparison of the 1970 versus the 2000 findings, people aged 60 and over were more likely over time to show concern for others in the event of their dying and were more likely than before to say that they had made out a will. Those who were younger and middle aged expressed a greater belief in the afterlife than in 1970, and middle-aged persons were more likely to express a preference for death at home than before.

The Hayslip and Peveto (2005) findings portray a complex picture regarding attitudes toward end-of-life issues that varied with ethnicity and cultural change as well as their interaction. The results suggest that people are more attuned (relative to 30 years earlier) to matters surrounding the quality of their lives and relationships with others as dying persons, the degree of control that they desire over the end of their lives, and the manner in which they would relate to others who are dying; however, this did vary somewhat by ethnicity. These shifts likely reflect experiences with death, hospice care, and shifting values regarding expectations of physicians' role in making end-of-life decisions and perhaps signal greater attention to both ethnic and age-related variations in such attitudes.

There also is an emerging, albeit limited, literature speaking to views and customs surrounding dying among culturally diverse subgroups. These groups include Native Americans (emphasizing the holistic nature of treatment via the shaman and the deterministic nature of death; see Carrese & Rhodes, 1995; Cox, 2003); Hindus (stressing the fulfillment of the physical body's purpose at death of being the medium through which life is experienced and its nonequivalence to one's true identity; see Rambachan, 2003); Muslims (stressing dying as a distinctly familial, exclusive of children, experience and emphasizing the confession of faith when death is near; see Sultan, 2003); Japanese (stressing the attempted resuscitation of the dying person; see Suzuki, 2003); Chinese (stressing the preparation of the body as key in determining soul satisfaction; see Crowder, 2003); and Jews (stressing the reduction of pain and suffering, subject to opposition to the artificial extension of life when it is clear that the physician can do no more to ease one's pain or cure one of a disease; see Schindler, 2003). This literature, though limited, reinforces the need to attend not only to the multiple aspects of cultural diversity and how they have an impact on the way the dying process is conceptualized but also to consider diversity in the context of cultural change.

□ The Influence of Culture on End-of-Life Choices

In examining research exploring the influence of culture on end-of-life choices, it is important to recognize that studies vary in terms of the specific nature of the issues addressed, and that some studies are purely descriptive (focusing on a single, and often small, sample), and others are comparative in nature, although these samples may also be small and unrepresentative. For example, Blackhall, Murphy, Frank, Michel, and Azen (1995) found that Korean Americans and Mexican Americans were more likely than were European Americans and African Americans to favor a family-centered decision-making model over a patient-centered autonomy model (i.e., the patient should be informed of a terminal diagnosis and make end-of-life treatment decisions) (see also Barrett & Heller,

2002). Hopp and Duffy (2000) and Torke, Garas, Sexson, and Branch (2005) found African Americans to favor, more than Whites, the use of any type of medical care to prolong life. Moseley et al. (2004) similarly found Whites to favor the withdrawal of life-sustaining treatment for an infant more than African Americans. Smith (2004) found African Americans to favor the primacy of the family in concert with the dying person's wishes regarding treatment near the end of life, often relying on their religious or spiritual beliefs to guide them in this process. Findings from SUPPORT (Study to Understand Prognoses and Preferences for Outcomes and Risks of Treatment) suggested that seriously ill African Americans are more likely to favor the use of cardiopulmonary resuscitation (CPR) in extending life than seriously ill White patients (Borum, Lynn, & Zhong, 2000). Kiely, Mitchell, Marlow, Murphy, and Morris (2001) found Whites, relative to minority groups, were more likely to have a living will or have a do not resuscitate (DNR) order (see also Murphy et al., 1996). Such differences between African Americans and Whites also have been reported in instances involving patients with Alzheimer's disease (Owen, Goode, & Haley, 2001).

Other research exploring end-of-life attitudes among a variety of minority subgroups, such as native-born Chinese or Chinese Americans (Fielding & Hung, 1996; Yick & Gupta, 2002), Greeks (Papadatou, Yfabtopoulos & Kosmidis, 2001), Latinos (Sullivan, 2001), Bosnian immigrants (Searight & Gafford, 2005), Hawaiians and Filipinos (Braun, Onaka, & Horiuchi, 2001; Braun, Tanji, & Heck, 2001), and Black Caribbeans (Koffman & Higginson, 2001) uniformly suggests rejection of a Western cultural emphasis on patient autonomy in decision making.

In addition to race, ethnicity, and culture, several other variables contribute to a sensitivity to individuals' preferences, values, and understanding as they relate to end-of-life decision making. In this context, we discuss the importance of age, gender, and sexual orientation.

Age

A fair amount of research has examined the possible influences of age on beliefs about end-of-life issues and decisions. Such work reflects the diversity that exists among older relative to younger persons (see Nelson & Dannefer, 1992), with the variability among older persons regarding end-of-life choices evident regarding (a) context (e.g., whether one is dying at home or in a hospice context vs. an institutional one such as a hospital or nursing home); (b) past experience with chronic or terminal illness; and (c) adherence to values that stress the transcendence of life in death (see Decker & Reed, 2005). Indeed, Schroepfer (2006) found terminally ill older persons to hold very diverse values regarding their readiness to die, which would likely have definite implications for end-of-life choices such persons might make.

Wellman and Sugarman (1999) explored differences between older and younger adults' views on treatment withdrawal (death following CPR attempt after the patient had earlier refused to continue medical treatment) and treatment withholding (death following CPR withholding pursuant to a request for no extraordinary measures for extending life) by randomly assigning younger and elder participants to one of five conditions. Each condition presented a different vignette describing a death after CPR failure that varied regarding the patient's preferences specific to end-of-life treatment options. Findings indicated that students judged the patient's actions as more suicidal and less intentional than did elders. The authors attributed this difference to elders being more understanding of patient's decisions to request no further treatment beyond a certain point. Elders were also less likely to hold negative attributions toward the more intentional (suicidal) actions of others at the end of life.These findings may have implications for the acceptability of DNR orders, living wills, and assisted suicide among different age groups. Many of these issues were considered extreme until the emergence of highly publicized cases like that of Terri Schiavo and the actions of Dr. Jack Kevorkian. These apparent age effects may therefore be alternatively interpreted as artifacts of historical changes in persons' exposure to high-profile cases involving end-of-life decision making, the acceptability and availability of hospice care, or the preference for life-extending treatments that were not available decades ago (see Hayslip & Peveto, 2005; Hayslip, Servaty, & Guarnaccia, 1999).

Hall, Gallagher, Gracely, Knowlton, and Weschules (2003), studying differences in age, gender, and cancer location on the amount of a final dose of opioids prescribed to terminally ill hospice patients, found a negative relationship between age and final dosage amount. The authors attributed such differences to less-severe and less-frequent pain complaints among older (vs. younger) adults, although there is debate about whether older adults are simply less sensitive to pain or have more tolerance to it. The finding that elders tend to be less likely to request pain relief, even in the face of significant pain, during the dying process has financial implications for such persons given the rising cost of pharmaceuticals. However, it may also be the case that offering more pain reduction medications would be greatly appreciated once cost is taken out of the discussion. Furthermore, elderly cancer patients may be harboring feelings that they are not worthy of more expensive medication aimed at decreasing their suffering; this again may reflect a possible cohort effect.

Cicirelli, MacLean, and Cox (2000) explored the role of age in hypothetical end-of-life decisions regarding extending life with all available medical treatment, preferring assisted suicide and refusing treatment, or refusing treatment only among a community-based sample of elderly adults. Although religiosity and two life values (quality and preservation of life) displayed the largest mean differences across scenarios and predicted the importance of refusing treatment (vs. extending life), age did not differentiate participants' endorsement of any of three end-of-life decisions (extending life, refusing treatment, and assisted suicide and refusal of treatment) after having read the scenarios. Age also did not correlate with whether respondents would use all available treatments to sustain life, refuse further treatment only, or a combination of preferring assisted suicide and refusing of treatment.

Some work has explored age differences in death meanings and death fears, which are likely to influence decisions about treatment at the end of life (see Turner, 2002). Cicirelli (2001), for instance, sought to document age and gender differences in these areas but found that of four death meaning subscales, only death as a motivator was related to age, with younger participants scoring higher than older participants. Younger participants also showed greater fear of the dying process, fear for significant others (after one's own death), and fear of the unknown than older participants. Cicirelli discussed these results in terms of older participants having less fear of dying because of greater acceptance of death as a result of having achieved their goals.

The Cicirelli (2001) and Cicirelli et al. (2000) studies lend further support for theories of death acceptance as a framework within which to understand older persons' end-of-life choices. It seems likely that as one ages, death becomes an increasingly salient issue and perhaps requires individuals to eventually accept the inevitable. To the extent to which one's competence to make such decisions has received some attention in the literature (e.g., Cohen, 2003; Condilis, Foti, & Holzer, 2004; Galbraith & Dobson, 2000; Nolan et al., 2005), it is clear that the lack of such competence would likely shift the burden of decision making to the physician or to the family, in which clear communication, understanding, and empathy would hopefully yield agreement regarding end-of-life matters.

The work mentioned seems to indicate that discussing end-of-life decisions may not be as sensitive an area for those of advanced age as formerly assumed and indicates that a person's religious/spiritual beliefs are likely to be salient influences on end-of-life choices among older adults (see Cicirelli, 1997, 1998). Interestingly, Moore and Sherman (1999) found that although older persons favored the completion of advance directives, discussing such issues with children and grandchildren proved to be more difficult. Spiritual and religious beliefs played a central role in such decisions, especially for elderly minority group members (Moore & Sherman).

However, as illustrated in Richard's story (Richard & Lyon, chapter 2, this volume), there can be a complex interaction of age, race, and spirituality. Despite the fact that Richard was young, he had already experienced the loss of his mother to AIDS and thus was not only ready to discuss advance care decision making but also demonstrated elements characteristic of older adults in that quality of life and futility were chief concerns for him. This is an important example of how elements of diversity and experience interact and rarely operate in isolation from one another.

Gender

There is considerable overlap among age and gender research in end-of-life decisions as age is often confounded with gender simply because of gender differences, currently favoring women, in life expectancy. Still, as women outlive men, gender is likely to play a central role in understanding end-of-life decisions. Gender takes on added significance when one considers choices faced by many elderly couples in light of the nature and length of their relationships prior to the death of one member. Therefore, although end-of-life decisions are likely to be different for men and women near the end of life, especially in later life, our review suggests that the empirical literature provides no evidence of a consistent gender effect.

As mentioned, death anxiety is often relevant to end-of-life decisions. Depaola, Griffin, Young, and Neimeyer (2003) compared the potential effects of gender, age, and ethnicity among older adults on the eight subscales of the Multidimensional Fear of Death Scale (MFODS). Only the Fear of the Dead subscale was sensitive to gender, with women reporting more fear of the dead. Cicirelli (2001) found that women tended to score higher on the Death as Extinction scale than did men, and women also reported more fear of the dying process and less fear of the unknown than did men. Indeed, women identified death as the end of one's existence, and thus it may be possible that they would have less fear of the unknown because, for women, death is not represented as embodying an unknown afterlife.

Bookwala, Coppola, and Fagerlin (2001) found that among four types of life-sustaining treatments, men tended to have significantly stronger preferences than women for (a) CPR and artificial nutrition and hydration; (b) life-sustaining treatments in three of nine hypothetical health situations; and (c) life-sustaining treatment when considering composite ratings across scenarios; however, women placed more value on the desire for a dignified death than men. Women, therefore, may be more likely to seek preventive and curative treatments. Gallagher-Thompson, Dillinger, and Gray (2006) argued that in exploring end-of-life concerns among older women, a multitude of influences on such decisions must be acknowledged: idiosyncratic life experiences, views regarding dying and death, degree of psychosocial adjustment, and cultural influences.

Sexual Orientation

There is some systematic work reporting the influence of sexual orientation on end-of-life issues, specifically with respect to patients with AIDS and clinicians who work with them (Bodnar, 1997; Eisold, 1997). Gay, lesbian, and bisexual individuals are likely to have differing views regarding end-of-life issues, such as fear of death; amount, duration, or rigor of treatments requested; and values concerning assisted suicide or withdrawal of treatment or DNR orders. Indeed, a person's diagnosis may serve as a moderating variable, such that specific diagnoses, given differing associated dying trajectories (Corr et al., 2006), allow for more or fewer opportunities to make end-of-life choices or express preferences for treatment. Thus, for those who are HIV positive, values regarding quality of life, dependency, and the sanctity of life are likely to have increasing impact on decisions to terminate treatment as the disease progresses and patients become weaker. Of course, the degree of centrality of sexual orientation (and ethnic identity) in terms of an individual's identity likely influences a person's decisions concerning end-of-life issues.

□ Physicians, Patients, and Families, and End-of-Life Care

A large majority of persons confronting end-of-life issues do so under the care of a physician, and in the context of end-of-life choices, the family's working relationship with their physician is crucial. To the extent that the patient's and the physician's attitudes toward end-of-life care differ, this discrepancy often results in patients and their families feeling disenfranchised relative to the physician in terms of making decisions regarding end-of-life care. Although physicians may assume that they know how to best care for a patient, families of dying persons do not always agree. Such barriers are often borne of uncertainty about what to do, perhaps based on one's personal values that compete with a lack of professional training (Levetown, Hayslip, & Peel, 1999–2000). Physicians who are anxious or uncertain about end-of-life treatment and discussion of this topic may be less likely to determine a plan of care that the patient would desire. Many physicians may believe that they lack alternatives, and because they are anxious, they often take sole responsibility for making treatment decisions, so that a pattern of paternalistic communication emerges between physician and patient as the physician engages in "telling" the patient about end-of-life issues with greater frequency than "asking" (Cohen et al., 2005).

Complicating matters are situations for which there is a need to make decisions for patients who lack decision-making capacity (see section above, The Influence of Culture on End-of-Life Choices). In these cases, physicians often develop a plan of care (Lang & Quill, 2004) independent of family involvement. Indeed, there is some evidence to suggest that physicians and other healthcare providers in the United States frequently neglect living wills, DNR orders, and other advance directives (Hilden, Louhiala, & Palo, 2004), believing that such patients do not understand their decision or are incapable of making an adequate decision. Variation across physicians interacts with patient characteristics such that dying persons who are older, female, depend on others for assistance with activities of daily living, and who perceive that their prognosis is poor have been found to prefer a DNR order (Covinsky et al., 2000).

The work discussed suggests that it is often the case that physicians do not attempt to determine end-of-life preferences of their patients, although most patients expect that the physician will do so, and prefer to frankly discuss changes in their health status and retain control over their situation (Kutner, Steiner, Corbett, Jahnigen, & Barton, 1999). If family members are overlooked by physicians, families feel marginalized in terms of having clear communication with their physicians (Russ & Kaufman, 2005), despite being a valuable source of objective information on the patient (see McPherson & Addington-Hall, 2004). Perhaps because they are not included, family members sometimes report a mistrust of physicians and their motives in treating loved ones (Leichtentritt & Rettig, 2002).

□ Conclusions and Recommendations

Being able to acknowledge the importance of cultural diversity and minority groups' preferences related to end-of-life decision making depends in part on understanding the construct of diversity itself in all of its complexity. Likewise, it is important to recognize that the cultural context in which such decisions are made also changes. Such variations affect (and are affected by) a person's perceived options for care near the end of life; the dynamics among physicians, families, and dying persons themselves; and the institutional context (e.g., nursing homes, hospitals, hospices) in which dying occurs.

In concert with cultural diversity, appreciating that interindividual variability should be considered along multiple parameters (e.g., age, gender, race/ethnicity, decision-making capacity, and sexual orientation) is also vitally important to understanding diversity as it relates to end-of-life care. Ultimately, realizing that multiple influences are operating when such decisions are made is key to understanding the barriers to creating an open context for communication (Glaser & Strauss, 1968). For example, the balance of power often favors physicians and lawyers in such matters, which can negatively affect openness and respect among participants. Clearly, a lack of understanding and sensitivity to diversity can interfere with clear and empathic communication with family members near the end of life.

Although Hallenbeck and Goldstein (1999) have argued that the acquisition of *cultural competence*—an appreciation for the differences between cultures and ethnic groups—is crucial in understanding preferences for end-of-life care (e.g., truth-telling, the use of informed consent, and advance directives), it is equally important to acknowledge the impact of negative dynamics created by a lack of sensitivity to individual differences. Some people desire an active role in such processes, whereas others prefer to defer to the physician or other healthcare professionals or other family members or loved ones; many families see themselves as responsible for protecting the dying individual from information that might be upsetting or undermine the hope of recovery or at least remission (see Turner, 2002). Thus, we argue that it is important to acknowledge diversity not only both within and across ethnic groups, but also within and across other groups, such as generational groups, wherein the importance of cultural change is likely to create cohort differences between both patients and family members and younger physicians. Similarly, awareness of diversity also needs to reflect differences across both gender and sexual orientation. In these respects, our knowledge base is more restricted, and thus examining more fully the impact of individual difference variables on end-of-life choices will be an important task confronting researchers and practitioners in the future.

In this context, as Turner (2002, p. 290) cogently stated, "If physicians ignore family requests, they risk alienating patients [and families] by communicating in a style that patients regard as blunt, harmful, uncaring, and unprofessional." However, Western cultural values emphasizing patient/person autonomy may not be understood or shared, and in fact may be rejected, by persons whose cultural heritage or individual life experiences (covarying with age, gender, or sexual orientation) to greater or lesser degrees emphasize respect for authority, collectivistic decision making, or peace at life's end (Barrett & Heller, 2002; Carrese & Rhodes, 1995; Hallenbeck & Goldstein, 1999).

One solution that has been proposed to such difficulties is to conduct a cultural ethnography with patients to explore their understanding of the illness, the nature of their understanding of suffering, and their values and goals given the limited time they have to live (see Krakauer, Crenner, & Fox, 2002). Kagawa-Singer and Blackhall (2001) recommended the physician ask culturally sensitive questions to understand the patient's identity. Such sensitivity can be understood along a number of dimensions:

(a) attitudes toward truth-telling; (b) religious or spiritual beliefs; (c) languages spoken, experience with poverty and discrimination, degree of integration into one's ethnic community; (d) whether decisions are patient centered or family centered; and (e) if resources are available to understand this person's cultural heritage and beliefs (e.g., interpreters, healthcare workers from similar backgrounds, family members, community or religious leaders). Such guidelines are consistent with the view of culture as a medium through which individual attitudes and behaviors are expressed (see Cole, 1999) versus an exclusive focus on an awareness of cultural differences per se. Similar recommendations regarding the culturalization of communication near the end of life have been made by Werth et al. (2002). In light of the cohort-specific life experiences regarding death and dying (see Hayslip & Peveto, 2005; Hayslip et al., 1999) that might differentiate younger professionals and older persons, exploring older patients' views on end-of-life issues is even more imperative, as is listening to persons of a different gender or sexual orientation. Such influences may be seen either as embedded in a cultural context or as forces with an impact on this context.

As Turner (2002) noted, avoiding communicative difficulties facilitates the patient's ability to provide informed consent regarding healthcare decisions near the end of life and, if desired, executing an advanced directive. One cannot make choices regarding issues about which one is ill-informed or if one's individual values, preferences, and opinions have not been explored, acknowledged, or validated, especially if such choices ultimately reflect the decision *not* to make a decision or allow someone else to make a decision about the quality of care one receives near the end of life (see Crow, chapter 4, this volume). Complicating interindividual communicative dilemmas are institutional barriers (lack of health insurance among minority groups, underrepresentation of minorities in medicine) that can only be addressed at the societal level (Krakauer et al., 2002). In addition, in view of the communicative difficulties that physicians and nurses often experience (see Levetown et al., 1999–2000) and recent failures to improve patient care outcomes and communication via purposeful interventions to enhance physician-patient communication (see, e.g., Borum et al., 2000), guidelines to improve such communication and restore decision-making power to patients and families when this is desired should be more forcefully enacted. We also advocate the use of flexible, patient-centered methods, especially in concert with more empathic and factual communication in the context of cultural competency to avoid the disenfranchisement of patients and families in making end-of-life choices. Indeed, adopting a "person-centered" approach in fact requires understanding, acknowledging, and encouraging diversity in the context of racial, ethnic, and other person-specific factors that influence what patients and families decide is best for them near the end of life.

References

American Health Decisions. (1997). *The quest to die with dignity.* Appleton, WI: American Health Decisions.

American Psychological Association. (2003). Guidelines on multicultural education, training, research, practice, and organizational change for psychologists. *American Psychologist, 58,* 377–402.

Barrett, R., & Heller, K. (2002). Death and dying in the black experience. *Journal of Palliative Medicine, 5,* 795–799.

Berry, J., Trimble, J., & Olmedo, E. (1986). Assessment of acculturation. In W. Lonner & J. Berry (Eds.), *Field methods in cross-cultural research* (pp. 291–324). Newbury Park, CA: Sage.

Blackhall, L., Murphy, S., Frank, G., Michel, V., & Azen, S. (1995). Ethnicity and attitudes toward patient autonomy. *Journal of the American Medical Association, 274,* 820–826.

Bodnar, S. (1997). Dances with men: The impact of multiple losses in my practice of psychoanalytically informed psychotherapy. In M. J. Belchner (Ed.), *Hope and mortality: Psychodynamic approaches to AIDS and HIV* (pp. 221–235). Hillsdale, NJ: Analytic Press.

Bookwala, J., Coppola, K., & Fagerlin, A. (2001). Gender differences in older adults' preferences for life-sustaining medical treatments and end-of-life values. *Death Studies, 25,* 127–149.

Borum, M., Lynn, J., & Zhong, Z. (2000). The effects of patient race on outcomes in seriously ill patients in SUPPORT: An overview of economic impact, medical intervention, and end-of-life decisions. *Journal of the American Geriatrics Society, 48,* S194–S198.

Braun, K., Onaka, A., & Horiuchi, B. (2001). Advance directive completion rates and end-of-life preferences in Hawaii. *Journal of the American Geriatrics Society, 49,* 1708–1713.

Braun, K., Tanji, V., & Heck, R. (2001). Support for physician assisted suicide: Exploring the impact of ethnicity and attitudes toward planning for death. *The Gerontologist, 41,* 51–60.

Brofenbrenner, U. (1979). *The ecology of human development: Experiments by nature and design.* Cambridge, MA: Harvard University Press.

Carr, D. (2003). A "good death" for whom? Quality of spouse's death and psychological distress among older widowed persons. *Journal of Health and Social Behavior, 44,* 215–232.

Carrese, J., & Rhodes, L. (1995). Western bioethics on the Navajo reservation. *Journal of the American Medical Association, 274,* 826–829.

Cicirelli, V. G. (1997). Relationship of psychosocial and background variables to older adults' end-of-life decisions. *Psychology and Aging, 12,* 72–83.

Cicirelli, V. G. (1998). Views of elderly people concerning end-of-life decisions. *Journal of Applied Gerontology, 17,* 186–203.

Cicirelli, V. G. (2001). Personal meanings of death in older adults and young adults in relation to their fears of death. *Death Studies, 25,* 663–683.

Cicirelli, V. G., MacLean, A. P., & Cox, L. S. (2000). Hastening death: A comparison of two end-of-life decisions. *Death Studies, 24,* 401–419.

Cohen, D. (2003). End of life issues for caregivers of individuals with Alzheimer's disease and related dementias. *Journal of Mental Health and Aging, 9*, 3–7.

Cohen, S., Sprung, C., Sjokvist, P., Lippert, A., Ricou, B., Baras, M., et al. (2005). Communication of end-of-life decisions in European intensive care units. *Intensive Care Medicine, 31*, 1215–1221.

Cole, M. (1999). Culture in development. In M. Bornstein & M. Lamb (Eds.), *Developmental psychology: An advanced textbook* (pp. 73–124). Mahwah, NJ: Erlbaum.

Condilis, P. J., Foti, M. E. G., & Holzer, J. C. (2004). End-of-life care and mental illness: A model for community psychiatry and beyond. *Community Mental Heath Journal, 40*, 3–6.

Connidis, I. (2001). *Family ties and aging.* Newbury Park, CA: Sage.

Corr, C., Nabe, C., & Corr, D. (2006). *Death and dying: Life and living.* Belmont, CA: Thomson.

Covinsky, K. E., Fuller, J. D., Yaffe, K., Johnston, C. B., Hamel, M. B., Lynn, J., et al. (2000). Communication and decision-making in seriously ill patients: findings of the support project. *Journal of the American Geriatrics Society, 48*, S187–S193.

Cox, G. R. (2003). The Native American way of death. In C. Bryant (Ed.), *The handbook of death and dying: Volume 2* (pp. 631–639). Thousand Oaks, CA: Sage.

Crowder, L. S. (2003). The Taoist (Chinese) way of death. In C. Bryant (Ed.), *The handbook of death and dying: Volume 2* (pp. 673–686). Thousand Oaks, CA: Sage.

Decker, I., & Reed, P. (2005). Developmental and contextual correlates of elders' anticipated end-of-life treatment decisions. *Death Studies, 29*, 827–846.

Depaola, S. J., Griffin, M., Young, J. R., & Neimeyer, R. A. (2003). Death anxiety and attitudes toward the elderly among older adults: The role of gender and ethnicity. *Death Studies, 27*, 335–354.

Doka, K. J. (2002). *Disenfranchised grief: New directions, challenges, and strategies for practice.* Champaign, IL: Research Press.

Eisold, B. K. (1997). Disease, death, and group process from a psychodynamic point of view. In M. J. Blechner (Ed.), *Hope and mortality: Psychodynamic approaches to AIDS and HIV* (pp. 175–191). Hillsdale, NJ: Analytic Press.

Fielding, R., & Hung, J. (1996). Preferences for information and involvement in decisions during cancer care among a Hong Kong Chinese population. *Psych-oncology, 5*, 321–329.

Fiske, S. T. (2004). *Social beings: A core motives approach to social psychology.* Hoboken, NJ: Wiley.

Galbraith, K. M., & Dobson, K. S. (2000). The role of the psychologist in determining competence for assisted suicide/euthanasia in the terminally ill. *Canadian Psychology, 41*, 174–183.

Gallagher-Thompson, D., Dillinger, J., & Gray, H. L. (2006). Women's issues at the end-of-life. In J. Worell & C. D. Goodheart (Eds.), *Handbook of girl's and women's psychological health: Gender and well-being across the lifespan* (pp. 406–415). New York: Oxford University Press.

Gallup Organization. (1996). *Knowledge and values related to hospice care.* Arlington, VA: National Hospice Organization.

Glaser, B., & Strauss, A. (1968). *Time for dying.* Chicago: Aldine.

Hall, S., Gallagher, R. M., Gracely, E., Knowlton, C., & Weschules, D. (2003). The terminal cancer patient: Effects of age, gender, and primary tumor site on opioid dose. *Pain Medicine, 4*, 125–134.

Hallenbeck, J., & Goldstein, M. (1999). Decisions at the end-of-life: Cultural considerations beyond medical ethics. *Generations, 23,* 24–29.
Hansson, R. O., & Stroebe, M. S. (2007). *Bereavement in late life: Coping, adaptation, and developmental influences.* Washington, DC: American Psychological Association.
Harvard Medical School Ad Hoc Committee to Examine the Definition of Brain Death. (1968). A definition of irreversible coma. *Journal of the American Medical Association, 205,* 337–340.
Hayslip, B., & Hansson, R. (2006). Hospice. In J. E. Birren (Ed.), *Encyclopedia of gerontology* (2nd ed., pp. 1–10). Oxford, England: Elsevier.
Hayslip, B., & Peveto, C. (2005). *Cultural changes in attitudes toward death, dying, and bereavement.* New York: Springer.
Hayslip, B., Servaty, H. L., & Guarnaccia, C. (1999). Age cohort differences in perceptions of funerals. In B. deVries (Ed.), *End-of-life issues: Interdisciplinary and multidimensional perspectives* (pp. 23–36). New York: Springer.
Health Communication Research Institute. (1996). *Telephone survey on end-of-life decision-making.* Sacramento, CA: Sacramental Health Care Decisions.
Hilden, H.-M., Louhiala, P., & Palo, J. (2004). End-of-life decisions: Attitudes of Finnish physicians. *Journal of Medical Ethics, 30,* 362–365.
Hopp, F., & Duffy, S. (2000). Racial variations in end-of-life care. *Journal of the American Geriatrics Society, 48,* 658–663.
Kagawa-Singer, M., & Blackhall, L. (2001). Negotiating cross cultural issues at the end-of-life. *Journal of the American Medical Association, 286,* 2993–3001.
Kalish, R. A., & Reynolds, D. K. (1976). *Death and ethnicity: A psychocultural study.* Los Angeles: University of Southern California Press.
Kastenbaum, R. (1998). *Death, society, and human experience.* Boston: Allyn & Bacon.
Kiely, D., Mitchell, S., Marlow, A., Murphy, K., & Morris, J. (2001). Racial and state differences in the designation of advanced directives in nursing home patients. *Journal of the American Geriatrics Society, 49,* 1346–1352.
Klass, D. (2001). Continuing bonds in the resolution of grief in Japan and North America. *American Behavioral Scientist, 44,* 742–763.
Koffman, J., & Higginson, I. (2001). Accounts of carers' satisfaction with health care at the end-of-life: A comparison of first generation black Caribbean's and white patients with advanced disease. *Palliative Medicine, 15,* 337–345.
Krakauer, E., Crenner, C., & Fox, K. (2002). Barriers to optimum end-of-life care for minority patients. *Journal of the American Geriatrics Society, 50,* 182–190.
Kutner, J. S., Steiner, J. F., Corbett, K. K., Jahnigen, D. W., & Barton, P. L. (1999). Information needs in terminal illness. *Social Science and Medicine, 48,* 1341–1352.
Lamb, V. L. (2003). Historical and epidemiological trends in mortality in the United States. In C. L. Bryant (Ed.), *Handbook of death and dying* (Vol. 1, pp. 185–197). Newbury Park, CA: Sage.
Lang, F., & Quill, T. (2004). Making decisions with families at the end-of-life. *American Family Physician, 70,* 719–723.
Leichtentritt, R. D., & Rettig, K. D. (2002). Family beliefs about end-of-life decisions: An interpersonal perspective. *Death Studies, 26,* 567–594.
Levetown, M., Hayslip, B., & Peel, J. (1999–2000). The development of the physicians' attitudes toward end-of-life attitude scale. *Omega: Journal of Death and Dying, 40,* 323–334.

McPherson, C. J., & Addington-Hall, J. M. (2004). Evaluating palliative care: Bereaved family members' evaluations of patients' pain, anxiety, and depression. *Journal of Pain and Symptom Management, 28,* 104–114.

Meyerowitz, B. E., Richardson, J., Hudson, S., & Leedham, B. (1998). Ethnicity and cancer outcomes: Behavioral and psychosocial considerations. *Psychological Bulletin, 123,* 47–70.

Moore, C., & Sherman, S. (1999). Factors that influence elders' decisions to formulate advanced directives. *Journal of Gerontological Social Work, 31,* 21–39.

Moseley, K., Chuch, A., Hempel, B., Yuan, H., Goold, S., & Freed, G. (2004). End-of-life choices for African American and white infants in a neonatal intensive care unit: A pilot study. *Journal of the National Medical Association, 96,* 117–124.

Mrozeck, D., Spiro, A., & Griffin, P. (2006). Personality and aging. In J. Birren & K. W. Schaie (Eds.), *Handbook of the psychology of aging* (pp. 357–379). San Diego, CA: Academic Press.

Murphy, S., Palmer, J., Azen, S., Frank, G., Michel, V., & Blackhall, L. (1996). Ethnicity and advanced care directives. *Journal of Law, Medicine, and Ethics, 24,* 108–117.

Nelson, E., & Dannefer, D. (1992). Aged heterogeneity: Fact or fiction? The fate of diversity in gerontological research. *The Gerontologist, 32,* 17–23.

Nolan, M. T., Hughes, M., Narendra, P., Sood, J. R., Terry, P. B., Atrow, A. B., et al. (2005). When patients lack capacity: the roles that patients with terminal diagnoses would choose for their physicians and loved ones in making medical decisions. *Journal of Pain and Symptom Management, 30,* 342–352.

Owen, J., Goode, K., & Haley, W. (2001). End-of-life care and reactions to death among African American and white family caregivers of relatives with Alzheimer's disease. *Omega: Journal of Death and Dying, 43,* 349–361.

Papadatou, D., Yfabtopoulos, J., & Kosmidis, H. (2001). Death of a child at home in hospital: Experiences of Greek mothers. *Death Studies, 20,* 215–235.

Patient Self-Determination Act of 1990, Publ. L. No. 101–508, 4206, 4751. of the Omnibus Reconciliation Act of 1990.

Phinney, J. S. (1990). Ethnic identity in adolescents and adults: Review of research. *Psychological Bulletin, 108,* 499–514.

Rambachan, A. (2003). The Hindu way of death. In C. Bryant (Ed.), *The handbook of death and dying* (Vol. 2, pp. 640–648). Thousand Oaks, CA: Sage.

Rosenblatt, P. C. (2001). A social constructionist perspective on cultural differences in grief. In M. S. Stroebe, R. O. Hansson, W. Stroebe, & H. Schut (Eds.), *Handbook of bereavement research: Consequences, coping and care* (pp. 285–300). Washington, DC: American Psychological Association.

Rosenblatt, P. C. (in press). Grief across cultures: A review and research agenda. In M. S. Stroebe, R. O. Hansson, H. Schut, & W. Stroebe (Eds.), *Handbook of bereavement research and practice: 21st century perspectives.* Washington, DC: American Psychological Association.

Russ, A. J., & Kaufman, S. R. (2005). Family perceptions of prognosis, silence and the "suddenness" of death. *Culture, Medicine, and Psychiatry, 29,* 103–123.

Schaie, K. W. (2005). *Developmental influences on adult intelligence.* New York: Oxford.

Schein, E. H. (2004). *Organizational culture and leadership* (3rd ed.). San Francisco: Jossey-Bass.

Schindler, R. (2003). The Jewish way of death. In C. Bryant (Ed.), *The handbook of death and dying* (Vol. 2, pp. 687–693). Thousand Oaks, CA: Sage.

Schroepfer, T. A. (2006). Mind frames toward dying and factors motivating their adoption by ill elders. *Journal of Gerontology: Social Sciences, 61B,* S129–S139.

Searight, H., & Gafford, J. (2005). "It's like playing with your destiny": Bosnian immigrants' views of advanced directives and end-of-life care decision-making. *Journal of Immigrant Health, 7,* 195–203.

Smith, S. (2004). End-of-life decision-making processes of African American families: Implications for culturally sensitive social work practice. *Journal of Ethnic and Cultural Diversity, 13,* 1–23.

Sternberg, R. J. (2004). Culture and intelligence. *American Psychologist, 59,* 325–338.

Sullivan, M. C. (2001). Lost in translation: How Latinos view end-of-life care. *Plastic Surgical Nursing, 21,* 90–91.

Sultan, D. H. (2003). The Muslim way of death. In C. Bryant (Ed.), *The handbook of death and dying* (Vol. 2, pp. 649–655). Thousand Oaks, CA: Sage.

Suzuki, H. (2003). The Japanese way of death. In C. Bryant (Ed.), *The handbook of death and dying* (Vol. 2, pp. 656–672). Thousand Oaks, CA: Sage.

Torke, A., Garas, N., Sexson, W., & Branch, W. (2005). Medical care at the end-of-life: Views of African American patients in an urban hospital. *Journal of Palliative Medicine, 8,* 593–602.

Turner, L. (2002). Bioethics and end-of-life care in multi-ethnic settings: Cultural diversity in Canada and the USA. *Mortality, 7,* 285–301.

Uhlenberg, P., & Kirby, J. B. (1998). Grandparent over time: Historical and demographic trends. In M. Szinovacz (Ed.), *Handbook on grandparenthood* (pp. 23–39). Westport, CT: Greenwood Press.

U.S. Census Bureau. (2001). *U.S. Census 2000, summary Files 1 and 2.* Retrieved May 13, 2003, from http://www.census.gov/main/www/cen2000.html

Values Near the End of Lives. (2001). *Grassroots perspectives and cultural diversity and end-of-life care.* Retrieved April 4, 2007, from http://www.ahd.org/ahd/library/position/ValuesEnd.html

Wellman, R. J., & Sugarman, D. B. (1999). Elder and young adults' perceptions of the decision to withdraw from medical treatment: A replication and extension. *Journal of Social Behavior and Personality, 14,* 287–298.

Werth, J. L., Jr., Blevins, D., Toussaint, K., & Durham, M. (2002). The influence of cultural diversity on end-of-life care decisions. *American Behavioral Scientist, 46,* 204–219.

Yick, A., & Gupta, R. (2002). Chinese cultural dimensions of death, dying, and bereavement: Focus group findings. *Journal of Cultural Diversity, 9,* 32–42.

18

CHAPTER

Decisions by and for Adults With Questionable Mental Capacity

Focus on Dementia

Ladislav Volicer

□ Introduction

Alzheimer's disease gradually impairs not only memory but also executive function (i.e., higher thought processes) of the affected individuals. Executive function is impaired even earlier in dementia. Progressive dementias also lead to development of language impairment that involves comprehension difficulties and speech deficits. These impairments eventually prevent individuals suffering from progressive dementias from making decisions regarding their finances and place of residence and ultimately decisions regarding their medical care. However, development of these impairments is gradual and insidious, and it is not easy to determine when an individual with dementia cannot make a specific decision. It is important to realize that decision-making capacity is decision specific, and individuals with dementia might be still able to make some simple choices while they are unable to make others that are more complicated. For example, the individual may be able to make appropriate choice about the clothes to wear while not understanding the complex issues involved in making decisions regarding medical versus surgical therapy of coronary artery disease.

□ Decision-Making Capacity

Healthcare providers may err by both overestimation and underestimation of capacity to make decisions regarding health care. Overestimation may occur because individuals are often not tested for their cognitive functioning and may be proficient in covering up their cognitive impairment. Overestimation of decision-making capacity is more common if the patient agrees with the healthcare provider (Pomerantz & de Nesnera, 1991). Underestimation of decision-making capacity may occur if an individual carries a diagnosis of Alzheimer's disease or another progressive dementia and a health practitioner erroneously assumes that the diagnosis itself makes the person unable to make decisions (Ganzini, Volicer, Nelson, Fox, & Derse, 2004). Underestimation of decision-making capacity is especially common in residents of long-term care facilities, who are often considered too impaired to make any decisions (Karlawish & Pearlman, 2003).

Myths Held by Clinicians

Ganzini and colleagues (2004) have identified 10 common myths that clinicians hold about decision-making capacity. They include the belief that decision-making capacity and competency are the same. Actually, competency is a legal determination, and an individual judged incompetent may still have capacity to make some decisions. Another belief is that when a patient makes decisions against medical advice, he or she is lacking decision-making capacity. It is important to explore the reasons for this decision because the patient may be able to rationally explain it. Some clinicians believe that once a person lacks decision-making capacity, he or she will never be able to make decisions again. However, cognitive ability fluctuates even in individuals with progressive dementia who may be temporarily impaired by another concurrent disease. Therefore, it is important to evaluate decision-making capacity whenever a decision has to be made. Another wrong belief is that only mental health experts can assess decision-making capacity. Actually, this assessment is best performed by the clinician who is responsible for the patient's care because he or she knows the patient the best (Markson, Kern, Annas, & Glantz, 1994).

Standards and Measurement

Depending on what perspective is adopted, four or five standards have been proposed as necessary to ensure that an individual possesses decision-making capacity (Table 18.1). Standards proposed by Marson's group (Earnst, Marson, & Harrell, 2000; Marson, Earnst, Jamil, Bartolucci, & Harrell, 2000) are more strict than standards proposed by Grisso and Appelbaum (1998), but Marson's standards are not uniformly accepted. One problem is that some cognitively intact elderly individuals do not meet all the standards proposed by Marson's group and would require a substitute decision maker. Another problem is that the requirement of "reasonable treatment choices" is open to different interpretations. It could be interpreted as "making decision that a reasonable person in like circumstances would make" (Marson et al., 2000, p. 917). However, this requirement would eliminate the possibility of an individual choice that differs from that of a majority of patients.

Many clinicians do not use the standards consistently in the determination of decision-making capacity of individuals with mild Alzheimer's disease. In one survey, clinicians involved in determining decision-making capacity were presented a vignette of an individual with mild Alzheimer's disease who developed colon cancer and had to decide about undergoing surgical treatment. They were asked which of Marson et al.'s (2000) standards they would consider necessary to determine whether the patient had decision-making capacity. The survey showed that only one third of respondents endorsed all five standards as necessary, and a small proportion of respondents endorsed only one or two elements (Volicer & Ganzini, 2003). These results indicated that clinicians do not use uniform standards for assessment of decision-making capacity.

An alternative recommendation for determining decision-making capacity postulates that not all standards are required for all treatment decisions. Drane (1984) proposed a sliding scale of decision-making capacity that specifies three different levels of standard requirements according to the nature of the decision (Table 18.1). The first level includes treatments that are clearly beneficial and do not pose serious danger—most commonly encountered in the treatment of acute conditions. Decision-making capacity for these treatments would just require awareness of the situation and assent from the patient. If the disease is chronic or the treatment is more dangerous or of less-definite benefit, the decision-making capacity would require understanding of the risks and outcomes of different options and a choice based on this understanding. The third level would apply for decisions that are dangerous and fly in the face of both professional and public rationality. In this situation, decision-making capacity would require appreciation of the consequences of the decision and the patient would have to provide reasons for his or her decisions.

The principle of a sliding scale was endorsed by the President's Commission (1982) and by some ethicists (Pearlman, 1997). However, other authors objected to this method because it is less objective than the strict application of specific standards (Kloezen, Fitten, & Steinberg, 1988). These other

TABLE 18.1 Standards Proposed for Evaluation of Decision-Making Capacity

Grisso et al., 1998	Marson et al., 2000	Drane, 1984
Ability to express a choice Ability to understand information relevant to treatment decision making Ability to appreciate the significance of that information for one's own situation Ability to reason with relevant information to engage in a logical process of weighing treatment options	Simply evidencing a treatment choice Making the reasonable treatment choice (when the alternative is unreasonable) Appreciating the consequences of a treatment choice Providing rational reasons for a choice Understanding the treatment situation on choices	Medical decisions that are not dangerous and objectively are in the patient's best interest: Awareness of situation, assent. Illness is chronic and treatment is more dangerous or has less-definite benefit: Understanding of risks and benefits, choosing based on this understanding Decisions very dangerous that are contrary to professional and public rationality: Appreciation of implications of this decision for one's life, ability to give subjective rational reasons for decision

authors argued that less stringency is achieved because different treatment situations present different levels of complexity for the patient to understand, so Marson et al.'s (2000) five standards should always be used.

Some authors have attempted to develop instruments for the determination of decision-making capacity. A study evaluated three of these instruments—MacArthur Competence Assessment Tool for Treatment (MacCAT-T; Grisso, Appelbaum, & Hill-Fotouhi, 1997; see also Appelbaum & Grisso, 2001), Hopemont Capacity Assessment Interview (HCAI; Edelstein, 2000), and Capacity to Consent to Treatment Instrument (CCTI; Marson, Ingram, Cody, & Harrell, 1995)—in a population of aged cognitively intact individuals and aged individuals with mild or moderate dementia (Moye, Karel, Azar, & Gurrera, 2004). These instruments evaluated decision-making capacity in four areas: understanding, appreciation, reasoning, and expressing a choice. All instruments differentiated between control and demented participants in understanding, but only the CCTI differentiated on appreciation, and only the MacCAT-T and CCTI differentiated on reasoning.

Despite these results, the MacCAT-T seems to be the most popular instrument for decision-making capacity determination. Moye, Karel, Gurrera, and Azar (2006) used it to show that decision-making capacity declines in individuals with dementia within 9 months and therefore should be frequently reevaluated. The MacCAT-T was also used in middle-aged and older patients with schizophrenia; it showed wide variability in performance that was unrelated to demographic characteristics and psychopathology rating (Palmer, Dunn, Appelbaum, & Jeste, 2004). This indicates that demographic characteristics and psychopathology ratings do not provide sufficient information about decision-making capacity in these patients.

Scoring of these instruments requires comparison of individual scores with performance of a cognitively intact control group, which raises a significant issue. It is not clear if the mean scores from the control group in one study could be used to determine decision-making capacity in general clinical practice. It is possible that moderately demented individuals, who do not have the ability to make decisions regarding their care, are still able to appoint a healthcare proxy (Mezey, Teresi, Ramsey, Mitty, & Bobrowitz, 2000).

□ Surrogate Decision Making

With the progression of dementia, all individuals eventually lose their decision-making capacity. It is very often after that point when difficult decisions regarding medical care have to be made. These decisions have to be made by a patient's surrogate or *proxy*. This person could be an individual designated previously by the patient, a guardian appointed by a court, a family member, or a significant friend. When a medical decision must be made after a person has lost decision-making capacity and a proxy has not been named, the U.S. Department of Veterans Affairs and some states have a specific roster that specifies the priority of individuals who can serve as a proxy. In Veterans Affairs hospitals, the hospital director may serve as a proxy for individuals who do not have anybody else, but in general healthcare providers should not serve as a proxy because that could be viewed as a conflict of interest. The proxies make decisions using one of two standards: substituted judgment or best interests (see Ditto, chapter 13, this volume).

Substituted Judgment Standard

Decisions made on the basis of substituted judgment rely on a patient's previous wishes that are known to the proxy. The proxy is supposed to act as if he or she is in the "patient's shoes." The previous wishes of the patient could be expressed either formally through a living will made before the patient became demented or informally through oral communication among the patient and the proxy or others about the patient's philosophy regarding medical interventions if he or she became demented. The problem with living wills and verbal statements is that they are very often quite general and do not cover advanced dementia. It has been reported that choices for other conditions predict poorly what the individual may want if he or she developed dementia (Reilly, Teasdale, & McCullough, 1994). An opportunity for formulation of advance directives is mandated at the time of admission into a nursing home and other healthcare facilities (see Patient Self Determination Act, 1990). Although not the intent of the law, in practice this discussion is often focused primarily on cardiopulmonary resuscitation (CPR) preference and reviewed only after the crisis of acute illness and hospitalization. Advance directive forms often contain inconsistent language and vague conditions for implementation. Therefore, the advance directives often have to be interpreted by the proxy.

If the advance directives are specific and refuse certain treatments, a conflict arises if the proxy does not agree with this treatment limitation. The President's Council on Bioethics (2006) concluded that "Advance instruction directives (or living wills), though valuable to some degree and in some circumstances, are a limited and flawed instrument for addressing most of the decisions caregivers must make for those entrusted to their care" (p. 214) and recommended that the proxies and courts should be able to override wishes expressed in advance directives. However, this recommendation was strongly rejected in a dissenting statement by Rowley (2006), who believed that an individual should have the right to make decisions about future medical care that would be honored without any reservations. The recommendation of the President's Council on Bioethics also does not take into consideration that some states require the existence of a specific advance directive if a proxy wants to discontinue tube feeding. Therefore, even though some advance directives may not be specific enough and have to be interpreted by a proxy, it is still better for both the patient and the proxy if the patient expressed previous wishes by executing advance directives.

The prevalence of advance directives/living wills among nursing home residents varies from state to state, with Ohio having almost a 10-fold higher prevalence than California, Massachusetts, and New York (Kiely, Mitchell, Marlow, Murphy, & Morris, 2001). There are some gender differences in end-of-life care preferences, with men preferring more life-sustaining treatments and women preferring a more dignified death (Bookwala et al., 2001). Age at which the individuals are asked about their preferences also plays a role, with individuals 70 years old or older stating that the most important factor for CPR decision is "I do not want to be a burden on my family," while younger individuals' most important factor is "I want to retain my capacity to think clearly" (Mead et al., 1995). The prevalence of advance directives in a nursing home is increased if the proxies have advance directives themselves, if the proxies are less religious, and if the residents are socially engaged (Allen et al., 2003).

Most of the research involving the healthcare team has focused on physicians' roles. Involvement of physicians is very important for establishment of advance directives. Physicians reported in a survey that 81% counseled their patients regarding advance planning issues, but only half of those discussed end-of-life care. Fewer than 20% provided advance care planning for their patients' caregivers, and again fewer than half of them discussed end-of-life care (Cavalieri, Latif, Cieselski, Ciervo, & Forman, 2002). Physicians themselves are in favor of palliative care if they develop advanced dementia (Marik, Varon, Lisbon, & Reich, 1999). Only 2% of the physicians wanted CPR, 87% of them indicated they would want all treatment withdrawn if death is imminent, and 95% would want treatment withdrawn should they be in a persistent vegetative state. Only 1% believed that healthcare providers should never remove or withhold life-sustaining therapy, and 38% of physicians indicated they would request that their life be ended (Marik et al.).

Physicians' attitudes are influenced by their race (Mebane, Oman, Kroonen, & Goldstein, 1999). Tube feeding in terminally ill patients was considered heroic by 58% of White physicians but by only 28% of Black physicians. White physicians were more likely to find physician-assisted suicide an acceptable treatment alternative than Black physicians. If they were in a persistent vegetative state, Black physicians were more than six times as likely to request aggressive treatment, while White physicians were three times more likely to want physician-assisted suicide. In a state of brain damage without terminal illness, 23% of Black and 5% of White physicians wanted aggressive treatment. A survey of nephrologists showed that they considered the medical benefits of treatment among dementia patients in decisions to discontinue renal dialysis, but 25% admitted difficulty with advance directives if the directives clashed with their beliefs (Rutecki, Cugino, Jarjoura, Kilner, & Whittier, 1997).

Best Interest Standard

Very often, appointed proxies or family members do not have any evidence of what the patient would want in a given medical situation (Karlawish & Pearlman, 2003). In such a case, they have to decide on the basis of the best interest of the patient from their own perspective. These decisions are very difficult, and the proxies may need guidance from the treatment team in this process. Otherwise, the proxies may feel overwhelmed and guilty if they decide to forgo some treatment modalities. This was the case for Crow (chapter 4, this volume) when she and her father had to make the difficult decision to withdraw treatment for Josh.

The proxy therefore has a difficult task determining what is in the patient's best interest. The caregivers of individuals with dementia, who are most often their proxies, generally more often select life-sustaining interventions than healthy older adults would want for themselves (Mezey, Kluger, Maislin, & Mittelman, 1996; Potkins et al., 2000). In one study, about half of spouses of Alzheimer's patients with moderate-to-severe dementia stated that they would opt for CPR, respirator, and a feeding tube. Only 10% of them would forgo antibiotics. The spouses were more likely to forgo treatments in the event of coma. Spouses were more likely to forgo CPR for patients with more severe dementia and were more likely to forgo tube feeding when patients were perceived to have a poorer quality of life (Mezey et al.). Similar results were obtained in a British study, in which 46% of family caregivers wanted CPR, 60% intravenous fluids, 52% intravenous antibiotics, and 60% oral antibiotics. In this study, presence of severe dementia resulted in a reduced wish for intravenous antibiotics (Potkins et al.). Spouses consenting to treatment were more comfortable with their decision than those forgoing treatment (Mezey et al.), indicating need for caregiver support during the decision process. It has been reported that family members are not well prepared for their decision-making roles and experience substantial burden, have limited understanding of dementia progression, are uncomfortable in setting the goals of care, have little experience with death, and are ambivalent about the anticipated death of their relative, considering the death both a tragedy and a blessing (Forbes, Bern-Klug, & Gessert, 2000). Unfortunately, caregivers often do not receive sufficient emotional support from healthcare professionals, although this support is improved if the patient is receiving home hospice services (Teno et al., 2004).

Proxy decisions are more limited than decisions individuals can make about their own care. In some states, the proxy is not authorized to decide that a feeding tube should be removed unless the patient had clearly stated and documented previous wishes indicating that he or she would not want to be put on tube feeding (Karlawish & Pearlman, 2003). Similarly, the assisted-suicide law in Oregon does not apply to individuals who cannot decide for themselves (Okie, 2005).

☐ Decisions About Medical Interventions

Individuals executing advance directives and proxies making decisions for individuals who lack decision-making capacity need accurate information about treatment options, including burdens and benefits. The

TABLE 18.2 Limitations of Medical Interventions

Intervention	Reasons for Limitations in Advanced Dementia
Cardiopulmonary resuscitation (CPR)	Very low probability of success (Finucane & Harper, 1999) Stress of the procedure and following treatment Increased impairment after successful resuscitation (Appelbaum et al., 1990)
Transfer to an acute care setting	Depressed psychophysiological functioning (Gillick et al., 1982) Better outcome if pneumonia treated without transfer (Fried et al., 1997; Thompson et al., 1997)
Tube feeding	No evidence of any beneficial effect (Finucane, Christmas, et al., 1999) Burden for the patient (discomfort, restraints, lack of tasting food, complications)
Antibiotic treatment of generalized infections	Lack of effectiveness in prolonging life (Fabiszewski et al., 1990; Luchins et al., 1997) Ability to maintain comfort without antibiotics (Hurley et al., 1993; Van der Steen et al., 2002) Prevention of unnecessary diagnostic workup and antibiotic adverse effects

burdens and benefits of the same treatments are often different in individuals who are cognitively intact and in individuals with moderate or severe dementia. The most common decisions that a proxy has to make are decisions about CPR, transfer to an acute care setting, tube feeding, and treatment of generalized infections with antibiotics. Proxies may also have to make decisions regarding treatment of behavioral symptoms of dementia with psychotropic medications.

Cardiopulmonary Resuscitation

The immediate survival of resuscitated nursing home residents is 18.5%, with only 3.4% discharged from the hospital alive (Finucane & Harper, 1999). Because there is a threefold reduction in the probability of successful CPR for persons with dementia (Ebell, Becker, Barry, & Hagen, 1998), only 1% of demented residents suffering cardiac arrest can be expected to be discharged alive from the hospital. Even this potential benefit may not be desirable in individuals with severe dementia because CPR is a stressful experience for those who survive given that they may experience CPR-related injuries such as broken ribs and often have to be on a respirator. The intensive care unit environment is not conducive to appropriate care for demented individuals, who are confused and often develop delirium. In addition, patients who are discharged alive from the hospital after CPR are much more impaired than they were before the arrest (Appelbaum, King, & Finucane, 1990).

Do not resuscitate (DNR) orders in nursing home populations are associated with advanced age, cognitive dysfunction, physical dependency, presence of advance directives, absence of Medicaid, and daily visitors (Zweig, 1997). The presence of a DNR order is also influenced by nursing home characteristics and the ethnicity of nursing home residents (Zweig). DNR decisions are affected by the language used to describe the CPR procedure and the probability of success presented to the resident. In a study of desire for CPR in a retirement village, 41% of residents opted for CPR if they had an acute illness before learning about survival statistics. When a 10–17% success rate was presented, only 22% desired CPR. The preference decreased to 5% when they were told that with a chronic illness present, the success rate of CPR is only 0–5% (Murphy et al., 1994).

Transfer to Acute Care Setting

Transfer of demented individuals to an emergency room or hospital exposes them to serious risks. Even cognitively intact hospitalized elderly individuals develop depressed psychological and physiological functioning that includes confusion, falling, not eating, and incontinence (Gillick, Serrell, & Gillick, 1982). These symptoms are often managed by medical interventions, such as psychotropic medications, restraints, nasogastric tubes (a tube inserted in the nose and mouth to primarily facilitate feeding), and catheters, which expose the patient to possible complications, including inflammation of veins (thrombophlebitis), blockage of an artery in the lungs (pulmonary embolus), inflammation of the lungs as a result of inhalation of foreign materials such as food (aspiration pneumonia), urinary tract infection, and infection-induced circulatory problems (septic shock).

Transfer of long-term care facility residents to an emergency room or hospital for treatment of infections and other conditions may not be optimal for management of these problems. Immediate survival after an episode of pneumonia is similar in residents receiving treatment in a long-term care facility and in a hospital (Mylotte, Naughton, Saludades, & Maszarovics, 1998). Longer-term outcomes are actually better in residents treated in a nursing home. It was reported that the 6-week mortality rate was 18.7% in nonhospitalized residents and 39.5% in hospitalized residents despite no significant differences between the hospitalized and nonhospitalized groups before diagnosis (Thompson, Hall, Szpiech, & Reisenberg, 1997). Similarly, a larger proportion of hospitalized individuals had worsening of their functional status or died at 2 months after the episode of pneumonia (Fried, Gillick, & Lipsitz, 1997). Thus, the available data indicate that transfer to an emergency room or hospital has a significant degree of risk and relatively few benefits for individuals with severe dementia. Therefore, this management strategy should be used only when it is consistent with overall goals of care and not as a default option.

Tube Feeding

Patients with severe dementia are unable to feed themselves and often develop swallowing difficulties that provoke choking on food and liquids. They may also start refusing food by not opening their mouth when they are fed. Choking and food refusal are often exhibited simultaneously. Swallowing difficulties and choking may be minimized by adjustment of diet texture and by replacing thin liquids with thick ones (e.g., yogurt instead of milk; Morris & Volicer, 2001), and food refusal often responds to antidepressant treatment (Volicer, Rheaume, & Cyr, 1994) or to administration of appetite stimulants (Volicer, Stelly, Morris, McLaughlin, & Volicer, 1997).

There is no evidence that long-term feeding tubes are beneficial in individuals with advanced dementia. Tube feeding does not prevent pneumonia resulting from inhalation of foreign materials such as food and actually might increase its incidence because it does not prevent aspiration of nasal drainage and of regurgitated stomach contents (Finucane, Christmas, & Travis, 1999). Tube feeding also does not prevent occurrence of other infections. A nasogastric tube may cause infections of sinuses and the middle ear, and gastrostomy tubes (tubes placed directly into the stomach for feeding) may cause skin aggravation and infections (e.g., cellulitis, abscesses, and even necrotizing fasciitis and myositis). Contaminated feeding solution may cause gastrointestinal symptoms and urinary tract infections (e.g., bacteriuria). Tube feeding does not prevent malnutrition, and it does not increase survival in individuals with progressive degenerative dementia. Insertion of a tube may actually cause death from cardiac complications during the surgical procedures required. Occurrence of pressure ulcers (e.g., bed sores) is not decreased by tube feeding, and it may actually be increased because of the use of restraints and increased production of urine and stool. There is also no evidence that tube feeding promotes healing of pressure ulcers or improved functional status of individuals with severe dementia (Gillick, 2000).

In addition to the lack of benefits, tube feeding has many adverse effects. Tube feeding increases discomfort of the patients by both the tube presence and by the use of restraints that are often necessary to prevent tube removal. Tube feeding also deprives the patient of the taste of food and contact with the caregivers during the feeding process. In addition to the adverse effects listed, feeding tubes may cause many local, respiratory, abdominal, and other complications (Finucane et al., 1999). This imbalance of burdens and benefits of tube feeding justifies recommendations that tube feeding should not be used in individuals with advanced dementia.

Decisions about tube feeding are highly emotional and often elicit court involvement. However, there is broad legal consensus in the United States that tube feeding is a medical procedure that may be discontinued if the patient or proxy so desires (Ashby & Mendelson, 2004). Discontinuation of tube feeding is also supported by most religious ethicists (Gillick, 2000; see Doka, chapter 16, this volume). The Orthodox Jewish position is that tube feeding should be given as long as it does not constitute undue danger, arouse serious opposition, or cause suffering to the patient (Rosin & Sonnenblick, 1998). A recent papal statement, supporting the use of tube feeding, was primarily targeted at maintaining tube feeding in individuals in a persistent vegetative state, who cannot perceive any suffering from tube feeding (Pope John Paul II, 2004). Because individuals with Alzheimer's disease very rarely, if ever, progress into the persistent vegetative state (Volicer, Berman, Cipolloni, & Mandell, 1997), this statement may not affect their care, although there could be differing opinions (Shannon & Walter, 2004).

The process of decision making regarding tube feeding is different across countries. A Netherlands study showed that advance care planning has taken place only in 68% of residents with dementia for whom a decision was made to forgo artificial nutrition and hydration, and in two thirds of all residents, the primary aim of forgoing artificial nutrition and hydration was to avoid unnecessary prolongation of life (Pasman et al., 2004). In this study, almost all physicians, nurses, and family members rated the decision-making process as "good" or "adequate," and the only dissatisfaction was with having to make the decision under the pressure of time constraints. In contrast, a Canadian study showed that only half of the decision makers believed that they had received adequate support from the healthcare team in making the decision, and often a physician spoke with them for only 15 minutes or less (37%) or not at all (28%; Mitchell & Lawson, 1999). Less than half of the proxies who agreed to initiate long-term tube feeding were confident that the patient would want to have tube feeding. The majority of proxies thought that they understood the benefits of tube feeding but believed that it prolongs life (84%) or prevents aspiration (67%). Fewer than half of the proxies thought that they understood the risks of tube feeding or believed that feeding tube had improved the patient's quality of life. Only a minority (38%) of proxies who agreed to initiate long-term tube feeding would want a feeding tube for themselves (Mitchell, Berkowitz, Lawson, & Lipsitz, 2000).

Antibiotic Therapy

Antibiotic therapy is quite effective in treating an isolated episode of pneumonia or other systemic infection. In most patients, it is possible to limit antibiotic therapy to oral preparations that are equally, if not more, effective as nonoral methods (Hirata-Dulas, Stein, Guay, Gruninger, & Peterson, 1991). It is preferable to limit the use of intravenous therapy in individuals with severe dementia who do not understand the need for intravenous catheters and consequently try to remove them and often have to be restrained or given psychotropic drugs to allow the treatment to continue. In patients who have poor oral intake, direct injections of antibiotics into the muscles can be used for treatment of infections.

However, the effectiveness of antibiotic therapy is limited by the recurrent nature of infections in advanced dementia. Antibiotic therapy does not prolong survival in cognitively impaired patients who are unable to ambulate, even with assistance, and may be mute (Fabiszewski, Volicer, & Volicer, 1990; Luchins, Hanrahan, & Murphy, 1997). Antibiotics are also not necessary for maintenance of comfort in demented individuals who can be maintained equally well with analgesics and antipyretics (fever-reducing drugs) and with oxygen if necessary (Hurley, Volicer, Mahoney, & Volicer, 1993; Van der Steen, Ooms, Van der Wal, & Ribbe, 2002). In addition, antibiotic use is not without adverse effects. Patients may develop gastrointestinal upset, diarrhea, allergic reactions, excessively high levels of potassium, and blood disorders. Diagnostic procedures such as blood drawing and sputum suctioning, which are necessary for appropriate use of antibiotics, cause discomfort and confusion in demented individuals who do not understand the need for them. Use of antibiotics in patients with advanced dementia should therefore take into consideration the recurrent nature of infections, which are caused by persistent swallowing difficulties with aspiration and by other factors predisposing them for the development of infections (Volicer, Brandeis, & Hurley, 1998), that significantly reduce the benefits of antibiotic treatment.

□ Decision-Making Procedure

A proxy who is making treatment decisions often feels stressed and guilty if the decision is to limit some medical interventions. Therefore, it is important to provide guidance and support. A program for shared decision-making regarding care of individuals with advanced dementia was implemented in a dementia special care unit at the E. N. Nourse Rogers Memorial Veterans Hospital in Bedford, Massachusetts (Volicer, Rheaume, Brown, Fabiszewski, & Brady, 1986).

In this program, recommendations for the proxy not only are made by the physician but also are developed as a consensus of the whole treatment team. It should be recognized that nursing staff are moral agents who have to be consulted before treatment decisions are made because they have to live with the residents and execute these decisions (Hurley, MacDonald, Fry, & Rempusheski, 1998). Several factors are important for the process of reaching consensus: patient decline, family coping, professional development of nursing staff, and nursing unit philosophy (Hurley, Volicer, Rempusheski, & Fry, 1995). Timing and trust are influential catalysts to family and staff readiness for achieving consensus.

Another program promoted advance care planning by education of nursing home social workers that included small-group workshops and role play/practice sessions for advance care planning discussions with residents and their proxy at admission, after any change in clinical status, and at yearly intervals; formal structured review of resident's goals at regular team meetings; flagging of advance directives on nursing home charts; and feedback to individual healthcare providers of the congruence of care they provided and the preferences specified in the advance care plan (Morrison et al., 2005). This program increased documentation of advance preferences for CPR (40% vs. 20%), artificial nutrition and hydration (47% vs. 9%), intravenous antibiotics (44% vs. 9%), and hospitalization (49% vs. 16%). The program also significantly decreased the occurrence of treatment discordant with previously stated wishes (5% vs. 18%) (Morrison et al.).

Treatment decisions should be made at a meeting of proxy and other family members or friends with the treatment team ahead of the time of crisis. The treatment team should include the physician or physician extender, nursing staff representative, and social worker, with the last serving as a meeting moderator. Presence of a chaplain is also useful for answering concerns regarding religious or ethical matters. This family conference is a good opportunity to answer all concerns expressed by the proxy and others close to the patient regarding the person's condition and treatment (Mahoney, Hurley, & Volicer, 1998). During the conference, the treatment team should clarify the patient's prognosis and describe options for management of complications and additional diseases that occur. Risks and benefits of all the management strategies should be clearly explained according to the evidence presented.

At the beginning of the discussion, it has to be determined if the patient expressed any wishes prior to losing decision-making capacity. The discussion may be framed as an opportunity for decisions regarding the goals of care—survival at all costs, maintenance of function, or comfort care (Gillick, Berkman, & Cullen, 1999). According to these goals, decisions are made to accept or forgo CPR, transfer to acute care setting, treatment with antibiotics, and tube feeding. These decisions (an advance proxy plan) are not permanent and may be changed by the proxy at any time. Therefore, it is necessary to maintain good communication between the treatment team and the proxy, notifying the proxy of any significant change in the patient's condition. The decisions should be reviewed periodically, and if the proxy dies or becomes incapacitated, a new proxy should update the plan. Volicer et al. (2002) developed a form that can be used to document an advance proxy plan.

Decisions about end-of-life care may be made easier by use of guidelines for clinicians and family members. Guideline use for palliative care in dementia has resulted in numerous positive outcomes. One study has shown decreases in inappropriately prescribed antibiotics and an increase in appropriately prescribed analgesics, including opiates (Lloyd-Williams & Payne, 2002). Guideline use has also led to the development of a checklist of considerations for decisions regarding treatment of pneumonia (Van der Steen, Ooms, Ribbe, & Van der Wal, 2001). There are two guidelines that specifically address the issue of tube feeding (Mitchell, Tetroe, & O'Connor, 2001; Rabeneck, McCullough, & Wray, 1997). Professional societies have also developed guidelines (e.g., Fisk et al., 1998) or published illustrative cases (e.g., Karlawish, Quill, & Meier, 1999) to improve care.

Existing guidelines were reviewed and their end-of-life care content evaluated (Mast, Salama, Silverman, & Arnold, 2004). In the area of dementia, of 56 possible guidelines, 24 were reviewed and 7 accepted for the study. The best 4 guidelines were issued by the American Medical Association (1999), American Psychiatric Association (1997), California Workgroup on Guidelines for Alzheimer's Disease Management (2002), and American Medical Directors Association (1998). More focused guidelines (e.g., end-of-life care in nursing homes) are currently in development through the Department of Veterans Affairs.

☐ Conclusion

Decision-making capacity is issue-specific and may fluctuate with time. Five standards for determination of decision-making capacity were presented, but not all of them are used in clinical practice. Clinicians are more likely to use a sliding scale concept that specifies three different standard requirements according to the nature of the decision. There are some instruments available for determination of decision-making capacity in a research setting, but none appear to have gained widespread acceptance in clinical settings.

When the individual lacks decision-making capacity, the choices have to be made by a proxy. Proxies should decide on the basis of the incapacitated individual's previous wishes or, if there is no evidence of any wishes, on the basis of the incapacitated individual's best interest. Proxies should develop an ongoing relationship that involves collaborative communication with the healthcare team and set goals for care before any crisis situation. This communication could result in the development of an advance proxy plan that specifies which medical interventions should be used or forgone in the future.

The proxy should have information about risk and benefits of medical interventions before deciding which should be used or forgone. This information should include the following: CPR is rarely successful and poses a great burden for an individual with dementia; it is often better to avoid transfer to a hospital and treat infections in a nursing home; tube feeding usually provides no benefit but decreased quality of life of an individual with dementia; and use of antibiotics for treatment of generalized infections is not necessarily prolonging life and increasing comfort in individuals with a terminal stage of dementia. Several societies have published guidelines for palliative care in dementia, and these could be used for education of both proxies and healthcare professionals.

☐ References

Allen, R. S., DeLaine, S. R., Chaplin, W. F., Marson, D. C., Bourgeois, M. S., Dijkstra, K., et al. (2003). Advance care planning in nursing homes: correlates of capacity and possession of advance directives. *The Gerontologist, 43,* 309–317.

American Medical Association. (1999). *Diagnosis, management and treatment of dementia: A practical guide for primary care physicians.* Chicago: Author.

American Medical Directors Association. (1998). *Dementia: Clinical practice guideline 1998.* Columbia, MD: Author.

American Psychiatric Association. (1997). Practice guideline for the treatment of patients with Alzheimer's disease and other dementias of late life. *American Journal of Psychiatry, 154,* 1–39.

Appelbaum, G. E., King, J. E., & Finucane, T. E. (1990). The outcome of CPR initiated in nursing homes. *Journal of the American Geriatrics Society, 38,* 197–200.

Appelbaum, P. S., & Grisso, T. (2001). *MacCAT-CR: MacArthur Competence Assessment Tool for Clinical Research.* Sarasota, FL: Professional Resource Press.

Ashby, M. A., & Mendelson, D. (2004). Gardner; re BWV: Victorian Supreme Court makes landmark Australian ruling on tube feeding. *Medical Journal of Australia, 181,* 442–445.

Bookwala, J., Coppola, K. M., Fagerlin, A., Ditto, P. H., Danks, J. H., & Smucker, W. D. (2001). Gender differences in older adults' preferences for life-sustaining medical treatments and end-of-life values. *Death Studies, 25,* 127–149.

California Workgroup on Guidelines for Alzheimer's Disease Management. (2002). *Guidelines for Alzheimer's disease management.* Los Angeles: Alzheimer's Association of Los Angeles, Riverside and San Bernardino Counties.

Cavalieri, T. A., Latif, W., Cieselski, J., Ciervo, C. A., Jr., & Forman, L. J. (2002). How physicians approach advance care planning in patients with mild to moderate Alzheimer's disease. *Journal of the American Osteopathic Association, 102,* 541–544.

Drane, J. F. (1984). Competency to give an informed consent: A model for making clinical assessments. *Journal of the American Medical Association, 252,* 925–927.

Earnst, K. S., Marson, D. C., & Harrell, L. E. (2000). Cognitive models of physicians' legal standard and personal judgments of competency in patients with Alzheimer's disease. *Journal of the American Geriatrics Society, 48,* 919–927.

Ebell, M. H., Becker, L. A., Barry, H. C., & Hagen, M. (1998). Survival after in-hospital cardiopulmonary resuscitation. A meta-analysis. *Journal of General Internal Medicine, 13,* 805–816.

Edelstein, B. (2000). Challenges in the assessment of decision-making capacity. *Journal of Aging Studies, 14,* 423–437.

Fabiszewski, K. J., Volicer, B., & Volicer, L. (1990). Effect of antibiotic treatment on outcome of fevers in institutionalized Alzheimer patients. *Journal of the American Medical Association, 263,* 3168–3172.

Finucane, T. E., Christmas, C., & Travis, K. (1999). Tube feeding in patients with advanced dementia: A review of the evidence. *Journal of the American Medical Association, 282,* 1365–1370.

Finucane, T. E., & Harper, G. M. (1999). Attempting resuscitation in nursing homes: policy considerations. *Journal of the American Geriatrics Society, 47,* 1261–1264.

Fisk, J. D., Sadovnick, A. D., Cohen, C. A., Gauthier, S., Dossetor, J., Eberhart, A., et al. (1998). Ethical guidelines of the Alzheimer society of Canada. *Canadian Journal of Neurological Sciences, 25,* 242–248.

Forbes, S., Bern-Klug, M., & Gessert, C. (2000). End-of-life decision-making for nursing home residents with dementia. *Journal of Nursing Scholarship, 32,* 251–258.

Fried, T. R., Gillick, M. R., & Lipsitz, L. A. (1997). Short-term functional outcomes of long-term care residents with pneumonia treated with and without hospital transfer. *Journal of the American Geriatrics Society, 45,* 302–306.

Ganzini, L., Volicer, L., Nelson, W. A., Fox, E., & Derse, A. R. (2004). Ten myths about decision-making capacity. *Journal of the American Medical Directors Association, 5,* 263–267.

Gillick, M., Berkman, S., & Cullen, L. (1999). A patient-centered approach to advance medical planning in the nursing home. *Journal of the American Geriatrics Society, 47,* 227–230.

Gillick, M. R. (2000). Sounding board—rethinking the role of tube feeding in patients with advanced dementia. *New England Journal of Medicine, 342,* 206–210.

Gillick, M. R., Serrell, N. A., & Gillick, L. S. (1982). Adverse consequences of hospitalization in the elderly. *Social Science and Medicine, 16,* 1033–1038.

Grisso, T., & Appelbaum, P. S. (1998). *Assessing competence to consent to treatment: A guide for physicians and other health professionals.* New York: Oxford University Press.

Grisso, T., Appelbaum, P. S., & Hill-Fotouhi, C. (1997). The MacCAT-T: a clinical tool to assess patient's capacities to make treatment decisions. *Psychiatric Services, 48,* 1415–1419.

Hirata-Dulas, C. A., Stein, D. J., Guay, D. R., Gruninger, R. P., & Peterson, P. K. (1991). A randomized study of ciprofloxacin versus ceftriaxone in the treatment of nursing home-acquired lower respiratory tract infections. *Journal of the American Geriatrics Society, 39,* 1040–1041.

Hurley, A. C., MacDonald, S. A., Fry, S. T., & Rempusheski, V. F. (1998). Nursing staff as moral agents. In L. Volicer & A. Hurley (Eds.), *Hospice care for patients with advanced progressive dementia* (pp. 155–168). New York: Springer.

Hurley, A. C., Volicer, B., Mahoney, M. A., & Volicer, L. (1993). Palliative fever management in Alzheimer patients: Quality plus fiscal responsibility. *Advances in Nursing Science, 16,* 21–32.

Hurley, A. C., Volicer, L., Rempusheski, V. F., & Fry, S. T. (1995). Reaching consensus: The process of recommending treatment decisions for Alzheimer's patients. *Advances in Nursing Science, 18*(2), 33–43.

Karlawish, J., Quill, T., & Meier, D. E. (1999). A consensus-based approach to providing palliative care to patients who lack decision-making capacity. ACP-ASIM End-of-Life Care Consensus Panel. *Annals of Internal Medicine, 130,* 835–840.

Karlawish, J. H. T., & Pearlman, R. A. (2003). Determination of decision-making capacity. In C. K. Cassel, R. Leipzig, H. J. Cohen, E. B. Larson, & D. E. Meier (Eds.), *Geriatric medicine* (4th ed., pp. 1233–1241). New York: Springer-Verlag.

Kiely, D. K., Mitchell, S. L., Marlow, A., Murphy, K. M., & Morris, J. N. (2001). Racial and state differences in the designation of advance directives in nursing home residents. *Journal of the American Geriatrics Society, 49,* 1346–1352.

Kloezen, S., Fitten, L. J., & Steinberg, A. (1988). Assessment of treatment decision-making capacity in a medically ill patient. *Journal of the American Geriatrics Society, 36,* 1055–1058.

Lloyd-Williams, M., & Payne, S. (2002). Can multidisciplinary guidelines improve the palliation of symptoms in the terminal phase of dementia? *International Journal of Palliative Care Nursing, 8,* 370–375.

Luchins, D. J., Hanrahan, P., & Murphy, K. (1997). Criteria for enrolling dementia patients in hospice. *Journal of the American Geriatrics Society, 45,* 1054–1059.

Mahoney, M. A., Hurley, A. C., & Volicer, L. (1998). Advance proxy planning. In L. Volicer & A. Hurley (Eds.), *Hospice care for patients with advanced progressive dementia* (pp. 169–188). New York: Springer.

Marik, P. E., Varon, J., Lisbon, A., & Reich, H. S. (1999). Physicians' own preferences to the limitation and withdrawal of life-sustaining therapy. *Resuscitation, 42,* 197–201.

Markson, L. J., Kern, D. C., Annas, G. J., & Glantz, L. H. (1994). Physician assessment of patient competence. *Journal of American Geriatrics Society, 42,* 1074–1080.

Marson, D. C., Earnst, K. S., Jamil, F., Bartolucci, A., & Harrell, L. E. (2000). Consistency of physicians' legal standard and personal judgments of competency in patients with Alzheimer's disease. *Journal of the American Geriatrics Society, 48,* 911–918.

Marson, D. C., Ingram, K. K., Cody, H. A., & Harrell, L. E. (1995). Assessing the competency of patients with Alzheimer's disease under different legal standards—a prototype instrument. *Archives of Neurology, 52,* 949–954.

Mast, K. R., Salama, M., Silverman, G. K., & Arnold, R. M. (2004). End-of-life content in treatment guidelines for life-limiting diseases. *Journal of Palliative Medicine, 7,* 754–773.

Mead, G. E., O'Keefe, S. T., Jack, C. I., Maestri-Banks, A. M., Playfer, J. R., & Lye, M. (1995). What factors influence patient preferences regarding cardiopulmonary resuscitation? *Journal of the Royal College of Physicians London, 29,* 295–298.

Mebane, E. W., Oman, R. F., Kroonen, L. T., & Goldstein, M. K. (1999). The influence of physician race, age, and gender on physician attitudes toward advance care directives and preferences for end-of-life decision-making. *Journal of the American Geriatrics Society, 47,* 579–591.

Mezey, M., Kluger, M., Maislin, G., & Mittelman, M. (1996). Life-sustaining treatment decisions by spouses of patients with Alzheimer's disease. *Journal of the American Geriatrics Society, 44,* 144–150.

Mezey, M., Teresi, J., Ramsey, G., Mitty, E., & Bobrowitz, T. (2000). Decision-making capacity to execute a health care proxy: Development and testing of guidelines. *Journal of the American Geriatrics Society, 48,* 179–187.

Mitchell, S. L., Berkowitz, R. E., Lawson, F. M., & Lipsitz, L. A. (2000). A cross-national survey of tube-feeding decisions in cognitively impaired older persons. *Journal of the American Geriatrics Society, 48,* 391–397.

Mitchell, S. L., & Lawson, F. M. (1999). Decision-making for long-term tube-feeding in cognitively impaired elderly people. *Canadian Medical Association Journal, 160,* 1705–1709.

Mitchell, S. L., Tetroe, J. M., & O'Connor, A. M. (2001). A decision aid for long-term tube feeding in cognitively impaired older adults. *Journal of American Geriatrics Society, 49,* 313–316.

Morris, J., & Volicer, L. (2001). Nutritional management of individuals with Alzheimer's disease and other progressive dementias. *Nutrition in Clinical Care, 4,* 148–155.

Morrison, R. S., Chichin, E., Carter, J., Burack, O., Lantz, M., & Meier, D. E. (2005). The effect of a social work intervention to enhance advance care planning documentation in the nursing home. *Journal of the American Geriatrics Society, 53,* 290–294.

Moye, J., Karel, M. J., Azar, A. R., & Gurrera, R. J. (2004). Capacity to consent to treatment: empirical comparison of three instruments in older adults with and without dementia. *The Gerontologist, 44,* 166–175.

Moye, J., Karel, M. J., Gurrera, R. J., & Azar, A. R. (2006). Neuropsychological predictors of decision-making capacity over 9 months in mild-to-moderate dementia. *Journal of Internal Medicine, 21,* 78–83.

Murphy, D. J., Burrows, D., Santilli, S., Kemp, A. W., Tenner, S., Kreling, B., et al. (1994). The influence of the probability of survival on patients' preferences regarding cardiopulmonary resuscitation. *New England Journal of Medicine, 330,* 545–549.

Mylotte, J. P., Naughton, B., Saludades, C., & Maszarovics, Z. (1998). Validation and application of the pneumonia prognosis index to nursing home residents with pneumonia. *Journal of the American Geriatrics Society, 46,* 1538–1544.

Okie, S. (2005) Physician-assisted suicide—Oregon and beyond. *New England Journal of Medicine, 352,* 1627–1630.

Palmer, B. W., Dunn, L. B., Appelbaum, P. S., & Jeste, D. V. (2004). Correlates of treatment-related decision-making capacity among middle-aged and older patients with schizophrenia. *Archives of General Psychiatry, 61,* 230–236.

Pasman, H. R. W., Onwuteaka-Philipsen, B. D., Ooms, M. E., van Wigcheren, P. T., Van der Wal, G., & Ribbe, M. W. (2004). Forgoing artificial nutrition and hydration in nursing home patients with dementia—patients, decision-making, and participants. *Alzheimer Disease and Associated Disorders, 18,* 154–162.

Patient Self-Determination Act of 1990, Publ. L. No. 101-508, 4206, 4751 of the Omnibus Reconciliation Act of 1990.

Pearlman, R. A. (1997). Determination of decision-making capacity. In C. K. Cassel, H. J. Cohen, E. B. Larson, & D. E. Meier. (Eds.), *Geriatric medicine* (3rd ed., pp. 201–209). New York: Springer.

Pomerantz, A. S., & de Nesnera, A. (1991). Informed consent, competency, and the illusion of rationality. *General Hospital Psychiatry, 13,* 138–142.

Pope John Paul II. (2004). Life-sustaining treatments and vegetative state: scientific advances and ethical dilemmas. *NeuroRehabilitation, 19,* 273–275.

Potkins, D., Bradley, S., Shrimanker, J., O'Brien, J., Swann, A., & Ballard, C. (2000). End of life treatment decisions in people with dementia: Carers' views and the factors which influence them. *International Journal of Geriatric Psychiatry, 15,* 1005–1008.

The President's Commission for the Study of Ethical Problems in Medicine and Biomedical and Behavioral Research. (1982). *Making health care decisions* (Vol. 1). Washington, DC: U.S. Government Printing Office.

President's Council on Bioethics. (2006). *Taking care: Ethical caregiving in our aging society.* Retrieved on April 30, 2007, from http://www.bioethics.gov/reports/taking_care/chapter5.html

Rabeneck, L., McCullough, L. B., & Wray, N. P. (1997). Ethically justified, clinically comprehensive guidelines for percutaneous endoscopic gastrostomy tube placement. *Lancet, 349,* 496–498.

Reilly, R. B., Teasdale, T. A., & McCullough, L. B. (1994). Projecting patients' preferences from living wills: An invalid strategy for management of dementia with life-threatening illness. *Journal of the American Geriatrics Society, 42,* 997–1003.

Rosin, A. J., & Sonnenblick, M. (1998). Autonomy and paternalism in geriatric medicine. The Jewish ethical approach to issues of feeding terminally ill patients, and to cardiopulmonary resuscitation. *Journal of Medical Ethics, 24,* 44–48.

Rowley, J. D. (2006). *Taking care: Ethical caregiving in our aging society.* Retrieved on April 30, 2007, from www.bioethics.gov/reports/taking_care/appendix.html

Rutecki, G. W., Cugino, A., Jarjoura, D., Kilner, J. F., & Whittier, F. C. (1997). Nephrologists' subjective attitudes towards end-of-life issues and the conduct of terminal care. *Clinical Nephrology, 48,* 173–180.

Shannon, T. A., & Walter, J. J. (2004). Implications of the papal allocution on feeding tubes. *Hastings Center Report, 34,* 18–20.

Teno, J. M., Clarridge, B. R., Casey, V., Welch, L. C., Wetle, T., Shield, R., et al. (2004). Family perspectives on end-of-life care at the last place of care. *Journal of the American Medical Association, 291,* 88–93.

Thompson, R. S., Hall, N. K., Szpiech, M., & Reisenberg, L. A. (1997). Treatments and outcomes of nursing-home-acquired pneumonia. *Journal of the American Board of Family Practitioners, 10,* 82–87.

Van der Steen, J. T., Ooms, M. E., Ribbe, M. W., & Van der Wal, G. (2001). Decisions to treat or not to treat pneumonia in demented psychogeriatric nursing home patients: Evaluation of a guideline. *Alzheimer Disease & Associated Disorders, 15,* 119–128.

Van der Steen, J. T., Ooms, M. E., Van der Wal, G., & Ribbe, M. W. (2002). Pneumonia: The demented patient's best friend? Discomfort after starting or withholding antibiotic treatment. *Journal of the American Geriatrics Society, 50,* 1681–1688.

Volicer, L., Berman, S. A., Cipolloni, P. B., & Mandell, A. (1997). Persistent vegetative state in Alzheimer disease—does it exist? *Archives of Neurology, 54,* 1382–1384.

Volicer, L., Brandeis, G., & Hurley, A. C. (1998). Infections in advanced dementia. In L. Volicer & A. Hurley (Eds.), *Hospice care for patients with advanced progressive dementia* (pp. 29–47). New York: Springery.

Volicer, L., Cantor, M. D., Derse, A. R., Edwards, D. M., Prudhomme, A. M., Gregory, D. C. R., et al. (2002). Advance care planning by proxy for residents of long-term care facilities who lack decision-making capacity. *Journal of the American Geriatrics Society, 50,* 761–767.

Volicer, L., & Ganzini, L. (2003). Health professionals' views on standards for decision-making capacity regarding refusal of medical treatment in mild Alzheimer's disease. *Journal of the American Geriatrics Society, 51,* 1270–1274.

Volicer, L., Rheaume, Y., Brown, J. Fabiszewski, K., & Brady, R. (1986). Hospice approach to the treatment of patients with advanced dementia of the Alzheimer type. *Journal of the American Medical Association, 256,* 2210–2213.

Volicer, L., Rheaume, Y., & Cyr, D. (1994). Treatment of depression in advanced Alzheimer's disease using sertraline. *Journal of Geriatric Psychiatry and Neurology, 7,* 227–229.

Volicer, L., Stelly, M., Morris, J., McLaughlin, J., & Volicer, B. J. (1997). Effects of dronabinol on anorexia and disturbed behavior in patients with Alzheimer's disease. *International Journal of Geriatric Psychiatry, 12,* 913–919.

Zweig, S. C. (1997). Cardiopulmonary resuscitation and do-not-resuscitate orders in nursing home. *Archives of Family Medicine, 6,* 424–42.

19

CHAPTER

Pediatric Patient-Oriented Problem Solving Near the End of Life

Chris Feudtner and Anne E. Kazak

Jessica was born an hour ago. Her mother was only in the fifth month of pregnancy when, the night before, the amniotic membranes ruptured. With a gush of fluid, a sequence of events unfolded so rapidly that both parents are in shocked disbelief. Because of premature lungs, Jessica was intubated and placed on a ventilator. Her condition has swiftly deteriorated because of presumed bacterial sepsis, and she requires medications to support her blood pressure.

□ Introduction

When an ill or injured child is approaching death, innumerable challenges arise (Bearison, 2005; Bluebond-Langner, 1978; Carter & Levetown, 2004; Feudtner, 2004; Field & Behrman, 2003; Hilden, Tobin, & Lindsey, 2003). Both good medical problem solving and sound decision making are paramount but often exceedingly difficult. In this chapter, we aim to examine these challenges within the broader framework of patient-oriented problem solving and decision making.

Our key points can be summarized briefly:

- Decisions involve deliberations about not only what to do but also how to best represent and interpret often complex and uncertain clinical situations.
- Because affective, as well as cognitive processes, affect the outcome of decision making, we need to develop effective ways to support people as they both feel and think their way through these situations.
- Although decisions that directly affect the way that children die are important, these decisions are a subset of the broader set of decisions that affects how children with severe life-limiting or life-threatening conditions live.

We base this chapter on several sources of information: published reports of primarily qualitative studies of pediatric patients living with life-threatening conditions or parents of children who are critically ill or who have died; published expert opinions or recommendations; findings from the general literature on decision making and problem solving; and our professional experience caring for dying children and their families. To better illustrate some of the main points that we wish to make, we have interwoven throughout the chapter four fictional vignettes of children with severe medical conditions that exemplify common aspects of pediatric end-of-life decision making.

☐ Overview of Childhood Death and the Place of Pediatric Palliative Care

> Isaac is in the newborn intensive care unit (NICU) bed next to Jessica. Born with a severe complex congenital heart malformation as well as a unique genetic syndrome that has never been described, Isaac has undergone two extensive heart operations during his 4 months of life and is now believed to have, from a structural perspective, a completely repaired heart. He has, however, continued to struggle with inadequate cardiac function, remains intubated, and on several occasions during the past month has required cardiopulmonary resuscitation.

Each year in the United States, approximately 55,000 infants, children, and adolescents die (Feudtner, 2001). Of these, most (52%) are less than a year of age, while one quarter (26%) are between 15 and 19 years of age when they die. Before the first birthday, medical conditions are the dominant cause of death; after the first year of life, trauma (accidents, homicide, and suicide) is the major cause of mortality. Among those children who died from medical conditions, just over a third (36%) died from what can be considered complex chronic conditions (CCCs; as opposed to sudden onset conditions or conditions that usually remit). These conditions include cancer (which is an exceedingly rare cause of death during infancy and only constitutes half of all CCC-related deaths during adolescence), as well as cardiovascular conditions (which across all age groups are the most common cause of CCC-related death and typically involve congenital heart malformations) and neuromuscular, genetic, respiratory, and a wide variety of other ailments. Across the nation, among the infants dying with CCCs, more than 90% die in hospitals; among the older children with CCCs, an increasing proportion are dying at home, rising from 16% in the early 1980s to 28% at the end of the 1990s (Feudtner, Feinstein, Satchell, Shabbout, & Kang, 2006).

What is far less certain is the number of dying children who, prior to their death, are considered—fleetingly or fully—as candidates for palliative care. Infants who die typically do so within hours or days of being born, and children who become gravely ill are often treated with every hope of reversing the disease process up to within moments of their death. Restricting the count then to just those children who die from a CCC (which is likely too small an estimate of the actual population in need), each year there are 15,000 infants, children, and adolescents who likely could have benefited from some degree of palliative care, and on any given day there are 5,000 such patients alive and potentially in need of this care, as in the case of Jessica or Isaac (Feudtner, 2001).

What kinds of care might such a child receive (see Figure 19.1)? Although many consider palliative care to be either incompatible or in competition with curative care (with either an abrupt or more ideally a gradual transition from curative to palliative care but with both concepts operating with some notion of a fixed sum of all care; Lynn, 1997), in reality there can be—and often is—far greater overlap of the components of a child's care. Broadly speaking, all of pediatric medical care can be viewed as serving four different goals: (a) Curative care aims to eradicate the cause of the disease and return the child to virtually full health (as was the initial goal for Jessica immediately after her birth); (b) life-extending care may concede that cure is not possible but endeavors to prolong life markedly, often by decades, but sometimes willing to settle for a few years or even months (which is the mode of care that Isaac is likely receiving); (c) comfort-promoting care focuses less on duration of life and more on the quality of a child's life considered holistically; and (d) family supportive care attends to the needs of parents and others.

Ideally, a pediatric palliative team is—perhaps ironically—not principally dedicated to the provision of palliative care per se but rather to the task of helping children and families understand their situation and the

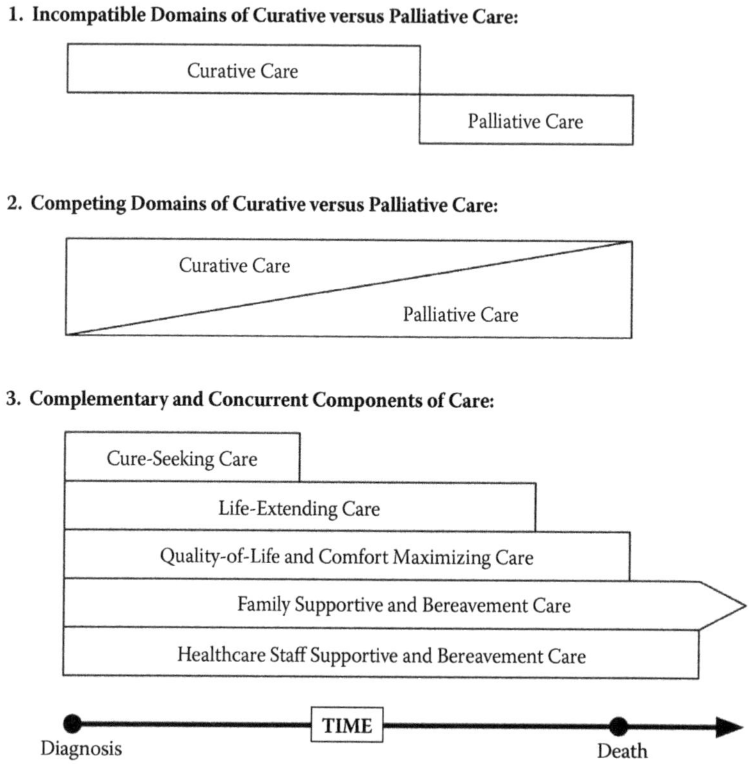

FIGURE 19.1 Tacit conceptual models of pediatric medical care. *Source:* Figure adapted from "Hospital Care for Children and Young Adults in the Last Year of Life: A Population-Based Study," by C. Feudtner, D. L. DiGiuseppe, and J. M. Neff, (2003), *BioMed Central: Medicine, 1,* 3.

vast permutations of ways in which they could be cared for, combining some mix of curative, life-extending, comfort-seeking or quality-enhancing, and family supportive care (Graham & Robinson, 2005; Robinson, Ravilly, Berde, & Wohl, 1997). Indeed, some children may undergo chemotherapy with the intent to cure while also receiving the same kinds of pastoral care and pain relief support that they would receive if cure were no longer possible. Other children may appropriately receive life-extending therapy, often until within hours of their clearly anticipated death. Because of this broader agenda—namely, to help patients and families with decision making not only within the palliative care experience but also about how to adjust the mix of care and the underlying sense of purpose and goals over time—some palliative care teams calls themselves pediatric advanced care teams (PACTs).

Like their counterparts in adult patient care, PACTs are often comprised of physicians, nurses, social workers, psychologists, and pastoral care workers and may also include child life therapists, art and music therapists, and bereavement therapists. Although there are many challenges that are similar to adult palliative care, the members of these teams confront some issues that are either distinctively pediatric or have a particular cast in the pediatric setting.

First, the normal developmental trajectory from decision-making incapacity during infancy to full capacity by young adulthood means that parents or other surrogates initially make all of the important health decisions for younger children. At some point during childhood, the child's own opinions and preferences need to be elicited and accounted for in the decision (through a still poorly defined procedure called *assent*). Sometime during the teenage years, the adolescent acquires full capacity to make complex decisions and is by 18 years of age (or younger if emancipated) granted the legal right to consent to or refuse treatment (American Academy of Pediatrics, Committee on Bioethics, 1995). Importantly, as emphasized by Lyon (Richard & Lyon, chapter 2, this volume), clinicians should not prematurely assume that adolescents lack the capacity to participate in medical decisions prior to their 18th birthday: Richard became very active in decision making and planning for his future care in collaboration with providers and his grandparents, notwithstanding the fact that some emotional and maturational processes that are characteristic of a person 16 years of age were quite evident. In brief, then, developmental considerations must guide pediatric decision-making processes, with care taken to avoid applying adult-oriented approaches to children without appropriate modification or presuming that adolescents lack substantial decision-making capacity or authority (American Psychological Association, 2005).

Second, the activities of problem solving and decision making are rarely individual or isolated as there is often a social network or ecology of people who are relevant to these processes, including the child, parents, other family members, the healthcare team of physicians, nurses, and other staff, and individuals from the community; all potentially influence the others through exchanges of information and the process of making decisions. These individuals then compose a variety of specific small communities within a hospital (such as intensive care units or a surgical service), with even larger conglomerations of hospitals within communities. Each of these layers of the social environment can exert very distinct influences on how problems are considered and decisions are made (Feudtner, 2005).

Third, perhaps even more so than in the care of dying adults, emotions have a powerful impact on how parents, patients, and healthcare providers conceive of the clinical situation, chart a subsequent course of therapeutic action, and perform the numerous and varied acts of care. Although feelings of grief and sadness are nearly universal, anger and more complex emotional states (such as hope, guilt, faith, and fierce determination) are common. These emotions may be triggered by, or targeted on, not only the child's health condition but also the behavior of other family members or the healthcare team or the manner in which medical care is provided. Regardless of their source, emotions often have a substantial influence on how decisions are made.

Fourth, prognosticating about which children are most likely to die and when is made difficult by the combination of the vast array of often-rare pediatric diseases and conditions and the remarkable robustness of children's health and ability to survive. Many children who do succumb to CCCs do so after several life-threatening crises, making prognostication complex and further confounding clear or certain predictions. For instance, with each crisis the following questions arise beyond the seemingly straightforward estimation of the likelihood of survival (see Figure 19.2): (a) What is the prior history of health crises? Has the child previously had a similar crisis and fully recovered? Is this "crisis" therefore perceived as routine or as life threatening? What were the assessments regarding the child's quality of life immediately preceding this crisis? How do these assessments vary among the patient, parents, family members, and healthcare providers? (b) How likely is the child to survive this crisis? (c) How much suffering will possible recovery entail and for how long? (d) What will the new quality-of-life baseline be and for how long? (e) How likely are future crises, and how bad will they be?

Fifth, the psychological outcome for surviving parents, siblings, and other family members is often viewed pessimistically, with expectations of family disintegration and psychopathology after the death of a child.

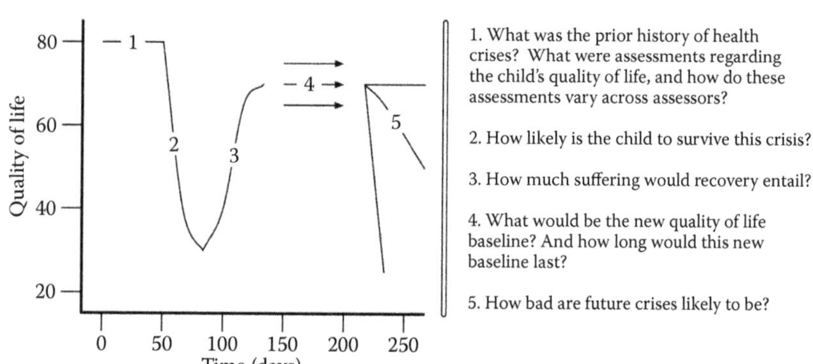

FIGURE 19.2 Prognostic uncertainty for medically fragile children with life-threatening conditions.

Much of the literature describing bereaved parents and siblings is derived from clinical samples of individuals or families seeking assistance after the death of a child. When considered from a broader public health perspective, a more adaptive and promising set of outcomes is observed, including a process of grieving, acceptance, support, and competence, despite loss for many families (Kazak & Noll, 2004).

Finally, although there is a general aversion to and denial of death in America, these tendencies are even more pronounced with regard to death during childhood, which is often a taboo subject. Various ethnic or cultural heritages may influence how particular families cope with the cognitive and emotional challenges of possible or impending death.

These general issues and many other patient- or family-specific factors inform how members of a PACT engage in the task of helping patients, parents, and healthcare providers make good decisions, aligned both with the deepest values of the child and family and with the clinical realities, constraints, and uncertainties imposed by the medical condition and our healthcare system. Before examining these decisions in detail, though, we wish to make the case for an expanded model of "decision making" in the context of pediatric life-threatening conditions.

☐ A Model of Clinical Decision Making and Problem Solving

> Gloria, who is 7, is lying propped up by pillows on the couch in her family's living room. Her brothers are watching TV while her mom and dad talk in the kitchen to the hospice nurse who is finishing up a visit. Next to Gloria, the feeding pump clicks away, slowly delivering the special formula that helps to control her otherwise intractable seizures. The flow of oxygen through her nasal cannula is constant and noiseless. Every few minutes, she coughs, and everyone turns to make sure she is okay, but no alarms go off because she is connected to no monitors.

How could a patient like Gloria and her family make decisions about her care that would enable everyone to achieve the apparent sense of peace in the midst of a highly emotional situation? At first, the resolution in this example may appear difficult to achieve, especially because modern Western medicine is dominated not only by the allopathic tradition (which tends to offer specific treatments, usually in the form of a drug, device, or surgical procedure for specific symptoms or diseases, as opposed to more holistic approaches) but also by a dominant notion of how people do (or at least, ought to) make decisions: the rational maximization of expected utility. This procedure has, across many prescriptions of how to decide "correctly" or "better" (Hammond, Keeney, & Raiffa, 1999; Keeney & Raiffa, 1993; Klein, 1998), a number of standard features:

- Define the problem
- Clarify goals, values, or objectives
- Generate or list options or possible courses of action
- Evaluate the pros and cons of each option and trade-offs across options
- Select the best option and implement the course of action

Although there are ample reasons to deem this scheme to be ideal, many other procedures of decision making have been described, depicted either as unfortunate aberrations or as legitimate alternatives with advantages and disadvantages when compared to the rational maximization of expected utility paradigm. Such as in Gloria's case, these alternative modes of decision making involve a variety of cognitive heuristics (such as availability, representativeness, anchoring, and adjustment; Gilovich, Griffin, & Kahneman, 2002; Kahneman, Slovic, & Tversky, 1982); affective heuristics (by which our evaluation of possible outcomes and treatment options is dramatically influenced by the feelings that we happen to associate with those outcomes or options; Slovic, Finucane, Peters, & MacGregor, 2002); and even broader paradigms of decision making as it actually unfolds in real life (in which, first and foremost, people have to decide which circumstances constitute a "problem" that warrants attention; Klein, 1998).

We view the challenges of decision making (and, as we are about to explain, the encompassing set of activities devoted to clinical problem solving) as requiring a hybrid model that locates the rational maximization of expected utility as a core procedure but within a context of other related tasks that in the end often dominate the decision and subsequent course of action (see Figure 19.3), which—as depicted in Gloria's case—does not always mean maximal medical intervention and treatment.

Past Experience

This model begins with the observation that individuals—patients, parents, and healthcare providers—experience their current situation under the influence of both an innate component (such as temperament and various forms of intelligence) and an acquired component (their past experiences, learned behaviors, and culturally mediated values). This observation is critical because these characteristics, whether fixed or modifiable, often

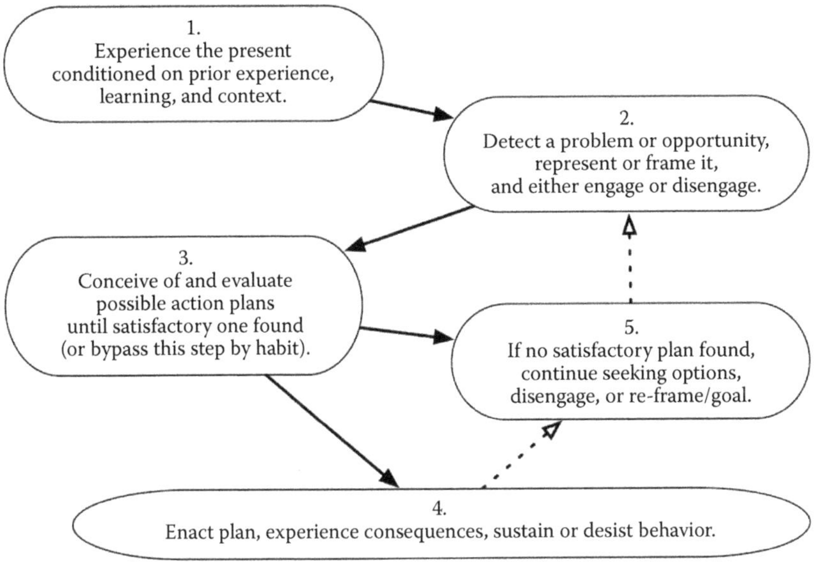

FIGURE 19.3 Problem-solving/decision-making model.

dramatically affect how people engage in problem solving and decision making. For parents of children with CCCs, much of the acquired component of the problem-solving cycle reflects prior experiences with the ups and downs of their child's condition and how healthcare providers responded to both the crises and remissions.

Clinical Pearl

Exploring this past history and what lessons or meaning parents or the child have extracted from their prior experience can greatly facilitate the process of grappling with current situations. Parents of children like Gloria have extensive experience both with their child and with the healthcare system, experience that has educated and informed their understanding of their child's situation and their approach regarding care.

Detection and Representation of Problems

Similar to the half-submerged flotsam that flows past the bank of a turbulent river, the day-to-day lives of ill patients and their parents and healthcare providers present dozens of possible problems (as is evident in the case narrative of Josh, presented by Crow in chapter 4 of this volume, and the family's attempt to understand all that occurred after Josh's devastating brain injury). The initial and ongoing task they confront is to detect that a problem exists that requires attention, formulate a mental representation of what exactly the problem is, and decide whether to engage in subsequent problem-solving activities (or to dismiss the problem as trivial or irrelevant). This process can be triggered (quite literally) by monitor alarms going off, by an internal reassessment, or by the warning of others. The ensuing mental representation of the problem takes perceptions, observations, or facts and turns them into a story or some other framework of meaning. This representation of the problem often entails certain priorities and goals, which in turn inform one of the most important decisions—made consciously or unconsciously—namely, whether to engage the problem. Once engaged, the representation of the problem provides the main framework through which an individual will understand not only the problem but also the range of possible responses to the problem.

Clinical Pearl

When clinical decision making seems to be generating substantial discord among the patient, parents, family members, or healthcare providers, one of the most useful activities is to explore how each person conceives of the situation, thereby clarifying how representations of the problem may differ radically. Questions similar to the following can be posed to each member of the decision-making team: How well do you think that the treatments are working? Do you think that the child is comfortable? How worried are you, and about what?

Other "Predecision" Decisions

In addition to decisions about whether a problem exists, how to represent it, and whether to engage it, patients and parents also often have preferences about who should be involved in making any clinical decisions and about how they and the healthcare team should work together to solve problems. Some want the extended family involved; others do not. Although our culture and the prevailing ethical standards suggest that clinical decisions need to be made in an autonomous manner by parents (or by emancipated minors or young adults), most empirical investigations of patients' or parents' expressed preferences about the manner of decision making have found that the majority desire a collaborative process, with the clinician providing not only factual information about the pros and cons of treatment options but also a treatment recommendation.

Clinical Pearl

Clinicians can ask patients and parents about who they think should be involved (or not involved) in helping them to make medical decisions and about how they want the clinician to help them, by providing information and letting them decide or by also providing clearly stated recommendations.

Habit-Based Decisions

When discussing how to address a problem that has arisen in the care of a child whose life is threatened by illness (such as impending respiratory failure or the relapse of a cancer that has proven refractory to all standard therapies), one often hears the comment, by parents and by healthcare providers alike, that "There really isn't a decision to be made—the choice is obvious." Whether the "obvious" choice involves intubation, enrollment in a Phase I clinical trial, or the initiation of palliative care, this type of comment reflects the fact that clinical problem-solving activity may or may not involve a conscious deliberative process. We believe that when confronted with major problems, parents and clinicians often bypass the idealized deliberative process and instead provide a more basic habitual response to the threat that the problem represents: In other words, the outcome of the decision of what to do in the context of a perceived grave threat is preprogrammed, based on prior learning and experience. The crucial decision in such instances is in fact the "predecision" about how to represent the problematic situation (such as which attributes to emphasize, which to ignore, and how the specific instance is quickly classified as a particular type of problematic situation) because this representation is critical in determining the subsequent response; the representation triggers the habitual course of action.

Clinical Pearl

If there is disagreement about how to respond to a clinical problem (especially ones that are deemed by parents or healthcare providers as threatening), clinicians may be able to help collective decision making not only by reviewing the facts of the problem but also by facilitating an examination (even briefly) of the various meanings that the problem might have for different people, outlining the range of possible treatment choices, and thus moving the decision-making dialogue beyond habit-based responses and into a more deliberative mode.

Deliberative Decision-Making Procedures

If a deliberative process is initiated, at least two different procedures appear to be used. The first procedure, which anecdotally appears to be far more common, involves the evaluation of options in series, searching for a satisfactory solution. The second procedure is more methodical, assessing a range of feasible options with a side-by-side comparison of the pros and cons of the options; this is the procedure codified in the informed consent process. Although some decisions clearly call for the methodical process (such as whether to undergo an invasive procedure or embark on a new course of medical treatment), we know little about either the factors that trigger decision makers, as individuals or a group, to use this approach when not dealing with the stereotypical decisions requiring informed consent or about exactly how methodically the procedure is carried out. The methodical procedure also—and imperatively—needs to have the various goals or objects that the problem solvers are seeking to achieve spelled out as explicitly as possible. This step is often omitted, much to the detriment of the subsequent dialogue, because different people often are prioritizing different goals.

Clinical Pearl

Although dealing with all clinical decisions in the more methodically deliberative manner would be far too time consuming, recognizing when decision making is not going smoothly and explicitly guiding the group of decision makers into this slower mode may help not only to forge a common representation of the problem and the available options but also to better manage a variety of heuristics that shape decision making in myriad ways.

Heuristics

Although the fully methodical deliberative process may appear to circumvent the limitations of decision making either by habit or by simply finding satisfactory (as opposed to more optimal) solutions, this process is still prone to bias because of a number of well-described heuristics used by people when making decisions under conditions of uncertainty. Heuristics are essentially "patterns of thinking" that make the process of judgment easier, often by substituting one question (such as estimating the probability of an intervention resulting in a good or bad outcome) with another question (how easily can we recall ever seeing this intervention result in a good or a bad outcome) (Kahneman & Frederick, 2002; Schwarz & Vaughn, 2002; Tversky & Kahneman, 1974). In the setting of end-of-life care, several of these heuristics are likely to be invoked. For instance, the "availability" heuristic just described influences how parents, based on their child's prior responses to therapy, estimate the likelihood that an intervention will (or will not) work; clinicians who present quantitative data should be mindful of this competing source of information. The same heuristic also can militate against palliative care because most children and families have no "available" experience with care resulting in greater comfort or peace.

Clinical Pearl

In such instances, with great tact, clinicians may need to provide enough of a vivid sense of how the option of palliative care can result in these outcomes to make them available for children or parents.

Affective Heuristic

A specific affective heuristic is also clearly important in how families consider palliative care options. Stated generally, this fundamental heuristic affects the process of decision evaluation by influencing the value that people attach to different characteristics of the options, with these values then influencing seemingly unrelated estimates of the magnitude of potential risk or benefit. For example, the sense of dread that typically accompanies the diagnosis of cancer appears to make people more likely to overestimate the likelihood of dying from cancer compared to the risk of dying from accidental trauma (the specter of which conveys less dread). The affective heuristic causes people to "base their judgments of an activity [such as palliative care] or a technology [such as a patient-controlled analgesic pump to deliver a narcotic for pain control] not only on what they *think* about it but also on what they *feel* about it" (Slovic et al., 2002, p. 410, emphasis original). Through the workings of the affective heuristic, strong negative or positive emotion will be interpreted as pertinent information, especially if the decision is being made under time pressure or other stress (Schwarz, 2002). To some degree, the sway that the affective heuristic holds over decision making can be modified and reduced by allowing more time for the decision-making process to unfold and perhaps by drawing people's attention directly to the various feelings (such as sadness, frustration, anger) that are likely influencing decision making. A process of this sort can be seen, elsewhere in this volume, in Jonathon Spannhake's account (chapter 3) of his ordeal of Gullian-Barre syndrome (GBS), as he grappled as much with pain and fear as with clinical information about GBS or his own personal clinical status.

Clinical Pearl

Clinicians must be mindful to help patients and families to manage not only factual information but also emotions and to provide time and to role model a language for doing so.

Enactment of Behavior or Plan

Clinical problem-solving activities do not stop once a decision has been made but instead continue into the phase of enacting the decision as either a simple behavior or a more complex plan. In clinical practice, we see three key aspects of problem solving during this phase. First, many decisions flounder because of poor implementation of the plan. Although this may be a sign of technical incompetence, far more often it is because of poor communication regarding not only the specific but comparatively superficial "to do" list but also more basically the thought process underlying the plan or (said differently) the intentionality of the decision. For example, a neonate with multiple congenital anomalies (also called "birth defects") who is dying may receive inadequate pain control if the implementation of an aggressive pain control plan does not include a discussion with the bedside nurse regarding the rationale or goals of care. Second, this is a phase of intensive learning on the part of the patient and family, and clinicians who help them to interpret the experience—good or bad—of new therapies or modes of care are vitally important. Otherwise, incorrect conclusions can be drawn that a drug or a treatment "doesn't work" (or the opposite). Third, as the patient or parents experience the consequences of the decision, they are evaluating—implicitly or explicitly, constrained to a lesser or greater extent by the disease and other circumstances—whether to continue the plan. Continued adherence, in other words, always hangs somewhat in the balance. At this point, the quality of the preceding decision-making process is often tested, especially regarding whether the new experiences can be incorporated, with some degree of continuity, harmony, or acceptance, into the developing framework of meaning about the child's life and illness.

Clinical Pearl

Clinicians who note that a decision is being enacted poorly should consider, in their differential diagnosis of the cause of the suboptimal performance, whether all members of the team understand the deepest goals that are guiding care; whether the patient or family is being sufficiently supported regarding the interpretation of new signs, symptoms, or other aspects of the dying experience; and whether motivation to adhere to the plan has dissipated because these new aspects of the experience threaten to obliterate the often already-frayed fabric of meaning for the patient or the family.

Reiteration, Revisiting, and Feedback Loops

The process of clinical problem solving that we have outlined here is nonlinear. Patients and family members (as well as healthcare providers) are frequently recasting their representation of the problem, detecting new problems, reevaluating old information or incorporating new information through a variety of learning feedback loops, and revisiting prior decisions. The recursive nature of this process is not a sign of suboptimal decision making; rather, we believe it is normative, in the senses of being both the most common pattern and the best pattern of confronting terrible situations and coping with the challenges of decision making under uncertainty.

Clinical Pearl

When grappling over time with a complex and often-evolving clinical predicament, one of the most useful words that a leader of a clinical team can possess is to *revisit*, as in, "Perhaps we should revisit this decision, and the thoughts and feelings that have guided our choices in the past because we may have learned something new that is changing how we think and feel about this decision." Explicitly stating the team's capacity to revisit previous decisions endows the decision-making process with flexibility and adaptability, characteristics that in turn help the team to confront an often-changing set of clinical problems and to make decisions in the face of uncertainty.

Children's Involvement in Decision Making

> Donald has the lights turned low in his hospital room as he quietly plays a video game while sitting in bed. The 14-year-old has leukemia that relapsed 3 months after a bone marrow transplant. During the past few weeks, Donald underwent another round of aggressive and highly toxic chemotherapy, but the cancer did not go away. His mother (who has the primary decision making after a bitter divorce and custody battle years ago), knitting at his bedside, has told the medical staff that she does not want to talk about the possibility of his death, and she adamantly does not want anyone to talk with Donald about his now-grim prognosis.

As most children progress from infancy through childhood into adolescence and young adulthood, they develop more complex preferences, acquire a greater understanding of short- and long-term consequences, and enhance their ability to contemplate trade-offs. They are, consequently, increasingly capable of participating in decisions about the health care that they receive. Other than the rather arbitrary definitions codified in law, there is no fine bright line that demarcates an abrupt transition from no capacity to full decision-making capacity; instead, there is a gradual ascension from incapacity to capacity (American Academy of Pediatrics, Committee on Bioethics, 1995). This typically progressive acquisition of ability creates two challenges when caring for sick children.

The first is assessment: Children must be assessed individually to determine their developmental (and not merely chronological) age and corresponding cognitive and emotional abilities pertaining to decision making because children differ in their capacity to participate in this process not only because of their different ages but also because of any cognitive impairments caused by their disease or by the treatment they have received.

This assessment should consider five child-specific characteristics, the first two being more specific to the realm of pediatric practice, although the last three are features used in the practice of adult medicine to determine capacity of patients to make autonomous decisions:

1. Their desire to participate in some capacity in the decision-making process. Whenever possible, clinicians need to ask the child directly words to the effect of, "We need to figure out how to take good care of you. Do you want to listen? Or tell us something?" For many children, this invitation (which—quite acceptably—might be refused) shows that the healthcare team respects them and may engender trust.
2. Their ability to express preferences regarding how they will be treated. Participating in a decision-making process might, for some children, consist not of making a choice per se but rather by informing the adult decision makers about their preferences for treatment (for example, to be awake or sedated for certain procedures, to be cared for in the hospital or at home), thus shaping the final treatment plan.

For the older adolescent and young adult, the assessment should be open to the possibility that the patient should have a major—and perhaps definitive—role in making a decision if the patient demonstrates the following characteristics (Appelbaum & Grisso, 1988):

3. Their ability to understand and appreciate on a personal level information about their condition and treatment options. This can be assessed by asking the patient to recount back to the clinician the key issues about the disease and the pros and cons of different treatment options (including the option of no further curative or life-prolonging treatment) and what this means for them.

4. Their ability to make a reasonable choice. Patients demonstrate this capacity if, when asked directly, "What do you think we should do?" the patient states a clear choice, and that choice falls within a range of "reasonable choices." Although admittedly vague, reasonable choices are perhaps best defined liberally as simply those choices for which the guiding rationale does not defy the basic rules of cause and effect or logic and the patient or care team has the means to carry out the choice. Great care must be taken not to label as "unreasonable" those choices with which we disagree.
5. Their ability to appreciate the consequences of a choice. If patients do indicate a clear choice, then the clinician should assess whether they appreciate, in terms specific to themselves, what will happen if the choice is enacted.

The assessment process sketched can only proceed if the child has been informed of his or her diagnosis or prognosis. Many parents and clinicians are, however, very reluctant to disclose what may be disturbing information to children or adolescents. The decision on the part of parents or healthcare providers to limit the child's awareness of their medical situation is, de facto, a decision to limit the child's participation in subsequent choices. Whether this approach of "shielding the child from the truth" is a good overarching strategy is debatable, especially in light of the reality that

- most cognitively intact children appear to have a much greater understanding of the seriousness of their medical condition, and even the likelihood of dying, than is openly discussed (Bluebond-Langner, 1978), and that
- the policy of keeping information secret can create a divide between the adults and the child, essentially isolating the child with his or her own awareness of the life-threatening implications of the disease, the possibility of dying, and myriad questions about death.

The second challenge is engagement: Once the child, parents, and healthcare team have assessed the ability and desire of the child to participate in the decision-making process, meaningful ways of engagement must occur. In this process, no promises—explicit or implicit—about their ability to control the therapeutic decisions should be made to the child or adolescent that cannot be met. In this regard, the healthcare team should be appropriately circumspect or wary of pursuing the child's assent to treatment if the child's refusal will not be honored or somehow accommodated. Instead, meaningful—and perhaps even health-promoting—engagement in the decision-making process can occur for some children with no need to engage in a quasi-formalized process of assent. Being invited to participate in the decision-making process, being listened to, and having their treatment preferences solicited and incorporated into the decision are equally important.

☐ Conclusions

The medical decisions that parents and young patients encounter when confronting life-threatening conditions are numerous and complex, often arising with a sense of urgency that belies the true subtlety of the decision-making process. We have described what we believe to be an appropriately nuanced model of clinical decision making and problem solving, one that we find to be both more accurate and useful than the currently pervasive view that is built entirely on notions of rational choice. Our core model and general precepts that we have described can inform the approach clinicians make as they grapple with common end-of-life care decisions, ranging from whether to enroll in a clinical trial or to adopt a palliative care approach, whether to withhold or withdraw life-sustaining treatments, or whether to manage symptoms of advanced illness aggressively to the point of deep sedation. As important, the model we propose also emphasizes that these particular decisions, even though they are so often cited, may not be the most influential decisions for dying pediatric patients but instead may be secondary to the history of events and prior decisions that have shaped the parents' and clinicians' underlying psychological representations of how a child's medical predicament is depicted and understood.

☐ References

American Academy of Pediatrics, Committee on Bioethics. (1995). Informed consent, parental permission, and assent in pediatric practice. *Pediatrics, 95,* 314–317.

American Psychological Association. (2005). *Report of the Children and Adolescents Task Force of the Ad Hoc Committee on End-of-Life Issues.* Washington, DC: Author.

Appelbaum, P. S., & Grisso, T. (1988). Assessing patients' capacities to consent to treatment. *New England Journal of Medicine, 319,* 1635–1638.

Bearison, D. J. (2005). *When treatment fails: How medicine cares for dying children.* New York: Oxford University Press.

Bluebond-Langner, M. (1978). *The private worlds of dying children.* Princeton, NJ: Princeton University Press.

Carter, B. S., & Levetown, M. (2004). *Palliative care for infants, children, and adolescents: A practical handbook.* Baltimore, MD: Johns Hopkins University Press.

Feudtner, C. (2001). Child advocacy and robust community-centered research. *Archives of Pediatric Adolescent Medicine, 155*, 438–439.

Feudtner, C. (2004). Perspectives on quality at the end of life. *Archives of Pediatric Adolescent Medicine, 158*, 415–418.

Feudtner, C. (2005). Hope and the prospects of healing at the end of life. *Journal of Alternative and Complementary Medicine, 11*(Suppl. 1), S23–S30.

Feudtner, C., DiGiuseppe, D. L., & Neff, J. M. (2003). Hospital care for children and young adults in the last year of life: A population-based study. *BioMed Central: Medicine, 1*, 3.

Feudtner, C., Feinstein, J., Satchell, M., Shabbout, M., & Kang, T. I. (2006, May). *Shifting site of death among children with complex chronic conditions in the United States, 1979–2002.* Paper presented at the Pediatric Academic Societies Annual Meeting, San Francisco.

Field, M. J., & Behrman, R. E. (Eds.). (2003). *When children die: Improving palliative and end-of-life care for children and their families.* Washington, DC: National Academy Press.

Gilovich, T., Griffin, D. W., & Kahneman, D. (2002). *Heuristics and biases: The psychology of intuitive judgment.* New York: Cambridge University Press.

Graham, R. J., & Robinson, W. M. (2005). Integrating palliative care into chronic care for children with severe neurodevelopmental disabilities. *Journal of Developmental and Behavioral Pediatrics, 26*, 361–365.

Hammond, J. S., Keeney, R. L., & Raiffa, H. (1999). *Smart choices: A practical guide to making better decisions.* Boston: Harvard Business School Press.

Hilden, J. M., Tobin, D. R., & Lindsey, K. (2003). *Shelter from the storm: Caring for a child with a life-threatening condition.* Cambridge, MA: Perseus.

Kahneman, D., & Frederick, S. (2002). Representativeness revisited: Attribute substitution in intuitive judgment. In T. Gilovich, D. W. Griffin, & D. Kahneman (Eds.), *Heuristics and biases: The psychology of intuitive judgment* (pp. 49–81). New York: Cambridge University Press.

Kahneman, D., Slovic, P., & Tversky, A. (1982). *Judgment under uncertainty: Heuristics and biases.* New York: Cambridge University Press.

Kazak, A., & Noll, R. (2004). Child death from pediatric illness: Conceptualizing intervention approaches from a family/systems and public health perspective. *Professional Psychology: Research and Practice, 35*, 219–226.

Keeney, R. L., & Raiffa, H. (1993). *Decisions with multiple objectives: Preferences and value tradeoffs.* New York: Cambridge University Press.

Klein, G. A. (1998). *Sources of power: How people make decisions.* Cambridge, MA: MIT Press.

Lynn, J. (1997). An 88-year-old woman facing the end of life. *Journal of the American Medical Association, 277*, 1633–1640.

Robinson, W. M., Ravilly, S., Berde, C., & Wohl, M. E. (1997). End-of-life care in cystic fibrosis [see comments]. *Pediatrics, 100*(2 Pt. 1), 205–209.

Schwarz, N. (2002). Feelings as information: Moods influence judgments and processing strategies. In T. Gilovich, D. W. Griffin, & D. Kahneman (Eds.), *Heuristics and biases: The psychology of intuitive judgment* (pp. 534–547). New York: Cambridge University Press.

Schwarz, N., & Vaughn, L. A. (2002). The availability heuristic revisited; ease of recall and content of recall as distinct sources of information. In T. Gilovich, D. W. Griffin, & D. Kahneman (Eds.), *Heuristics and biases: The psychology of intuitive judgment* (pp. 103–119). New York: Cambridge University Press.

Slovic, P., Finucane, M., Peters, E., & MacGregor, D. G. (2002). The affective heuristic. In T. Gilovich, D. Griffin, & D. Kahneman (Eds.), *Heuristics and biases: The psychology of intuitive judgment* (pp. 397–420). New York: Cambridge University Press.

Tversky, A., & Kahneman, D. (1974). Judgment under uncertainty: Heuristics and biases. *Science, 185,* 1124–1131.

Index

A

B

C

D

E

F

I

J

K

L

N

O

P

Q

R

T

U

V

W

Y

For Product Safety Concerns and Information please contact our EU representative GPSR@taylorandfrancis.com
Taylor & Francis Verlag GmbH, Kaufingerstraße 24, 80331 München, Germany

www.ingramcontent.com/pod-product-compliance
Ingram Content Group UK Ltd.
Pitfield, Milton Keynes, MK11 3LW, UK
UKHW022004180926
475701UK00003B/194

* 9 7 8 1 1 3 8 9 6 7 2 5 0 *